# Whole Person Healthcare

# WHOLE PERSON HEALTHCARE

## Volume 3

## The Arts and Health

Ilene A. Serlin, PhD, ADTR, General Editor

Jill Sonke-Henderson, BA, Rusti Brandman, PhD,
Ilene A. Serlin, PhD, ADTR, and John Graham-Pole, MD,
Volume Editors

Praeger Perspectives

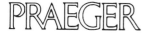

Westport, Connecticut
London

**Library of Congress Cataloging-in-Publication Data**

Whole person healthcare / Ilene A. Serlin, general editor.
    p. ; cm.
  Includes bibliographical references and index.
  ISBN-13: 978–0–275–99231–6 (set : alk. paper)
  ISBN-13: 978–0–275–99232–3 (v. 1 : alk. paper)
  ISBN-13: 978–0–275–99233–0 (v. 2 : alk. paper)
  ISBN-13: 978–0–275–99234–7 (v. 3 : alk. paper)
  1. Integrative medicine. I. Serlin, Ilene A. [DNLM: 1. Mind-Body and
Relaxation Techniques. 2. Behavioral Medicine—methods. 3. Health Behavior.
4. Holistic Health. WB 880 W628 2007]
  R733.W489 2007
  610—dc22     2007013444

British Library Cataloguing in Publication Data is available.

Library of Congress Catalog Card Number: 2007013444
ISBN-10: 0–275–99231–4 (set)    ISBN-13: 978–0–275–99231–6 (set)
        0–275–99232–2 (vol. 1)          978–0–275–99232–3 (vol. 1)
        0–275–99233–0 (vol. 2)          978–0–275–99233–0 (vol. 2)
        0–275–99234–9 (vol. 3)          978–0–275–99234–7 (vol. 3)

First published in 2007

Praeger Publishers, 88 Post Road West, Westport, CT 06881
An imprint of Greenwood Publishing Group, Inc.
www.praeger.com

Printed in the United States of America

The paper used in this book complies with the
Permanent Paper Standard issued by the National
Information Standards Organization (Z39.48–1984).

10 9 8 7 6 5 4 3 2 1

# VOLUME 3:
# THE ARTS AND HEALTH
# CONTENTS

# FOREWORD

When I was a senior resident in internal medicine, I was a little startled to hear one of the most respected senior physicians say to me one day, "You know, Dean, the mind doesn't really affect the body very much. I'm surprised that you believe that it does. And it can't be studied anyway."

This was not *that* long ago—in 1984. And it was at Harvard Medical School's Massachusetts General Hospital, which goes to show how much the field of behavioral medicine has evolved since then.

Because behavioral medicine is a relatively new field, it can be challenging to sort out what is most effective. This three-volume series does a lot of that work for you. It has assembled a group of accomplished experts in the field who can help guide you to understand better what works and what does not, for whom and under what circumstances.

We tend to think of advances in medicine as a new drug, laser, or other high-tech device. It can sometimes be hard for people to believe that relatively simple changes in behaviors, such as diet and lifestyle, can make such a powerful difference in our health and well-being, but they often do.

During the past 30 years, my colleagues and I at the nonprofit Preventive Medicine Research Institute and the School of Medicine, University of California, San Francisco (UCSF), have conducted a series of randomized controlled trials and demonstration projects demonstrating how powerful behavioral medicine approaches can be. We used the latest in high-tech, state-of-the-art diagnostic technology (including quantitative coronary arteriography and cardiac PET scans) to prove the power of low-tech, low-cost, and often ancient interventions.

At the time the conventional wisdom was that the progression of coronary heart disease could only get worse and worse. At best, you might be able to slow the rate at which the disease progressed, but that was about it. We were able to show, for the first time, that the progression of even severe coronary heart disease may begin to reverse using a multifactorial behavioral medicine program of comprehensive lifestyle changes. These included eating a whole-foods, low-fat diet rich in fruits, vegetables, whole grains, legumes, and soy products; getting moderate exercise; practicing stress management techniques, including yoga and meditation; and using support groups to build community and enhance love, intimacy, and healthier communication.

What did we find? Within a month, there was a 91 percent reduction in the frequency of angina, and most patients became essentially pain-free. These patients not only *felt* better, they *were* better; their hearts received more blood flow, and they pumped blood more efficiently. Within a year, we found that even severely blocked coronary arteries became measurably less occluded, and there was even more reversal of their coronary artery disease after five years than after one year. In contrast, coronary artery disease continued to worsen in patients in the usual-care control group. After five years, 99 percent of patients were able to stop or reverse the progression of their heart disease as measured by cardiac PET scans, and there were 2.5 times fewer cardiac events. These findings were published in the *Journal of the American Medical Association.*

Last year, we published the first randomized controlled trial (in collaboration with Dr. Peter Carroll at UCSF and Dr. William Fair at Memorial Sloan-Kettering Cancer Center) showing that the progression of prostate cancer may be affected by a similar behavioral medicine intervention. This study was published in the *Journal of Urology.*

After completing these randomized controlled trials showing how medically effective these behavioral medicine approaches could be, we conducted a series of three demonstration projects showing that these approaches are not only medically effective, but also cost-effective, in people with coronary heart disease. Through our nonprofit institute we began training hospitals throughout the country in our behavioral medicine program that integrates the best of traditional and complementary interventions. Mutual of Omaha found that almost 80 percent of people who went through this program and were eligible for coronary bypass surgery or angioplasty were able to safely avoid it, saving almost $30,000 per patient in the first year. In a second demonstration project, Highmark Blue Cross Blue Shield found that they were able to reduce their costs by 50 percent in the first year and by an additional 20 percent to 30 percent in subsequent years.

On the basis of these findings, Medicare conducted a demonstration project of our approach and another behavioral medicine program based on our work by Dr. Herbert Benson, a pioneer in behavioral medicine who conducted research documenting the power of meditation to elicit what he termed the "relaxation response." Our data were peer reviewed in an all-day hearing at the Centers for Medicare and Medicaid Services by 16 experts, who concluded in a national coverage determination that Medicare should now cover cardiac rehabilitation programs that include behavioral medicine interventions. Since reimbursement is a major determinant of medical practice, this Medicare coverage may help to increase the demand for behavioral medicine practitioners and thus help make the field more sustainable.

Also, medical care costs are reaching a tipping point. Many corporations are beginning to find that their employees' medical care costs are exceeding their entire net profits, which is clearly not sustainable. For example, Starbucks spends more for healthcare for their employees than for coffee beans, and General Motors spends more on healthcare than on steel. As a result, there is a growing receptivity for behavioral medicine programs that have been shown to reduce costs and improve health.

At a time when the power of behavioral medicine approaches is becoming increasingly well documented, the limitations of high-tech medicine are becoming more evident. For example, tens of billions of dollars each year are spent on angioplasty and cardiac stents, even though a recent meta-analysis of all the randomized controlled trials showed that these approaches do not prolong life, or even prevent heart attacks, in stable patients with coronary heart disease. Newer, more expensive technologies, such as coated stents, actually *increased* the risk of having a heart attack. There is a growing realization that it often makes more sense to pay for behavioral medicine interventions than for ones, such as angioplasty, that are dangerous, invasive, expensive, and largely ineffective.

In contrast, the landmark Interheart study examined almost 30,000 people in 52 different countries throughout the world. The investigators found that heart attacks can be prevented in more than 90 percent of people simply by changing nine easily measured risk factors (smoking, lipids, hypertension, diabetes, obesity, diet, physical activity, alcohol consumption, and psychosocial factors), all of which are the focus of behavioral medicine.

Ultimately, behavioral medicine is about transforming our lives, not just our behaviors. Meditation, for example, can be presented as a stress management technique, which it is, but it can be even more powerful if used to help people quiet down their minds and bodies enough to rediscover and experience an inner sense of peace, joy, and well-being.

In our studies, we found that it was not enough to focus on behaviors; we had to work at a deeper level. Many people smoke, overeat, drink too much, abuse other substances, and work too hard as a way of numbing their pain, depression, and loneliness. We found that when we work at that level, people are more likely to make and maintain comprehensive lifestyle changes that are life enhancing rather than self-destructive.

*Dean Ornish, MD*

*Founder and President, Preventive Medicine Research Institute Clinical Professor of Medicine, University of California, San Francisco*

# PREFACE

Minding the body and embodying the mind are two challenges that face medicine, psychology, and related healthcare disciplines. The better we get—and we are indeed getting better—at treating life-threatening illness, the more we convert previously terminal diseases like cancer and heart disease into chronic illnesses. As life expectancy increases, we expect more from medical care and life itself. The technology that has brought us elegant noninvasive imaging, monoclonal antibodies in the treatment of cancer, statins to lower cholesterol, microsurgery, antidepressant and antipsychotic medication, and microarrays of gene expression, has, oddly enough, created a greater demand than ever for mental methods of controlling and understanding our bodies. It is as though the technological advances in medicine provide not just methods but processes that inspire us to find other ways to manage our bodies better from a psychosocial as well as a biotechnological perspective.

Indeed, the public appetite for integrative approaches to healthcare has grown remarkably. In the past decade the use of integrative services has grown by 1 percent of the population per year (Eisenberg et al., 1993, Eisenberg, Davis, & Ettner, 1997). Americans now spend more money on alternative and complementary medical care than they spend out of pocket on doctors or hospital care. They make more appointments with such practitioners than with primary care doctors. They are clearly seeking something they do not find in modern high-tech medicine. In the past, such contacts were something of a secret—two-thirds of patients did not tell their doctors they were availing themselves of herbal, meditative, or physical treatments such as acupuncture, yoga, and massage. But physicians are increasingly accepting of what is now being called integrative care, and more patients are open about their bimedicality, which is good for both kinds of care.

Another force driving those with medical illnesses to integrative care is the fact that, by and large, integrative services are outside the grasp of health insurers. This means that good old-fashioned market forces drive the development of services. People pay out of pocket for what they want, rather than running the thicket of regulations, approvals, copayments, limitations, and other artificial bureaucracy that plagues healthcare in the United States. People feel more in control of their integrative treatment than of their mainstream medical care. This is a crucial and helpful dimension, since the essence of serious stress is helplessness—the inability to do anything about the stressor. Feeling in charge of a treatment elicits cooperation and a sense of competence. In a classic study of the effect of patient involvement in treatment, Ralph Horwitz and colleagues (Horwitz et al., 1990) examined the effects of beta blockers in reducing risk of death after a heart attack. These widely used drugs, which block arousal of the sympathetic nervous system, are now standard care. Horwitz and colleagues' study demonstrated that these drugs were indeed effective in reducing mortality and that better adherence to the medication regimen was associated with lower mortality. But the surprise in this large randomized trial was that better adherence was also associated with reduced mortality among those receiving *placebo* medication. Apparently, it was their adherence that kept them alive, as much as the medication.

I was asked to see the CEO of a large corporation in the coronary care unit because he was suffering from intractable hiccups. He had suffered a myocardial infarction, and the heart injury may have been irritating his diaphragm. But he had been unresponsive to medication, so they asked me to try hypnosis with him. I saw this man, accustomed to controlling everything around him, flat on his back, wearing little, with tubes going in and out of every orifice. He felt demoralized and helpless. He turned out not to be hypnotizable, but I taught him a relaxation exercise to try to minimize his reactive muscle tension that accompanied the frustration he felt about his illness and annoying symptom. I returned the next day to see how he was doing, and his wife greeted me excitedly, saying he had felt much better after seeing me and was eager to have another visit. Surprised, I asked about his symptom. "Oh, he still has the hiccoughs but just felt so much better after talking to you," she said. When I asked him why, he said, "I have been flat on my back for a week having things done to me. You were the first person who told me there was something I could do for myself." So while objectively I didn't help him with the symptom, finding a way that he could participate in his recovery made a difference to him.

The average doctor spends some 7 minutes with a patient; the average practitioner of integrative medicine 30 minutes per patient. These numbers suggest what is missing in high-tech medical care: attention to the person with the disease. Sir William Osler said that it is more important to know the person who has the disease than the disease the person has. The twentieth century ushered in the era of scientific medicine with the Flexner report, which recommended that medicine be taught in organized curricula emphasizing two years of basic training in the fundamental sciences of medicine, including biochemistry, pathology, anatomy, immunology, and pharmacology. This was a departure from the apprenticeships that had dominated medical training until that time. The Flexner report promoted tremendous advances in healthcare, emphasizing more the science rather than the art of medicine, which was needed, since we were not far from the era of purgatives and blood-letting, which had often inflicted more harm than good. The oldest adage of medicine had been, "to cure rarely, to relieve suffering often, to comfort always." However, in the twentieth century we rewrote that job description to be, "to cure always, relieve suffering if you have the time, and let someone else do the comforting." This was a swing of the medical pendulum too far in the other direction. No matter how good we get at medical treatment, the death rate will always be one per person. Medicine and medical intervention will have to help us live with dying as well as cure diseases.

*Whole Person Healthcare* addresses this need, presenting in a lively and scholarly way a variety of approaches to helping the person with the disease learn to live better with it. Interventions ranging from essentials of mind-body medicine through psychological and spiritual approaches to art, music, dance, writing, and other applications of creative expression to healthcare are presented by experts in these areas. These experts provide a varied and authoritative review of methods to harness the human in the service of better health. We ignore what is most human in us at our peril. The science and art of psychologically, socially, emotionally, spiritually, and physically expressive intervention in healthcare is growing rapidly and is much needed. These volumes address that need, both for those with medical illnesses and for those who treat them. They are timely and timeless. Enjoy them.

*David Spiegel, MD*

*Willson Professor and Associate Chair of Psychiatry & Behavioral Sciences*
*Medical Director, Center for Integrative Medicine*
*Stanford University School of Medicine*
*Stanford, California*

## REFERENCES

Eisenberg, D., Davis, R., & Ettner, S. (1997). Trends in alternative medicine use in the United States, 1990–1997. *Journal of the American Medical Association, 280,* 1569–1575.

Eisenberg, D. M., Kessler, R. C., Foster, C., Norlock, F. E., Calkins D. R., & Delbanco, T. L. (1993). Unconventional medicine in the United States. Prevalence, costs, and patterns of use. *New England Journal of Medicine, 328,* 246–252.

Horwitz, R. I., Viscoli, C. M., Berkman, L., Donaldson, R. M., Horwitz, S. M., Murray, C. J., et al. (1990). Treatment adherence and risk of death after a myocardial infarction. *Lancet, 336*(8714), 542–545.

# ACKNOWLEDGMENTS

Many people have served as inspiration, believed in this project, and read drafts of various sections. First, our editor at Praeger, Debora Caravalko, has encouraged and supported us through three years of gestation to give birth to these "triplets." Second, I want to thank my family, Florence, Barbara and Erica Serlin, and Jeff Saperstein for putting up with my preoccupation all these years. Friends and mentors, Kirk Schneider, Tobi Zausner, Stan Krippner, and Pat DeLeon were always there with wise advice. Fellow editors, with whom I have collaborated on projects over many years, Marie DiCowden, Kirwan Rockefeller, Stephen S. Brown, Jill Sonke-Henderson, Rusti Brandman, and John Graham-Pole, have been unflagging believers and collaborators in this work. Thanks to Dean Ornish and David Spiegel for supporting the work with their foreword and preface. Finally, all the editors and contributors, whose names appear in each volume, have given generously of themselves and shared their work and expertise.

*Ilene A. Serlin, PhD, ADTR*

# INTRODUCTION

Mind-body therapies offer an exciting new healthcare frontier. This series introduces the public, healthcare professionals, and students to this future. Mind-body therapies address the complex interaction of mental, physical, and spiritual dimensions of health and illness. Because these therapies deal with the whole person in his or her setting, rather than in terms of isolated disease entities or body parts, this integrative approach is referred to as whole person healthcare. Each volume of this series demonstrates the application of mind-body therapies in a variety of contexts, showing their relevance across a wide range of settings and disciplines. Healthcare practices are expanding from traditional medical settings into new areas such as rehabilitation, wellness programs, and community education—offering practitioners new opportunities and challenges.

These developments are consistent with a variety of recent trends within psychology, such as the "Year of the Whole Person" (Serlin, 2001–2002; Serlin, Levant et al. 2001) and the addition of the word *health* into the mission statement of the American Psychological Association (APA) in 2001. An APA Health Care for the Whole Person Task Force in 2004, under the leadership of APA's president Ron Levant, began to gather evidence of the effectiveness and best practices of integrative collaborative care.

This series presents theory and clinical instruction for bringing a *whole person* perspective to healthcare. Each volume features chapters written by experts in various areas of mind-body healthcare, with case examples and a Tool Kit that lays out basic principles of clinical practice in this area. The afterword for each volume is by a renowned expert in the interface of psychology and healthcare, including the director of the APA Practice Directorate, the director of the APA Education Directorate, a member of the APA Board of Directors, and a former APA president. The preface is written by David Spiegel, Medical Director of the Center for Integrative Medicine at Stanford University Medical Center, and the foreword is by Dean Ornish, Founder and President of the Preventive Medicine Research Institute. This series has been blessed with contributions from some of the most inspired and creative leaders of the psychology and healthcare community.

What is whole person healthcare? Whole person healthcare integrates the best of medical and psychological practices into a biopsychosocialspiritual model. While traditional psychology has celebrated the Decade of Behavior and the Year of Cognition, it is now time for a psychology of the whole person, which integrates behavior, cognition, and consciousness—body, mind, and spirit. It takes into account the impact of life-style on health issues and educates patients to be informed consumers who practice prevention and make changes in their lives toward self-care and health. It relies on experiential as well as theoretical learning and utilizes symbolic and nonverbal as well as linear and verbal modes of expression, data gathering, and verification. Cynthia Belar, APA's Executive Director for Education, called for an integrative psychology:

> I have spent years educating physicians and other health professionals that psychology had a scientific knowledge base and practice relevant to both "mental" and "physical" health…the biopsychosocial model cannot be segmented into its component parts without attention to interactive efforts. (Belar, 2000, p. 49)

Russ Newman, Executive Director of the APA Practice Directorate, used the term "strategic resilience" to describe a new collaboration of psychology with healthcare in which lifestyle plays an important aspect of psychological and physical health.

The whole person approach considers the person in the context of his or her world. It seeks to understand the *meaning* of symptoms, as well as their biological and behavioral causes. Adapting a whole person model is becoming critical for healthcare professionals as an increasingly educated public demands integrative approaches. Growing numbers of people are turning to integrative practitioners for the treatment of a broad spectrum of medical conditions, as well as to reduce stress and enhance personal effectiveness through methods such as meditation, yoga, and acupuncture. These techniques are far less effective if applied mechanically and require a new way of thinking about integration. Psychologists and other healthcare practitioners who hold a whole person perspective are showing how to integrate them into the therapeutic process. The enormous popularity of Bill Moyers's television series "Healing and the

Mind" and the revelation in the January 28, 1993, issue of the *New England Journal of Medicine* that over one-third of Americans utilize unconventional medicine, yet do not tell their doctors, signaled a major shift in public attitudes toward healing (Eisenberg et al., 1998). The trend is growing; a rigorous study done in 2004 shows that 80 percent of cancer patients use complementary, alternative, and integrative therapies (Dittman, 2004; Dossey, 1991, 1992). With its emphasis on prevention and education, integrative healthcare is also cost effective (DeLeon, Newman, Serlin, Di Cowden, et al., 1998; Gazella, 2004, p. 83). The National Institutes of Health (NIH) funded a National Center of Complementary and Alternative Medicine to support research into alternative approaches, and the center's budget and prominence have been growing yearly. NIH also issued a "Roadmap" with an emphasis on prevention and education. The Consortium of Academic Medical Centers for Integrative Medicine consists of 23 medical schools with programs in integrative medicine that include education, research, and clinical training.

Mind and body are interrelated (Rossi, 1986). Candace Pert's groundbreaking work on psychoneuroimmunology demonstrated that the processing of emotions often affects physical illnesses and the ability to heal. Research on healthy humans, as well cancer and HIV-positive patients, has shown that significant increases in immune function and positive health outcomes correlate with constructive emotional expression (Pert, 1997). Holistic perspectives on the self can be found in humanistic psychology, humanistic medicine, preventive medicine, health psychology, and wellness practices.

Integrative healthcare addresses a three-fold crisis in our medical systems: (1) the "completely disgruntled health care consumer," (2) the "disenfranchised, disillusioned physician," and (3) the growing perception that our approach to healthcare "is a broken model" (Gazella, 2004, p. 86). Combining whole person psychology with healthcare practices will revive the morale and effectiveness of healthcare practitioners while opening a wide range of opportunities. Since so many Americans already utilize integrative healthcare, but do so with little useful information for quality control or sound decision making, healthcare practitioners can make a large contribution simply by offering a systematic whole person evaluation and providing listings of available resources. This series goes beyond this, building upon state-of-the-art practices and existing literature to describe how a whole person model can be applied in a wide range of settings and areas of practice.

Beyond making sound theoretical sense, an integrative whole person approach is urgent as we face ever-more complex health issues. For example, one-third of California's 2 million teens are very overweight or obese and are at risk for life-threatening illnesses by the time they reach age 30. The highest rates of these at-risk teens are among Latin Americans and African Americans. In a study carried out by the U.S. Department of Agriculture, over one-half of all American adults are considered overweight or obese, spending about $33 billion each year on diet books, diet pills, and weight loss programs (Squires, 2001). Both losing weight and keeping weight off are psychological issues that require understanding of motivation, stress factors, coping mechanisms, and social support. An encouraging study at the University of California, San Francisco, suggests positive results from an approach to weight loss (PRNewswire, 2000) in which sustained weight loss resulted from training people in two basic internal skills of self-nurturing and limit setting. Psychological interventions give people more conscious control over their lives while improving their self-esteem and sense of meaning (Yalom, 1980). Integrative therapies are also cross-cultural, opening healthcare to diverse, disabled, and marginalized populations.

Psychosocial support groups have proven to be a significant whole person intervention in healthcare. They have increased quality of life and survival time in cancer patients (Fawzy, Fawzy, et al., 1993; Spiegel, Bloom, et al., 1989). Supportive-expressive group therapies are existentially based and aim to help patients live their lives more fully in the face of a life-threatening illness. A wellness model would focus on how to help ordinary individuals cope with such extraordinary circumstances, while support groups address questions of meaning, mortality, and expression.

## A NEW INTEGRATIVE PARADIGM

A new healthcare approach must move away from the culture's "scientific materialism"—with its fragmentation of mind, body, and spirit—to a new integrative paradigm. Nobel laureate Roger Sperry described the coming paradigm shift as moving from this scientific materialism to an integrative, holistic, non-mechanistic, bidirectional model. Scientific materialism is based on the Cartesian dualism of mind and body. The new paradigm would provide "a more realistic realm of knowledge and truth, consistent with science and empiric verification" (Sperry, 1991, p. 255), while including the "ultimate moral basis" (Sperry, 1995, p. 9) of environmental and population sustainability. In Sperry's interactionist, nondualistic model of mental and physical states, causation is determined upward from physical states as well as downward from mental states. In this model, the mind affects the body, just as the body affects the mind.

Consciousness, which brings together the physical and mental aspects of experience, comprises the area of meaning, beliefs, and existential choice. An illness such as breast cancer, for example, might involve the symbolic aspects of a woman's body, her attitudes and sensibilities about her life's meaning, and her understanding of the spiritual dimensions of her existence, as well as a confrontation with her mortality. Out of such confrontations can come a renewed will to live, hardiness, and optimism (Maddi & Hightower, 1999).

Stories of death and rebirth descend into sadness and ascend to joy. Disconnection and reconnection are ancient themes reflected in the myths common to all humankind. With the courage to create (May, 1975), new narratives move the self from deconstruction to reconstruction (Feinstein & Krippner, 1988; Gergen, 1991; May, 1989; Sarbin, 1986). These healing narratives are experienced as coherent and meaningful and have been gaining attention in many areas of clinical practice, including family therapy (Epstein, White, & Murray, 1992; Howard, 1991; Omer & Alon, 1997; Polkinghorne, 1988; Rotenberg, 1987). The act of telling stories has always helped humans deal with the threat of nonbeing, and sometimes the expressive act itself has a healing effect (Pennebaker, 1990). Not all expressive acts are verbal, however. Whole person healthcare embraces diversity of technique and approaches that include nonverbal and multimodal modalities such as the expressive therapies and mindfulness meditation (Kabat-Zinn, 1994). The arts are a particularly effective way to bring symbolic expression and coping mechanisms to people who cannot express trauma verbally or cognitively. From a humanistic whole person perspective, the creative act is a courageous affirmation of life in face of the void of death. Art comes from the basic human need to create, communicate, create coherence, and symbolize. The arts are also transcultural, expressing archetypal symbols that are universal throughout history and across cultures. By bringing the body, ritual, and community back into healthcare, diversity is served by countering the dominance of a white, individualistic European male verbal psychological and medical tradition. Whole person healthcare goals include achieving a gender and culture balance of emotional empathy, self-awareness, assertiveness, instrumental problem solving, and expressiveness (Levant, 2001).

The religious and spiritual dimensions of human nature and human fate are ultimate questions that are integrally related to whole person healthcare. Although long banished by Western medicine, spiritual concerns are proving vital in whole person healthcare. One of the three major themes the National Multicultural Conference and Summit sponsored by the APA in 1999, for example, was "spirituality as a basic dimension of the human condition." It recommended that

> psychology must break away from being a unidimensional science, that it must recognize the multifaceted layers of existence, that spirituality and meaning in the life context are important, and that psychology must balance its reductionistic tendencies with the knowledge that the whole is greater than the sum of its parts. Understanding that people are cultural and spiritual beings is a necessary condition for a psychology of human existence. (Sue, Bingham, Porche-Burke, & Vasquez, 1999, p. 1065)

A healthcare system that separates science from spirit is culturally narrow and "may not be shared by three quarters of the world nor by the emerging culturally diverse groups in the United States" (Sue et al., 1999, p. 1065). Spiritually based rituals have been shown to be effective coping strategies for dealing with life stresses (Pargament, 1997) and serious trauma (Frankl, 1959). However, while a national survey showed that 92 percent of all American reported that "my religious faith is the most important influence in my life" (Bergin & Jensen, 1990, p. 5), most healthcare professionals are unprepared to deal with these issues (Shafranske & Malony, 1990). Learning to deal professionally and objectively with these issues is, in fact, an ethical concern (APA, 2003).

## STRUCTURE OF THE SERIES

Each volume of this series is designed to guide readers into a different area of whole person healthcare, and each provides a coherent overview of the field. The contributions are transdisciplinary, from practitioners and programs in psychology, medicine, clergy, public policy, and the arts.

- **Volume 1: Humanizing Healthcare,** edited by Marie Di Cowden, lays a foundation of definitions and practices of integrative healthcare for the twenty-first century. It helps practitioners develop protocols and assess efficacy of alternative practices, emphasizes the relevance of integrative healthcare for marginalized populations, and discusses risk prevention, policy, and issues of patient protection.
- **Volume 2: Psychology, Spirituality, and Healthcare,** edited by Kirwan Rockefeller and Stephen S. Brown, focuses on issues of meaning in illness; the role of spirituality; health and mental health; chaplaincy and pastoral care; and research and practice in yoga, meditation, imagery, QiGong, prayer, ritual, and death and dying.
- **Volume 3: The Art of Health,** edited by Jill Sonke-Henderson, Rusti Brandman, Ilene Serlin, and John Graham-Pole, introduces readers to the history and practices of art and healthcare throughout the ages. It presents the history of art and health in ancient healing rituals; shows the relevance of rituals in the growing number of international contemporary art-in-health programs; and discusses applications of art, music, dance, drama, and poetry therapy programs at the bedside, in groups, and in cross-cultural conflict.

## SUMMARY

The Year of the Whole Person provides a timely focus for a much-needed collaboration among healthcare professionals. This collaboration can bring together the best practices from psychology and medicine for a comprehensive treatment approach. The current unsustainable U.S. healthcare system urgently needs a more efficient utilization of services; the underserved patients are demanding that their healthcare professionals talk to each other and combine quality traditional and complementary practices—an experience through which healthcare professionals can rediscover their modern yet ancient roles as healers of the mind, body, and spirit.

# REFERENCES

American Psychological Association. (2003). Guidelines for multicultural education, training, research, practice and organizational change for psychologists. *American Psychologist, 58*(5), 377–402.

Belar, C. (2000, September). Learning about APA. *APA Monitor, 31*(8), 49.

Bergin, A. E., & Jensen, J. P. (1990) Religiosity of psychotherapists: A national survey. *Psychotherapy, 27*(1), 3–7.

De Leon, P., Newman, R., Serlin, I., Di Cowden, M., et al. (1998, August). *Integrated health care.* Town Hall symposium conducted at the meeting of the American Psychological Association, San Francisco, CA.

Dittman, M. (2004). Alternative health care gains steam. *American Psychological Association Monitor, 35*(6), 42.

Dossey, L. (1991). *Meaning and medicine.* New York: Bantam.

Dossey, L. (1992). Era III medicine: The next frontier. *ReVision: A Journal of Consciousness and Transformation, 14*(3), 128–139.

Eisenberg, D., Davis R., Ettner, S., Appel, S., Wilkey, S., Van Rompay, M., & Kessler, R. (1998). Trends in alternative medicine use in the United States, 1990–1997; Results of a follow-up national survey. *Journal of the American Medical Association, 280*(18), 1569–1575.

Epstein, D., White, M., & Murray, K. (1992). A proposal for the authoring therapy. In S. McNamee & K. J. Gergen (Eds.), *Therapy as social construction.* London: Sage.

Fawzy, F. I., Fawzy, N. W., et al. (1993). Malignant melanoma: Effects of an early structured psychiatric intervention, coping, and affective state on recurrence and survival 6 years later. *Archives of General Psychiatry, 50*(9): 681–689.

Feinstein, D., & Krippner, S. (1988). *Personal mythology.* Los Angeles: Tarcher.

Frankl, V. (1959). *Man's search for meaning.* New York: Praeger.

Gazella, K. (2004, July/August). Mark Hyman, MD. Practicing medicine for the future. *Alternative Therapies, 10*(4), 83–89.

Gergen, K. (1991) *The saturated self.* New York: Basic Books.

Howard, G. (1991). Culture tales: A narrative approach to thinking, cross-cultural psychology, and psychotherapy. *American Psychologist, 46,* 187–197.

Kabat-Zinn, J. (1994). Foreword. In M. Lerner, *Choices in healing* (pp. xi–xvii). Cambridge, MA: MIT Press.

Levant, R. (2001). *We are not from Mars and Venus!* Paper presented to the American Psychological Association, San Francisco, CA.

Maddi, S., and Hightower, M. (1999). Hardiness and optimism as expressed in coping patterns. *Consulting Psychology Journal: Practice and Research, 51*(2), 95–105.

May, R. (1975). *The courage to create.* New York: Bantam Books.

May, R. (1989). *The art of counseling.* New York: Gardner Press.

Omer, H., & Alon, N. (1997). *Constructing therapeutic narratives.* Northvale, NJ: Aronson.

Pargament, K. I.(1997). *The psychology of religion and coping.* New York: Guilford Press.

Pennebaker, J. W. (1990). *Opening up: The healing power of expressing emotions.* New York: Guilford Press.

Pert, C. B.(1997). *Molecules of emotion.* New York: Scribner.

Polkinghorne, D. E. (1988). *Narrative knowing and the human sciences.* Albany: State University of New York Press.

PRNewswire. (2000, October 18). First obesity treatment to report sustained weight loss-skill training vs. drugs and diets.

Rossi, E. L. (1986). *The psychobiology of mind-body healing.* New York: Norton.

Rotenberg, M. (1987). Re-biographing and deviance: Psychotherapeutic narrativism and the Midrash. New York: Praeger.

Sarbin, T. (Ed.). (1986). *Narrative psychology: The storied nature of human conduct.* New York: Praeger.

Serlin, I. A. (2001–2002). Year of the whole person. *Somatics,* Fall/Winter, 4–7.

Serlin, I., Levant, R., Kaslow, N., Patterson, T., Criswell, E., & Schmitt, R. (2001). *Healthy families: A dialogue between holistic and systemic-contextual approaches.* Paper presented to the American Psychology Association, San Francisco, CA.

Shafranske, E. P., & Maloney, H. N. (1990). Clinical psychologists' religious and spiritual orientations and their practice of psychotherapy. *Psychotherapy, 27,* 72–78.

Sperry, R. W. (1991). Search for beliefs to live by consistent with science. *Zygon, Journal of Religion and Science, 26,* 237–258.

Sperry, R. W. (1995). The riddle of consciousness and the changing scientific worldview. *Journal of Humanistic Psychology, 35*(2), 7–34.

Spiegel, D., Bloom, J. R., et al. (1989). Effect of psychosocial treatment on survival of patients with metastatic breast cancer. *Lancet, 2*(8668): 888–891.

Squires, S. (2001, 10 January). Only high-carb, modest-fat diets work for long. *San Francisco Chronicle,* A2.

Sue, D. W., Bingham, R. P., Porche-Burke, L., &Vasquez, M. (1999). The diversification of psychology: A multicultural revolution. *American Psychologist, 54*(12), 1061–1069.

Yalom, I. D. (1980). *Existential psychotherapy.* New York: Basic Books.

# VOLUME EDITORS' NOTES

*John Graham-Pole, MD, Jill Sonke-Henderson, BA,
Rusti Brandman, PhD, and Ilene A. Serlin, PhD, ADTR*

Poets...drink at streams which we have not yet made accessible to science.
—Sigmund Freud.

Florida State Governor Jeb Bush's wife, Columba, paints flowers on a Shands Hospital mural as guest of the University of Florida's Arts in Medicine program. Kenyan ethnomusicologist David Akombo joins patients and families in a tribal healing ritual of music, dance and story. A teenage girl in excruciating sickle cell pain crisis tells her doctor: "Don't give me any more pain meds—I want to dance." And at the Society for the Arts in Healthcare 2006 conference, the White Ribbon Alliance's Theresa Shaver presents African and Asian mothers' birthing stories from the Ubumama project.

Evidence-based medicine (EBM) evolved from the ever more specialized focus of medical science, with quantitative data, especially the randomized clinical trial, as its gold standard. But in trying to eliminate biases, it came to discount a wealth of narrative, psychosociospiritual, "subjective" experience. Qualitative research accedes to its participants' need to bring these socially and culturally determined biases and positions with them; so it embraces them and puts them to work as evidence. Quantitative and qualitative research complement each other in healthcare, not least through the marriage of science and art. Any apparent dichotomy between them must be seen as false.

### Cell Shed

I lean in among the tubes besetting you,
my breath voluntary, yours urged. Our cells

mingle each with the other's, spilled in
spindrift of air-water-ice between mouths.
You, going, dying, take my life to rest. I,
living, left, draw in, exhale your seed. (Graham-Pole, 2002, p. 41)

This poem describes the last 36 hours of a patient dying on a ventilator. EBM and I had done all we could, but I could give this young woman other things: my time, physical comfort, a little music, a safe death. Her gift to me was to let my mind set aside the *objective* of biomedical knowledge, reality, and value in favor of the *subjective* of narrative epistemology, ontology, and axiology. I could ask different questions: Why is this happening? What does she understand? Were we right to let her die like this? Is she at peace? Of what value am I here? Research questions all. And she gave me another research subject's gift: her experience of transition as evidence to translate into poetry.

Science is, at bottom, knowledge; in classical Greece, art referred to anything that could be learned. The bedside practice of every physician is founded in observations—*clinical signs*—gathered over several hundred years and systematically recorded for every medical school classroom. It is no accident we use *art* to describe both creating works of beauty and offering loving service to those in need. One sure achievement of modern biomedicine is to show that an exact picture of human experience is unattainable. So art, with its economical ability to condense certain irreducible human happenings, offers instead ineffable truths as evidence. Between science and art there will always be the space of T. S. Eliot's "stillness between two waves of the sea" (Eliot, 1962, p. 145). We try in the volume to offer a bridge to walk across.

## REFERENCES

Eliot, T. S. (1962). *The complete poems and plays.* Orlando, FL: Harcourt, Brace, Jovanovich.
Graham-Pole, J. (2002). *Quick: A pediatrician's illustrated poetry.* Lincoln, NE: Writer's Club Press.

Chapter One

# APPLICATIONS OF ART TO HEALTH

*John Graham-Pole, MD*

Forget the news and the radio and the blurred screen.
This is the time of loaves and fishes.
People are hungry, and one good word is bread for a thousand.

—David Whyte

## INTRODUCTION

The quickly expanding fields of art for health and the arts therapies are finding their long overdue place in three areas of modern Western healthcare: (1) *clinical practice:* the care of patients and their families; (2) *education:* of both professional and nonprofessional groups; and (3) *research:* into the efficacy of art and the arts therapies as holistic healing modalities. Any work of artistic creativity carried out in a healthcare setting can be seen as a piece of art, and/ or a description of bedside clinical activity, and/or a healing experience for a patient and her caregivers, and/or a story included in a qualitative research study (Lander & Graham-Pole, 2006).

In an attempt to integrate these diverse but crosscutting expressions of our human potential, I will briefly describe applications of all three in this chapter—clinical practice, professional and lay pedagogy, and quantitative and qualitative research. I will set my review in the context of the subjects covered in far greater detail in other chapters. Included there are series editor Ilene Serlin's excellent introduction to the expressive arts therapies as one aspect of mind-body medicine, coeditor Jill Sonke-Henderson's in-depth review of the history and scientific rationale of this evolving discipline, and my other coeditor Rusti Brandman's comprehensive coverage of world trends in the art-for-health field. Specific chapters are devoted to the visual arts, music, dance, drama, narrative, and poetry therapies respectively, each seen from clinical, educational, and research perspectives. I will briefly introduce these three primary topics.

*(1) Clinical practice:* The most conspicuous aspect of healing art is its contribution to the aesthetics of physical healthcare environments, through architecture, signage, and installations of art and sculpture. Clinical psychologist Mihaly Czikszentmihalyi, in his book *Creativity* (1991), proposes that a harmonious and meaningful environment fosters individual creativity and a sense of control and calm. Often quoted to justify the modern renaissance of art for health is the randomized clinical trial conducted by architect Roger Ulrich more than 20 years ago (Ulrich, 1984) showing that patients recovered from surgery significantly faster when offered a view of nature through their hospital window, when compared with control subjects. Of more significance, however, are the clinical practices of artists and expressive arts therapists at the hospital bedside and other health settings, which make use of a constellation of arts media (Graham-Pole, 2000; McNiff, 1992; Samuels & Lane, 1998). Artists thrive on a kind of deconstruction and reconstruction of chaos, bringing fearlessness to their work in healthcare in the face of the kind of chaos that every seriously ill person's life has become.

*(2) Professional and lay education:* Art is being used to educate students of healthcare, through medical humanities programs (Charon & Montello, 2002), which are widespread in medical and nursing training, and which incorporate the literary, visual, musical, and dramatic arts. Educational courses in the healing arts are also attracting the attention of a wide diversity of healthcare and related professionals. Art and education is addressed extensively by Camic in chapter 14, as it applies to clinical psychologists, and a broad overview is included in this chapter. Art also plays a central role in educating wider lay communities, through delivering health promotion messages, including billboards and public performance (Lander, 2005).

*(3) Quantitative and qualitative research:* A large body of research related to art for health, both quantitative and qualitative in scope, has emerged over the past 50 years. The science of creativity and health that underlies all assessment of art as therapy is fully reviewed by Evans in chapter 5. The gold standard of efficacy in modern medicine remains evidence-based, often taken to indicate quantitative data collection and interpretation that tests hypotheses. However, art, by its essential nature a subjective and ubiquitous form of human expression, does not lend itself well to the narrow focus of the randomized clinical trial. Just as the more defined discipline of the creative arts therapies, and the more free-ranging art-for-health movement, are finding synergistic expression, so quantitative, or objective, and qualitative, or subjective, evaluations of

the healing effects of art and art therapy are increasingly coming to complement each other.

Before covering each of these three connections to the application of art to human health further, I offer a context to this evolving modern phenomenon.

## EVOLUTION OF APPLICATIONS OF ART TO HEALTH

Recently, I took three colleagues to meet a 14-year-old patient whom I will call Isolde. Isolde has had diabetes since infancy, and underwent a below-knee amputation because her foot had become gangrenous as a result of poor circulation and superimposed infection. When we entered her room in the Pediatric Intensive Care Unit she was awake but drugged with morphine for the pain. At first, she remained sullen and took little interest in us, but she gradually became more animated when we asked her about her favorite bands.

"You know Tim McGraw's '*Live Like You Were Dying*'? Well, I can sing that in sign language," she announced. We asked her how come she knew signing. "My boyfriend's deaf and dumb, so I learned it." One of my colleagues asked: "Can you sign 'I love you?'" "Sure." Isolde promptly pointed to her face, then crossed her hands over her heart, then spread them wide in an expansive gesture that embraced all four of us. After watching her create this rhythm with her hands, we began to imitate her, picking up this new language as we did so. Soon we had what amounted to a four-part harmony going as we silently signaled these timeless words back to Isolde, then to each other.

Until this unexpected development, we had been no more than professional colleagues at a patient's bedside. It had taken only a few moments of exchanging this ancient, artful greeting to bring down the artificial barrier between the patient, Isolde, and a diverse group of artist caregivers.

As reviewed extensively by Sonke-Henderson in chapter 1, art-making has been a healing force since prehistory. Asian, African, American, and Australasian shamans all used art to evoke natural and divine forces of healing. Isolde's signing from her bed in an isolation room of a modern intensive care unit seemed to me to evoke these ancient rituals. To our forebears, art and creativity were a source of power and connection (Fox, 2004; Samuels & Samuels, 1990); witness the prehistoric cave art of Africa and Europe, telling evidence that our forebears lived at the interface of visible and invisible, physical and spiritual. Art was the primordial way of making sense of the universe; it must have personified health for them, if they thought about it, and perhaps it does for some today.

The earliest known examples of art being used as visualization, to heighten the senses and inner awareness, are the wall paintings of Ice Age cave dwellers in central Africa, France, Spain, and Scandinavia (Samuels & Samuels, 1990). This antedated the development of language; once verbal discourse became widely used for communication, people were able to distance themselves from their essentially sensual experience of the world about them. With the gradual domination of vision, dream, and sensation by thought and analysis came the emergence of science, and what has been called the birth of civilization.

Art, though, has stayed an essential nutrient of human culture, of our very humanity, since its prehistoric application to visioning, dreaming, and worshiping. Every human society has used art to express its ideas and its faith, and to make sense of its world. Art educates us, uplifts us, and beautifies us. There is no world as boundless as that of the imagination; and it is its magical use that marks us out from other earthly creatures. Today, Asclepius remains the patron of Western medicine: Apollo's mortal son, his healing temples in Delphi, Epidaurus, and elsewhere were witness to dreams, visualization, music, dance, and theater—all in the service of health and healing (see Sonke-Henderson, chapter 2). The biomedical model of modern medicine had its origins in the Hippocratic scientific corpus that examined every facet of the origin of treatments for disease. But today it is firmly yoked with the holistic and artistic concepts of Asclepius. This interdependency is the essential ingredient of art for health.

## LINKS WITH OTHER HEALING ARTS

In exploring the multitude of ways in which we can improve our well-being individually and collectively, this movement has natural links to other disciplines. (1) Most relevant to this book is the evolving synergism between art for health and the creative arts therapies, many of which are extensively reviewed in later chapters. (2) Art as a healing force is inextricably linked to the even larger discipline of holistic health and mind/body therapies, which are central to this three-volume series. (3) A third connection is to the movement that has emerged over the past two decades linking spirituality and human health. I will briefly review each.

### Creative Arts Therapies

> The blessings experienced in therapy can reach further: they can remind artists everywhere what the function of art has always been and will always be.
> —Rudolph Arnheim

Art therapist Shaun McNiff states in the introduction to his book *Art as Medicine* (1992) that the making of art as a medicine moves through different phases of creation and reflection, but the medicinal agent is art itself, which releases the psyche's intrinsic therapeutic forces. As extensively described in the chapters by Aldridge, Fox, Goodill, Krantz and Pennebaker, Landy, McNiff, and Serlin, the creative arts therapies—art, dance, drama, music, narrative, and poetry—have established a place for themselves in many countries over the past 50 years. Each uses art modalities for intentional therapeutic and rehabilitative intervention, and for promoting the integration of physical, emotional, cognitive, and social functioning. Each discipline has established professional training standards, including an approval and monitoring process, a code of ethics, standards of clinical practice, and a credentialing protocol. The creative arts therapists usually have training in psychological diagnosis and therapy. Although unique and distinct from one another, each shares related processes and goals that provide people who have special needs, most often psychosocial, new ways to express themselves with healing intent, perhaps unavailable through standard medical therapies. An organization created in 1979, the National Alliance of Creative Arts Therapies Association, represents an alliance between six separate creative arts therapies associations (www.ncata.org).

More recently, art for health has emerged side by side with the continuing evolution of the creative arts therapies, and has brought art making into a range of clinical settings, including hospitals, nursing homes, hospices, and communities of every kind. Creative arts therapists and artist in residence often work together. Although there are areas of overlap, it is best to think of them as complementing and learning from each other. Artists in residence are careful not to claim as their intent any psychological interpretation or specific benefit for the individual, and avoid using the word *therapy*, although it is implicit in their endeavors (see chapter 4 by Sonke-Henderson and Brandman). Rather, they seek to expand the worldview of medicine and healthcare, to lighten and uplift the environment, and to offer individual and collective healing in the most holistic sense.

## Holistic Movement

In order to understand how healing happens, in the 21st Century, we shall look not only at our atoms and molecules but at consciousness as well. In so doing, we shall reinvent medicine, adding an ancient wisdom to modern science.

—Larry Dossey

The holistic health movement has also emerged in the past several decades as an integral component of healthcare, with the primary goal of optimizing the body-mind-spirit health of both individual and community. The terms *alternative* and *complementary* are inadequate to capture the sense that the integrated whole has a reality greater than the sum of its parts. Art for health is at core holistic, because it consciously pursues the highest level of functioning and balance of the physical, environmental, mental, emotional, social, and spiritual aspects of human experience. The intention is to achieve a dynamic state of being *fully alive,* ideally creating a condition of well-being, regardless of the presence or absence of physical disease.

A holistic approach to a patient's life systems optimizes present and future health; all life experiences, including birth and death, are seen holistically as learning opportunities for both patient and practitioner. Believing that all people have innate powers of healing in their bodies, minds and spirits, holistic health practitioners view people as the unity of body, mind, spirit, and the systems in which they live; and they enable patients to use these powers to affect the healing process. Leading organizations in the United States include the American Holistic Medical Association (www.holisticmedicine.org), the International Society for the Study of Subtle Energies (www.issseem.org), and the Institute of Noetic Sciences (www.ions.org).

While some psychologists continue to explore the possible links between creativity and mental illness, others have made a strong case for the importance of our creative intelligence to leadership in the world. It seems inherently likely that the artistic temperament, rather than conforming to the stereotype of emotional instability, is one of an increased sensitivity that renders us more open to both suffering and joy. Many people never fulfill this creative potential, and this may be a root cause of the prevalence of psychological distress in our culture. Peak human experiences, when we are said to be at our healthiest, have been characterized as being an almost effortless, yet highly focused, state of consciousness (Czikszentmihalyi, 1997). The several hundred artists that I have come to know in the 15 years since we established our Shands Arts in Medicine program at Shands Hospital, University of Florida, know this state of consciousness well; and they seem to me to be among the most holistically healthy group of people I have known.

## Spirituality Movement

> This is indeed the Spirit's work—to awaken all things. That is the artist's work also: to resurrect and awaken all that is and all we perceive.
>
> —Matthew Fox

People have probably always used spiritual practice to enhance their own and others' health. Almost half the Americans asked in a large survey said that they had used prayer for health reasons (Dossey, 1993). Relevant to art for health, those drawn to the use of art and art therapies, under the duress of personal or family illness, often find it spiritually as well as emotionally and physically beneficial. The theologian Matthew Fox sees creativity as tapping into our most elemental and spiritual being. The subtitle of his book, *Creativity* (2004), is *Where the Divine and the Human Meet.* Its central thesis is that the highest communion with the original source of our being comes through simple expression of creativity, which is key to our individual and collective health. He proposes that our society's redemption lies in releasing our widespread fear of creativity's innate and eternal wisdom.

Philosophers, psychologists, and poets have also argued that this urge to create is at the core of our humanity, and that in the act of creating we are giving birth to our authentic selves. T. S. Eliot saw every artistic endeavor as an act of personal re-creation. The arts and healing movement is therefore insep-arable from the movement to bring spirituality into the forefront of healing practice. Both art therapy and spiritual practice focus on ways to promote pos-itive psychological states, which may in turn lead to better health. The advan-tage of focusing on positive psychology, such as greater meaning and personal growth, is that people can learn to enhance these states in a measurable way. The National Center for Complementary and Alternative Medicine (www. nccam.nih.gov) and other funding agencies have begun to support scientific investigation of spiritually based practices, to better understand whether they have health benefits, and if so, how, and for what conditions and populations.

## APPLICATIONS TO CLINICAL MEDICINE

The creating process...seems the best way to give the world a bit of sanity.
—Teenage cancer patient

The incorporation of art for health into modern care was formalized with the founding of the Society for the Arts in Healthcare (www.thesah.org) in 1991. In modern clinical practice with patients and their families, art has made inroads into two broad areas. First, it contends that enhancing the physical environment of healthcare facilities through aesthetic architectural design and signage, installations, sculptures, and live performances in public and private spaces improves the holistic well-being of all who experience them. It is there-fore committed to using art to transform barren, depersonalized settings to an interactive healing ambience, complete with color, texture, sound, movement, and conversation.

In the United Kingdom, Paintings in Hospitals (www.paintinginhospitals. org.uk), a registered charity founded in 1959, loans 4,000 pictures to more than 250 hospitals, hospices, and other healthcare facilities. The University of Michigan Hospital's Art that Heals program, initiated in 1987 (www.med. umich.edu/goa/), offers performing and visual arts activities, including an art cart, with a traveling library of framed poster prints from which patients select and exchange art work for their rooms. The Healing Wall in the Atrium of Shands Hospital at the University of Florida is a 30-foot structure, con-sisting of more than 800 ceramic tiles painted by patients of all kinds, their families, and the Shands Hospital staff (www.shandsartsinmedicine.com). The messages and images on the tiles often start up conversations between strangers. A grand piano is a permanent feature of the Atrium, and a musi-cal performance takes place every Friday during the noon hour. Three other healing walls have since been erected in the Shands Hospital Cancer Center and the Pediatric and Neonatal Intensive Care Units.

Performance art offers a similar aesthetic appeal for patients, family members, and health professionals alike. *Lilian,* a rock musical written by Michael Bishop and community members in Tasmania in 1989, about the visible yet invisible presence of people with mental health problems, has been performed several times over the last 15 years throughout Australia. The production has moved out of hospital settings into the wider community, and has been combined with discussion groups and workshops to engage audiences in critical reflection and action plans to reduce the stigma of psychological illness. The play *Wit,* by Margaret Edson (1999), concerning the final illness of a woman university professor, and her interactions with her medical and nursing staff, has been widely used as a teaching tool in U.S. medical humanities programs.

Art at the bedside of patients, as well as in communal hospital spaces that involve family members and professional caregivers, has become the second major focus of art for health and the arts therapies. These consist of either the passive enjoyment of art created by others, or the active participation of a patient or group of patients in making art. The purposeful involvement of patients in the creative process has the goal of enhancing emotional self-expression, self-esteem, autonomy, and the ability to take charge of decision making in critical situations.

The latter activity is increasingly led, not only by specially trained creative art therapists, but by professional artists of all kinds, who are becoming part of the healthcare team in many hospitals. Dr. Patch Adams, portrayed by Robin Williams in the 1998 film of the same name, has been a pioneer in this movement. His Gesundheit Institute (www.patchadams.org) grew out of the recognition of the healthcare crisis in the United States, promoting an alternative people-not-profit approach. His mission statement sees such activities as art for health as a growing activism that promotes optimal health for both individuals and communities.

The term *artist in residence* refers to artists who work in healthcare facilities of all kinds, who call on medical, nursing, and social work staff to identify suitable patients: for example, those who may be hospitalized for long periods, those who have severe symptoms susceptible to nonpharmaceutical therapeutic approaches, and those who are facing critical medical situations. The artist then explores different art forms (visual, music, poetry, dance, magic, clowning) that will best meet the patient's need and creative energies, and involves the patient passively or actively in a creative process.

Healing art is not a domain restricted to established artists and art therapists, nor to patients and their immediate families. But its use for self-care by the professional caregiver is a quite new innovation. An example is Days of Renewal, organized by the University of Florida's Center for the Arts in

Healthcare Research and Education (CAHRE: www.arts.ufl.edu/cahre), which offers a whole-day experiential, arts-based workshop for nurses and other caregivers, and is the subject of ongoing research into its measurable benefits. Including the professional caregiver is a way to build community and break down apparent barriers between giver and recipient. An example is a gathering one recent Thanksgiving Eve on the Shands Hospital inpatient cancer unit. At the end of the weekly Arts in Medicine workshop, 10 patients and volunteers, realizing the staff at the nurses' station would also much sooner be home for this family celebration, serenaded them with an impromptu rendering of "America the Beautiful." There was a lot of laughter, and not a few tears, among the nurses and other staff—which led to thanksgiving being exchanged on all sides.

There are now large numbers of artist-in-residence programs in North America. The program at Shands Hospital, University of Florida, is among the largest: since its founding in 1991, at least 300 artists and several thousand students from all branches of healthcare and the arts have worked in this program. Our mission is to personalize and "de-professionalize" the arts in healthcare venues, taking the approach that every human is an artist. A key component has been to involve not only artists from the university and community, but also those emerging from among patients, families, staff, and volunteers.

An inherent limitation of any artist-in-residence program is that there are always more potential recipients than there are artists to supply this need. A recent innovation that approaches this problem is the marriage of art and technology at the bedside. At Shands Hospital, we are exploring the use of state-of-the-art computer technology to offer hospitalized patients access to online multimedia environments of virtual-reality visual art and music, in an attempt to give nonpharmacological relief from physical and psychological symptoms. The system is integrated into patient rooms via existing hospital LAN and PC-compatible patient computers installed at the onset of the project. Flat-screen monitors and surround sound create an easily accessible environment for the patient, who can activate the system on demand through a menu-driven interface with a wireless tablet. The system also allows investigators to track patient usage and outcomes—focusing on physical pain, anxiety, and degree of relaxation—through on-screen visual analog scales to obtain quantitative patient reports of these symptoms (Klein, Graham-Pole, Sonke-Henderson, & Haun, 2006).

## APPLICATIONS TO PALLIATIVE CARE SETTINGS

Palliative medicine is the emerging discipline of giving comfort and relieving the symptoms of body, mind, and spirit of patients who are usually very seriously ill, although not necessarily fatally so. The arts are ideally suited to this task.

The executive director of Hospice King-Aurora in Ontario Canada tells the story of hospice volunteers responding to a dying woman's dream of a trip to Paris with her husband. They created a café in the couple's living room, and shortly before her death set up tables with red-checkered cloths, played Edith Piaf, served French food, and so transported the couple off to their evening in Paris. A patient I know learned in his late sixties that he had advanced cancer. After forced retirement from his workaholic job, he started to commandeer the kitchen at home, buying gourmet cookbooks and immersing himself in the culinary arts. He tried out these increasingly delicious experiments on friends and family, before venturing into catering a couple of dinner parties. He lived a little over a year from the time he first knew his diagnosis; his wife said after his death that it was the best year of their long married life. A third example of art as palliative care is the fashion show described by Dorothy Lander that she and her stepdaughter put on for her dying husband (Lander, Napier, Fry, Bradoner, & Acton, 2005). The author is six feet tall, while her stepdaughter stands only five feet. Despite the deep sadness of their situation, they made this a fairly lighthearted experience for all, by the simple expedient of the two "models" trading clothes while the husband-father-patient was able to rouse sufficiently to capture the scene through photographs.

There are several reasons why art lends itself to palliative and end-of-life care, well summarized in a recent publication of the British organization Help the Hospices (www.helpthehospices.org.uk). The word *palliate* means literally to comfort and relieve suffering, very much in line with art for health. Patients with advanced illness or severe disability have a particular need to sense some control and autonomy, to explore psychological and spiritual issues, and ideally (as in the second example above) to learn new skills. If one is restricted in mobility, or bed-bound, an aesthetically pleasing environment becomes especially important. Hospices mostly recognize this, and focus on enhancing the physical setting with art of all kinds, from sculpture and murals to beautiful architecture and landscaping. Teresa Schroeder-Sheker's "prescriptive music" for dying people has created a whole new art form, with its own training and licensure—that of playing harp music continuously for those at the very end of their lives (Shroeder-Sheker, 1993).

Although palliative care settings tend to highlight the passive enjoyment of visual, musical, and performance art, more active involvement in individual or group activities can be facilitated by artists, for example, storytelling, quilting, poetry, and journaling, and the use of musical instruments such as a portable keyboard. The Web site Rosetta Life (www.rosettalife.org) was created by an organization of English professional artists, to enable people with life-limiting illness to explore important experiences through photography, video, poetry, drama, and other creative art forms. A current Rosetta Life project is seeking to provide specially "prescribed" original musical compositions to young people in Third World settings.

The enduring power of art in palliative and end-of-life care has been beautifully documented in Sandra Bertman's book, *Grief and the Healing Arts* (1999). Perhaps art's most important aspect in this setting is the close connection between our creativity and our spirituality, as discussed in depth by Matthew Fox (2004). A poem by the Sufi poet Rumi speaks eloquently to this:

> I saw grief drinking a cup of sorrow.
> "It tastes good, does it not?"
> "You've caught me," grief answered,
> "and you've ruined my business.
> How can I sell grief when
> you know it's a blessing."

To summarize, art for health and the arts therapies highlight the healing potential of the relationship established between patient and caregiver, linked to the often unspoken acknowledgment that we are all fully and equally *human*. This modern social movement is still in its early stages. The rest of this chapter will be devoted to discussing some of the growing educational, research, and social applications.

## APPLICATIONS TO EDUCATION

A colleague and I recently taught a class to senior medical students on the healing arts. We had them write for 10 minutes about an encounter with a seriously ill patient that had proved to be an uplifting or learning experience. Wanting this to be an exercise for their *right* brains, we asked them to then identify a color, a gesture, and an animal that came to them in reflecting on their stories, stressing the need to "grab" the first images that came to mind. Although much accustomed to the objectivity of the "H and P" (*history and physical*) that is omnipresent in so many doctor-patient encounters, none of these students had difficulty in this unaccustomed journey into the subjective aspect of their work: the *patient story*—something that is always at the center of their work as doctors, despite the increasingly sophisticated and technical nature of modern medicine.

Because art reflects every aspect of the world we live in and know—nature, society, ideas, emotions, relationships—it is uniquely situated to help in interpreting our whole learning experience, whether as health practitioners or as members of the lay public. As Evans illustrates elegantly in chapter 5, creativity is a multicontextual, multidimensional concept, explored by educators, scientists, and philosophers for millennia. Piaget may have seen it as something essential only to children's early development, to be put aside with the onset of adulthood; but holistic approaches to education, pioneered by Rousseau and later Montessori, champion a vital and enduring role for creativity, imagination, and play throughout our lives (Czikszentmihalyi, 1991; Gardner, 1983; Kane, 2004). In chapter 14, Camic gives a valuable description of the place of art in clinical and counseling psychology education and career opportunities. Two more applications of its use in healthcare education are also evolving, which I will summarize.

First, art is used in medical humanities programming, to educate students of healthcare, doctors, nurses, and others, and to change the way healthcare practitioners interact with patients (Charon & Montello, 2002). One of our Shands AIM artists, Gail Ellison, teaches a course in creative writing to first- and second-year medical students that is always oversubscribed, and often described in evaluations as the best experience of their four-year training. Life drawing classes are also increasingly used to help students of healthcare "see" their patients with a greater visual awareness. AIM's cofounder, Mary Rockwood Lane, who is on the faculty of the University of Florida (UF) College of Nursing, teaches a course for undergraduate and graduate nursing students that explores the connections between art and spirituality in healthcare.

CAHRE's mission at UF is to identify the many connections that exist between the creative and healing arts in an academic medical setting. This university center currently has for-credit courses in fine arts, dance and theater, music, writing, and spirituality. Students are drawn from our undergraduate and postgraduate body and from local, regional, and national health and other practitioners of all kinds. A particularly popular feature is the Arts in Healthcare Summer Intensive—a comprehensive three-week "how-to" course offering both didactic and hands-on information on how to establish, fund, maintain, and evaluate an art-for-health program.

Second, community education very often makes use of art to deliver health promotion messages to wider communities, and to have a positive impact on the well-being of the population, an application often unacknowledged and even unnoticed. For example, antismoking billboards, AIDS educational pamphlets, and popular theater performances in shopping centers and public squares are only as effective as their artistic appeal allows. Lander (2005) points out that artists have long been popular educators, citing the example of Hogarth's engravings, *Gin Lane* and *Beer Street*, which shaped the public policy of eighteenth-century Britain.

The art-for-health movement can be thought of as a second renaissance, arising some 700 years after the first, and celebrating the marriage of art and science in healthcare. It is vital to maintain a balance between the two as testimony to the gradual opening up of the biomedical model to this alliance, coexistent with the global exploration of body-mind-spirit connections as adjuncts to mainstream medicine. While conventional medicine has sometimes criticized and even actively suppressed this exploration, claiming it lacks the support of strong scientific evidence, advocates of holistic approaches can be overly dismissive of the extraordinary achievements of medical science. A balanced viewpoint sees the expansion of the domains of both as equally and essentially creative acts, vital to the future health of our global society.

## APPLICATIONS TO RESEARCH

There is ample scientific evidence that art and art therapy serve human health, ranging across physical, cognitive, emotional, social, and spiritual domains. These are addressed widely in several chapters that explore the scientific constructs of human creativity, and their relevance to human health. These effects include self-expression and catharsis, self-efficacy, awareness and problem-solving, and the relaxation response. Mechanisms underlying these effects are less understood, although they probably affect many body-mind systems. I include a few introductory comments.

Our culture is recognizing the vital coalition between art and science. The theory that every human being possesses multiple intelligences, first expounded by Gardener (1983), is widely accepted, and offers inspiration to the modern renaissance *uomo universale* aspirant. Leonardo da Vinci is the enduring exemplar of multisystem genius. It would have been unthinkable for Italian Renaissance thinkers and visionaries to separate science from art, yet this has been until recently the fate of modern society. An excellent example of renewal of the art-science alliance is the United Kingdom's well-funded National Endowment for Science, Technology, and the Arts (www.nesta.org.uk), which promotes "innovation nation" through subsidy of creativity and experiment across and between science and art (Kane, 2004, p. 9).

The visual arts have been shown to have powerful healing effects in people with widely diverse conditions and disabilities. The evidence supporting art therapy was brought together in two books by art therapist Cathy Malchiodi (1999a, 1999b). Paint, clay, and other materials have long been used by patients of all kinds by occupational and physical therapists to help recovery from strokes and injuries, and by psychotherapists and hospice workers to deal with psychological and end-of-life issues. Architect Roger Ulrich showed more than 20 years ago that views of nature from a patient's hospital bed after a surgical procedure caused them to report less anxiety, need less pain medication, and make a significantly faster postoperative recovery than those not exposed to these views (Ulrich, 1984). He and others have gone on to investigate in a series of studies the visual experiences and stimuli that produce the greatest benefit to patients with different conditions and in different situations (Ulrich, 1992).

Our HeArts & Hope studies at Shands Hospital, University of Florida, referred to earlier (Klein et al., 2006), explore the use of state-of-the-art computer technology at the bedside, to test the efficacy of offering hospitalized patients access to online multimedia environments of virtual-reality visual art accompanied by surround-sound music. Our hypothesis is that patients will not only use these media often, but that their use will prove an effective nonpharmacological approach to the relief of physical and psychological symptoms. This sophisticated electronic system allows researchers to record every patient usage of the varied menu of media available at the bedside, and to instantly analyze their online recordings of change in symptoms. In our current National Cancer Institute-funded study, we are collecting detailed data for 28 consecutive days from patients undergoing stem cell transplantation—a form of treatment that inevitably causes at least as severe effects as the underlying condition for which it is used. Simple on-screen visual analogue scales quantify the degrees of physical pain, anxiety, and relaxation the patient is experiencing, which are compared with simultaneous standard paper-and-pencil measurements to establish the statistical validity of the electronic recordings.

As described above, caregivers and hospital administrators are recognizing the importance of aesthetically pleasing environments in speeding the patient's recovery from different illnesses. Physicians at New York's Sloan Kettering Hospital reported that many cancer patients who visited the Museum of Modern Art to view Monet's *Water Lilies* described their emotional state afterward as a letting go of their concerns. A study of live music performed in the waiting room of an outpatient clinic in London's Chelsea and Westminster Hospital revealed lower blood pressures; duration of subsequent labor and delivery was also over two hours shorter than that of historical controls (Staricoff & Loppert, 2003). Healing gardens and other natural environments have been shown to have relaxing and restorative effects, and improve overall outcomes (Cooper-Marcus & Barnes, 1995). Cooper-Marcus and her colleagues conducted postoccupancy evaluations on patients, their families, and healthcare workers, showing positive mood changes, improved quality of care, and greater patient and family satisfaction.

The many benefits of music therapy have been studied by modern caregivers for more than half a century, reviewed by Aldridge in chapter 10, with a particular emphasis on palliative care. Music and sound have been used to lighten the effects of physical and psychological disorders and disabilities that affect people throughout life, ranging from the newborn nursery, where it speeds growth and development in newborn babies (Standley, 2005), to the end of life, where it is known to relieve pain and anxiety (Aldridge, 1998).

The health effects of reading and writing, including poetry, journaling, and other composition, are reviewed fully in chapters 9 (Fox) and 11 (Krantz & Pennebaker). Self-composition and journal writing have been subject to extensive quantitative research. Clinical psychologist James Pennebaker and his colleagues have led research in this field, with conclusive evidence of the power of the written word on improving health (Pennebaker, 1997). The initial research was conducted on undergraduate students, with the remarkable finding that journaling produced not only significant benefits to psychological but also to physical well-being. Later studies with people with widely diverse health issues have confirmed that the recording in a journal of stressful and traumatic events improves overall health.

Performance art (dance and drama) also benefits health, for which Goodill and Dulicai (chapter 7), Landy (chapter 8), and Krantz and Pennebaker (chapter 11) offer ample documenting evidence. Laughter-inducing spontaneous play has been claimed to be as beneficial as aerobic exercise (Cousins, 1991; Kane, 2004); as with all creative activity, benefits are probably mediated through the immune system. Listening to humorous audiotapes significantly increases salivary immunoglobulin (IgA), our first line of defense against infection, and other studies corroborate the benefits of clowning on the immune system (Berk, 1989).

Haya Rubin and her colleagues published a comprehensive analysis of the effects of the visual and auditory environment of healthcare facilities on medical outcomes of patients of all kinds, from newborns to elders and people with advanced illnesses (Rubin et al., 1998). Their focus was on strictly quantitative studies that proved or disproved a particular hypothesis. An even more comprehensive study of the role of the physical and aesthetic design of a hospital was conducted by Ulrich and his colleagues for the Center for Health Design (Ulrich, 1992).

New research to explore the health effects of art and art therapy must balance the merits of quantitative and qualitative design. The effect of changing the aesthetics of healthcare environments does not lend itself easily to quantitative methodology, particularly randomized clinical trials, which by definition focus on a specific narrow outcome. No artist, working with any art form, sets out with this intention. A simple example is the possible effect on individual passers-by or a whole community, whether overtly ill or well, of viewing an art installation in a hospital atrium: a randomized clinical trial exploring all the possible benefits of this experience would be impossible to design. Yet such features are becoming ubiquitous in modern healthcare facilities, in the wide belief that they promote physical, psychological, and probably spiritual health benefits.

Assessing the experience of viewing a mural or sculpture, or listening to ambient music while on the way to a clinic appointment, or strolling through a healing garden outside a cancer center, is more accessible to qualitative research (Denzin & Lincoln, 2005), which examines the subjective, or experiential, rather than the objective, or strictly quantifiable, the hallmark of quantitative research.

Recent healthcare research has made the case that qualitative narrative-based studies are as evidence-based as strictly quantitative studies, for decades the gold standard of medical therapeutic research (Kearney, 2000). Qualitative research was developed in the social sciences to uncover a deeper understanding of people and the social and cultural contexts in which they live. Data sources include participant observation (fieldwork), in-depth subject interviews and narratives, documents and texts, and the researcher's impressions and reactions. Future investigation of the health effects of the creative arts therapies will benefit from combining qualitative with quantitative research methods in the same study (triangulation: Kaplan, 2001).

A simple example is a study we conducted 15 years ago, a year after AIM's initiation at Shands Hospital. We collected one thousand questionnaires from patients, family members, and health practitioners, asking for both quantifiable information about the effects of the program on their physical, emotional, and sociospiritual health, and for open-ended (qualitative) feedback about how the various art forms had affected their stay, visit, or work. Both quantitative and narrative data were used as evidence to convince the hospital's administration to fund this previously volunteer artists-in-residence program ever since. My colleagues and I have embarked on a qualitative study of the application of the arts to palliative care, gathering the stories of professional and personal caregivers drawn from several countries.

Probably the primary mechanism whereby the arts and arts therapies affect our health is through strengthening of the immune, hormonal, autonomic, and other systems of the body. This is linked to the established field of psychoneuroimmunology, a term first coined by Robert Ader in 1975 to describe how mental processes directly affect the body's physiology (Ader, Felter, & Cohen, 2001). Candace Pert later showed the existence of endogenous polypeptide neurotransmitters that originate in the hypothalamus, and send messages to every cell in the body so far studied (Pert, 1997). Similar effects are seen with meditation, guided imagery, and prayer: new brain wave patterns are produced and the body's physiology changes from one of stress to one of relaxation, from one of fear to one of creativity and inspiration. These mechanisms are explored further in later chapters.

Research in this field is expanding quickly. Assessment of professional and family caregiver support through use of art is a compelling issue, given the huge stresses and burdens that often arise over the long term. In 2002, the Society for the Arts in Healthcare (SAH) in the United States initiated a research program with its counterpart in Japan, the initial findings of which were published in a recent monograph (Kable, 2003).The effect of art in recruiting and retaining staff and volunteers also requires study, as do studies on cultural differences and social inclusion related to class, gender, religion, race, ethnicity, age, and generation. The importance of art as a response to collective trauma experiences, such as the AIDS pandemic in Africa, the September 11 terrorist attacks, the victims of earthquakes in Pakistan, and the victims of Hurricane Katrina in New Orleans, has only recently captured public attention, and is reviewed by Speiser and Speiser (chapter 13).

## APPLICATIONS TO SOCIAL CHANGE

> I want all of my work to engage and to empower people to speak, to strengthen themselves into who they most want and need to be and then to act…the function of us all, as creative artists, is to make the truth as we see it irresistible.
>
> —Audre Lorde

That art should occupy a central role in the service of irresistible truth, as envisioned by an African-American lesbian poet-activist, is an aptly lofty goal for societal health education and promotion. For three centuries, art has been relegated to the sidelines: aesthetically pleasing but essentially irrelevant, frivolous, and dispensable. The truth is it is vital to our human welfare, an enduring psychosociospiritual resource underlying innovation and progress, as relevant to our health as any scientific endeavor, and a basic prescription for the ills of our society. If the twentieth century was the age of machines, the twenty-first is that of integrative systems of modern human endeavor (Kelly, 1996): scientific, artistic, educational, corporate, cultural, geographic, spiritual, work- and/or class-based. We inhabit a complex and chaotic world; engaging with it takes a special human intelligence: one of imaginative, flexible, optimistic, and ardent experiment. This is the central place of art; the universe is enduringly creative, and we humans co-evolve, with it and with each other, as part of its unfolding drama.

Artists have been engaged through history in social and political movements that affect our societal health. They have been leaders not only in public education but in upholding unpopular political positions and inspiring popular struggles: witness Hogarth's satirical prints, the literature of Charles Dickens and other Victorian writers, the use of homemade banners, flowers, posters, and ribbons by temperance activists and suffragettes, the long-suppressed works of many Asian, South and Central American, and Eastern European poets, and the AIDS Memorial Quilt. The homespun visual media of women temperance activists (Lander, 2005) can be thought of as prelude to the modern art for health movement, especially because it highlighted the use of crafts for a social purpose, as opposed to artworks hung in galleries. The mission of the AIDS Memorial Quilt, preserved and cared for by the Names

Project Foundation, is to raise public awareness about the enormity of the pandemic, to inspire action in the struggle against HIV and AIDS, and to offer a highly creative means of remembrance and collective healing (www. aidsquilt.org).

## CONCLUSION

Art has become a potent holistic force for human healing, of individuals and of our global community, and its value in healthcare pedagogy and research is expanding exponentially. The reason is that human creativity, in the final analysis, is the only resource we have to achieve social change. Today, the most ubiquitous tool available is the World Wide Web. Global access has created, in an astonishingly short time, an infinitely creative, free-moving, and unrestrained "democracy" of self-expression through universal online networks such as blogs and Wikipedia.

In his book, *The Play Ethic*, Pat Kane welcomes the Internet's potential for long-established institutions to "deconstruct themselves into new forms: a new way for parents and children to be with each other, a new way for technology's benefits to be accessible and empowering" (Kane, 2004, p. 351). These trends will inevitably impact our personal and collective short-term and long-term social and psychological health, for good or ill. For a balanced, whole-person approach to holistic health practice, pedagogy, and research to take its proper place in modern society, the Da Vincian principles of *arte/scienza* must find lasting renaissance.

## TOOL KIT FOR CHANGE

### Role and Perspective of the Healthcare Professional

1. As artists and health practitioners, we explore the vital and enduring links of art, holism, and spirituality to personal and collective human health.
2. Through art and the expressive arts therapies, we help every giver and receiver of care reap the benefits of human creativity.
3. As artists and health practitioners, we are activists for an essential social evolution that has its origins in human prehistory.

### Role and Perspective of the Participant

1. As one challenged by illness or disability in yourself or a loved one, your life story is at the heart of your aptitude for creative and artistic expression.
2. Art and art-making have the potential to improve every aspect of your physical, psychological, social, and spiritual health.
3. Art for health is a social movement for change that enables you to connect deeply with every other participant in art and art-making activities.

## Interconnection: The Global Perspective

1. Art for health and the expressive arts therapies are at once practice (service to others through art), pedagogy (teaching and learning about art for health), and research (discovery of the healing benefits of art and the expressive arts therapies).
2. Art and science are equal and complementary partners in our human evolution.
3. Art and the expressive arts therapies have always been and will always be vital to our individual, societal, and global health.

### Relevant Web Sites

www.aidsquilt.org
www.artsintherapy.com
www.arts.ufl.edu/cahre
www.helpthehospices.org.uk
www.holisticmedicine.org
www.ions.org
www.issseem.org
www.med.umich.edu/goa/
www.nccam.nih.gov
www.paintingsinhospitals.org.uk
www.patchadams.org
www.rosettalife.org
www.shandsartsinmedicine.com
www.thesah.org
www.nesta.org.uk

## REFERENCES

Ader, R., Felter, D., & Cohen, N. (2001). *Psychoneuroimmunology* (3rd ed.). New York: Academic Press.

Aldridge, D. (1998). *Music therapy in palliative care: New voices.* London: Jessica Kingsley.

Arnheim, R. (1972). *Toward a psychology of art: Collected essays.* Berkeley: University of California Press.

Berk, L. (1989). Neuroendocrine and stress hormone changes during mirthful laughter. *American Journal of Medical Science, 298,* 390–396.

Bertman, S. (1999). *Grief and the healing arts: Creativity as therapy.* Amityville, NY: Baywood.

Charon, R., & Montello, M. (2002). *Stories matter: The role of narrative in medical ethics.* London: Routledge.

Cooper-Marcus, C., & Barnes, M. (1995). *Gardens in healthcare facilities: Uses, therapeutic benefits, and design recommendations.* Concord, CA: Center for Health Design.

Cousins, N. (1991). *Anatomy of an illness.* New York: Bantam.

Czikszentmihalyi, M. (1991). *Flow: The psychology of optimal experience.* San Francisco: HarperPerennial.

Czikszentmihalyi, M. (1997). *Creativity: Flow and the psychology of discovery and invention.* San Francisco: HarperPerennial.

Denzin, N., & Lincoln, Y. (2005). *The SAGE handbook of qualitative research* (3rd ed.). Thousand Oaks, CA: Sage.

Dossey, L. (1993). *Healing words: The power of prayer and the practice of medicine.* New York: HarperSanFrancisco.

Dossey, L. (1999). *Reinventing medicine: Beyond mind-body to a new era of healing.* New York: HarperCollins.

Edson, M. (1999). *Wit: A play.* London: Faber & Faber.

Fox, M. (2004). *Creativity: Where the divine and the human meet.* New York: Jeremy Tarcher.

Gardner, H. (1983). *Frames of mind: The theory of multiple intelligences.* New York: Basic Books.

Graham-Pole, J. R. (2000). *Illness and the art of creative self-expression.* Oakland, CA: New Harbinger.

Kable, L. (Ed.). (2003). *Caring for caregivers: A grassroots US-Japan initiative.* Washington, DC: Society for the Arts in Healthcare (SAH).

Kane, P. (2004). *The play ethic.* London: Macmillan.

Kaplan, B. (2001). Evaluating informatics applications—social interactionism and call for methodological pluralism. *International Journal of Medical Informatics, 64,* 39–56.

Kearney, M. (2000). *A place for healing: Working with suffering in living and dying.* Oxford: Oxford University Press.

Kelly, K. (1996). *Out of control: The new biology of humans and machines.* London: Fourth Estate.

Klein, J., Graham-Pole, J., Sonke-Henderson, J., & Haun, J. (in press). Assessment of bedside computerized audiovisual programming for hospitalized patients. *Cancer Nursing.*

Lander, D. (2005). The ribbon workers as popular educators. Re-presenting the colours of the Crusades. *Studies in the Education of Adults, 37,* 47–62.

Lander, D., Napier, S., Fry, B., Brander, H., & Acton, J. (2005). Memoirs of loss as popular education: Five palliative caregivers re-member through the healing art of hope and love. *Convergence, 38,* 121–139.

Lander, D., & Graham-Pole, J. (2006). The appreciative pedagogy of palliative care: Arts-based or evidence-based?. *Journal for Learning through the Arts: A Research Journal on Arts Integration in Schools & Communities, 2.* Retrieved September, 2006, from http: repositories.cdlib.org/clta/lta/vol2/iss1/art15.

Lorde, A. *Quoted in* Charles Rowell (1991). Above the wind: An interview with Audre Lorde. *Callaloo, 14,* 83–95.

Malchiodi, C. (1999a). *Medical art therapy with adults.* London: Jessica Kingsley.

Malchiodi, C. (1999b). *Medical art therapy with children.* London: Jessica Kingsley.

McNiff, S. (1992). *Art as medicine.* Boston: Shambala.

Pennebaker, J. (1997). *Opening up: The healing power of expressing emotions.* New York: Guilford Press.

Pert, C. (1997). *Molecules of emotion.* New York: Scribner.

Rubin, H., Owens, A., & Golden, G. (1998). *Status report—An investigation to determine whether the built environment affects patients' medical outcomes.* Martinez, CA: The Center for Health Design Press.

Samuels, M., & Samuels, L. (1990). *Seeing with the mind's eye: The history, techniques, and uses of visualization.* New York: Random House.

Samuels, M., & Lane, M. R. (1998). *Creative healing: How to heal yourself by tapping your hidden creativity.* San Francisco: HarperCollins.

Shroeder-Sheker, T. (1993). Music for the dying: A personal account of the new field of music thanatology. *Journal of Mind-Body Health, 9,* 36–48.

Standley, J. (2005). *Medical music therapy: A model program for clinical practice, education, training, and research.* Silver Springs, MD: American Music Therapy Association.

Staricoff, R., & Loppert, S. (2003). Integrating the arts into healthcare: Can we affect clinical outcomes? In X. Kirklin & B. Richardson (Eds.), *The healing environment: Without and within* (pp. 63–80). London: Royal College of Physicians.

Ulrich, R. (1984).View through a window may influence recovery from surgery. *Science, 220,* 420–421.

Ulrich, R. (1992). How design impacts wellness. *Health Care Forum Journal,* 20–25.

Whyte, D. (1997). *The house of belonging.* Langley, WA: Many Rivers Press.

Chapter Two

# HISTORY OF THE ARTS AND HEALTH ACROSS CULTURES

*Jill Sonke-Henderson, BA*

Ancient cave drawings and paintings link us to the experiences of our early human ancestors. These images provide insight into the nature of early human experience as it relates to creativity and art, to spirituality and healing, and to the interconnectedness among these aspects of early human life. Artworks found in the caves at Chauvet in Northern France and in the caves at Bhimbetka in Central India depict the presence of body art and jewelry created and worn by people over 30,000 years ago. This desire to elaborate on the natural human form suggests that the human ability and desire to create beauty and meaning is a defining characteristic of humans (see Dissanayake, 2000).

The caves at Lascaux in Southern France contain exquisite works of art dating from approximately 20,000 B.C.E. Joseph Campbell (1990), in his book *Transformations of Myth through Time*, describes the discovery of the ancient tools found near the caves at Lascaux. Amidst the clearly useful objects, there was found an object of "divinely superfluous beauty" (p. 6), an object of art that for Campbell represents an emergence of spiritual awareness in man. This object had no apparent use, but had some quality that led it to be deemed a work of art, and something about it reflected a spiritual experience as well. The question that arises here is, what is it that differentiates art from tools, or from anything else for that matter? More essentially, what is art and how is it that we recognize it as such? Dissanayake (1988) asserts that it became possible to "differentiate between artifacts and experiences that were concerned with ordinary daily maintenance and those that were for some reason appeared or were made to be special" (p. 128) as early as, and likely before, early hominid development with Homo erectus.

It was the Greeks who, in the Classical Era, first defined the arts as disciplines in the way that we know them today; but creativity and art have, since long before the Classical Era, been used by human beings to express the divine and the human experience and to transform levels of consciousness. Although it may not be so in the West today, over most of our human history, the arts were not separated from the basic aspects of living; they were simply a part of life's common functions. In many cultures, they held primary roles in communication, healing, fertility, hunting, food production, and even in combat. In Australia, elders educated the young through storytelling; men in ancient Greece practiced choreographed dances to prepare for battle; even now in Haiti, painted vodoun flags invoke the spirits of love and safety, and Yoruba women in Africa sing and dance to please the Orishas (spirits) of fertility and sustenance. Today in many developed nations, however, the arts are perceived as separate from the essentials of life. They are largely practiced by specialists known as artists and are seen as luxuries.

The essential link between the arts and spirituality is clearly represented in the recognition of historians and scholars that one representation of a spiritual awareness in man is the impulse to create, to express the divine mysteries. Modern as well as early humans have recognized the transcendent quality of the arts. In the design of holy places, the visual arts and music have long been used to shift one's state of consciousness from the mundane to the sacred. Holy grounds, temples, and churches are places of beauty, filled with music, art, and architecture designed to quiet the mind and prepare the individual to better connect to the spirit realm, to him or herself, to wisdom, and to others. Throughout history, humanity has recognized the power of art to inform, inspire and transform; and in turn, has recognized the power of transcendent experiences in facilitating the production of great art. In the fourth century B.C.E. in the Cults of Dionysus, thousands of people sang and danced every night until a state of ecstasy was achieved. Interestingly, Dionysus was not only the god of wine, known for leading these great drunken and dancing orgies, but was also known as the god of the generative forces in world. Since the eighth century, the Sufis, or Whirling Dervishes as they are also known, have danced to achieve ecstasy and spiritual insight. Sufi poets Rumi and Kabir harnessed the transcendent energy of the rituals to create some of the world's greatest poetry.

It is not only great artists who can experience the transcendent qualities of art. Anyone can engage in a creative process and reap the benefits. Not unlike Dionysian cult members, many people today go to night clubs to drink and dance. Like our predecessors, we find ecstasy in this experience, feel uplifted and connected to our peers. Children draw, dance, sing, and act out dramas every day. This impulse to express through creative artistic media is innately human, and we see it clearly in children. Those who maintain this connection to creative expression go on to develop technical artistic proficiency and become professional artists, while others create for the experience and not the outcome. Many people choose to participate in the arts as audience members or viewers, but still find the experience of art transcendent. So, what differentiates art from other objects, or from entertainment? Creation is a divine act. It evokes a sense of wonder, of limitlessness, of inspiration, and of knowing. It changes us. This is true of both the creative process and of resulting works of art; both artist and viewer are affected. This is what can be seen to connect art to spirituality and, in turn, to healing.

## THE ARTS AND HEALTH

Until the sixteenth century c.e., illness and health were considered by every known culture to be primarily spiritual matters. It was many centuries after Hippocrates developed the seeds of rational medicine that the reductionist ideals of Western medicine formally separated mind, body, and spirit, reducing illness to a physical matter and establishing medicine as a physical science. Until this time and even throughout much of the world today, the healing rituals of most cultures have been firmly rooted in faith and tradition. Animistic indigenous cultures, which still exist on every continent, hold that disease and pain represent disruptions of various sorts in the harmonious relationships between man and the spirit world. Illness is a spiritual matter and is approached as such. Within healing rituals, the arts provide the means for transcendence into the spiritual realm, and also create tangible and meaningful representations for the belief systems and healing systems of each culture.

Archaeological findings as well as paintings, sculpture, and bas reliefs found in animistic regions suggest great similarities among the culture and belief systems of early animistic peoples of Africa, Asia, the Americas, Oceania, and Europe. Among these images are many depicting characters known as shamans. Shamans are the healers of these communities, and significant among their tools for healing are the arts and the imagination. The shaman, a "manipulator of the sacred" and "great master of ecstasy" (Eliade, 1964, p. 4), acts as the intermediary between the visible, ordinary world and the spirit world, journeying through the imagination to the spirit world to bring healing to individuals and the community. Shamanic rituals involve music, dance, drama, and visual and sometimes written forms of art. Community members are often active in these rituals, assisting the shaman in his journey to the outer realms of consciousness. Medical performances by shamans, individuals, and communities aid in reestablishing the balance between the human and spirit worlds.

The following three sections, focused on Africa, Native America, and Asia, will interchangeably refer to various cultures as animistic, traditional, aboriginal, or indigenous. All of these terms refer to the original populations of a particular area. These sections are not intended to represent a chronological look at these cultures, but will acknowledge that they span history and will explore just a few examples of the changing and unchanging relationships between the arts and healing throughout our human history.

## AFRICA: CREATIVITY AND HEALING AS A WAY OF LIFE

Africa provides us with rich examples of the roles of the arts in healing. Traditional African cultures are filled with long-established healing rituals and, while African culture is quite diverse, traditional belief systems are consistently based in animistic principles that hold that everything in the universe is animated or contains spirit. In Africa today, up to 80 percent of the population uses traditional medicine for primary healthcare (World Health Organization, 2005). These traditions include visual, creative, herbal, and mystical methods that are unique to various geographic areas. Throughout Africa, alchemical transmutation is found in ritual works of art such as sculpture and masks associated with healing (Ghent, 1994). Traditional healers, including shamans and medicine men, imbibe healing powers into the materials used in the creation of sacred and healing art. These pieces themselves are believed to have the power to heal, prevent disease, protect individuals and communities from harm, enhance fertility, cure mental illness, and even to bring atonement for moral transgressions. Images depicting the preparation of healing artworks and healing rituals involving these objects can be found in prehistoric cave paintings throughout sub-Saharan Africa.

The !Kung San of the Adobe region of South Africa, also known as the Kalahari Bushmen, are one of the oldest and most documented foraging societies in the world. The !Kung believe that ghosts, or *gangwasi*, are responsible for illnesses and other misfortunes. The most potent response that the !Kung have to illness is *num*, the healing energy that allows one to enter a trance and while in this state, to effect a cure (Kottak, 1998).

Many !Kung aspire to become healers, or shaman, and as many as half of the men and one-third of the women are known to have the power to heal. The art of healing is passed from one healer to another through rigorous ritual and training. Healing among the !Kung is most often accomplished through the !Kai Dance. The all-night ritual is held several times a week beginning at sundown. The healing power of the !Kai Dance depends upon the activation of *num*, which resides in the belly of the shaman. Through sustained ecstatic dancing, the substance heats up to a boil and travels up the healer's spine, exploding with healing power in the brain. In this state, they can heal themselves and others.

To the Tambuka speaking people of northern Malawi, dance and musical experience are "the structural nexus where healer, patient and spirit meet" (Friedson, 1996, p. xvi). A healer in Tambuka society is recognized when he, or occasionally she, is afflicted with the "disease of the prophets" (*nthenda ya uchimi*) which manifests as a physical disease and is diagnosed by another prophet healer, or *nchimi*. Interestingly, the maturation of the disease is considered to be the transition from patient to healer. One might speculate that every medical system could be stronger if its healers were initiated through the process of disease itself.

The ontological basis of Tambula culture holds that diseases, as well as their cures, are generally brought about by spirits, most notably *vimbuza* (a broad term encompassing a class of spirits, diseases they cause, and the music and dance used to cure them). Both diagnosis and cure are achieved through *vimbuza* dances, which are inextricably connected to music and drumming. *Vimbuza* rituals are practiced several nights a week in Tambuka communities. In each healing ritual the entire community, as well as the individual, benefits. This belief, which lies in stark contrast to contemporary Western healthcare values that focus primarily on the individual, is central to many African societies and is reflected in the folk saying, "To heal a sick child, the entire village must be cured."

Not entirely dissimilar to the !Kai dance tradition, the Tambuka view dance as a means for heating and cooling the spirits that occupy both patient and healer. An important part of the practice of the adept healer is the cooling of the *vimbuza*, just to the point where the *mizimu*, the spirits that allow the healer to "see," can "go on top." The process can be described as follows. "Instead of possessing the dancer, the *vimbuza* act as a source of energy that pushes the *mizimu* up, thus creating the necessary conditions for seeing" (Friedson, 1996, p. 30). Within the *vimbuza* ritual, the *nchimi* dances to the rhythm of drums to enter a trance-like state wherein he or she can access the spirit realm. Within this state the healer does not lose his or her sense of self, but speaks and acts from the influence of contact with the *vimbuza* spirits. A diagnosis is made and curing actions including dance or applications of herbal remedies may follow. For the Tambuka people, a clinical reality is constructed with the healing rituals. Music and dance blur the boundary between the human and spirit realms. Rather than being a passive participant in a healing practice as in Western medicine, the Tambuka patient is typically the active center of the ritual. The clinical reality for the Tambuka people is just as vivid and real for them as for those who seek Western medical treatment, perhaps more so because of the longstanding cultural roots and active experiences imbedded in the tradition.

## NATIVE AMERICA: RITUAL AND FAITH

Inside a tent in the Pacific Northwest more than ten thousand years ago, a group of people sit around a fire drumming and singing. At the center of the circle a man, dressed in ornate regalia including an animal mask, dances. The intent of the group is to assist the man, who is the tribe's shaman, into a trance state so that he can heal a member of the tribe. The shaman dances in a sunwise direction around the fire, all the time looking upward toward the tent's smoke hole. Some of the other participants play drums, others chant, and others yield weapons in movements reflecting pursuit. Periodically, the shaman's movements mimic a particular animal, thus bringing the spirit of that animal to the circle. The shaman suddenly stands still and screams, which is the sign that a spirit has entered his body. The tent becomes silent and, speaking through the shaman, the spirit animal reveals the patient's diagnosis. With abandoned yet ritualized dance movements, the shaman withdraws an imaginary spear-like object from the patient's body. He then performs convulsive movements and gestures for the patient to run with him around the fire in both directions. Finally, he declares the patient healed. (See Hultkrantz, 1992)

Throughout the many different Native American tribes that have inhabited the continent, healing traditions and practices vary greatly in appearance, but only mildly in meaning. Rituals such as the one described above are commonplace and central to ways of life. At the core of these values is spiritual development and harmony with nature and the spirit world (Csordas, 2002). Illness is generally considered to be either an invasion of a malevolent spirit or the representation of a lack of harmony or balance with nature or the spirit world. Shamanic healing rituals often involve sand painting, dance, drumming, and chanting, and are centered on the use of symbols that hold deep cultural meaning. These modalities are used either as representation or transformation. A painting or a dance might be done to represent the desired balance with the universe and to maintain health, or might be done to facilitate the shaman's or the patient's transcendence into the spirit world in order to seek the aid of a spirit to assist in returning balance.

Sand painting is a common element in Navajo healing rituals. It is an intricate process that engages shaman and patient together in a healing intention and ritual. The sand paintings created by the shaman contain images symbolizing origin myths that assist the patient in identifying with the forces of creation and in re-creating himself into a state of wholeness and health (Sandner, 1977). In the ritual, the patient sits or lies in the middle of the tribal circle next to a person who chants and sings. During the long ritual, the patient is encouraged to develop and focus on healing images. At the same time the shaman creates a sand painting on the ground next to him representing "the spiritual and physical landscape in which a patient and illness exist, the etiology of the disease and the mythology chosen for the cure" (Achterberg, 1985, p. 49).

The Sun Dance, perhaps the most famous of all Native American rituals, is a ritual of sacrifice and renewal performed by all tribes of the High Plains.

Within the dance, the tribe's people seek renewal for the living earth and all of its components, renewal of spirit and of health (Liberty, 1980). The ritual, generally lasting for three days and nights, was essentially a thanksgiving ritual to praise the supreme being, *Tam Apo* ("our father") for the past year, to ask for blessings for the coming year, and to induce a state of very profound and extended suffering for the purpose of purification. During the ritual, the shaman performs dances to cure those who are ill. Dancers are treated by the shaman, who uses an eagle wing to brush off their illness, while infusing them with fresh power. An important aspect of the Sun Dance is that of faith. Faith in the success of the Sun Dance and in strenuous dancing itself is essential. The ritual and dancing can bring and sustain health, but the dancer can further improve his health if his faith is strong. The arts themselves act to quiet and focus the mind, and allow the practitioner to connect deeply with the intention of the ritual. The images used are familiar to the practitioners as they have been passed down through generations and are deeply ingrained in the cultures. They are strong and clear representations of the Native American belief systems.

## ASIA: IMAGERY AND MEANING

Asia is a vast and diverse continent with a rich history of indigenous mystical and healing traditions. Asian cultures have traditionally viewed illness in spiritual terms, while many, such as the Chinese, have enduring ancient healing traditions with sophisticated scientific bases. Chinese medicine, which originally viewed illness as the doing of an evil spirit (Lee, 1980), has for thousands of years attended to both the spiritual and physical aspects of illness and health (Huang & Williams, 1999).

Traditional Malaysian healing is rooted in the Malay religion and involves either the *pawang* (shaman or medicine man) or the *bomoh* (spirit medium). In Malaysia as well as in Thailand, dance, drama and music have been and are still commonly used to excise evil spirits from the body. Perhaps the most significant of all creative healing practices in these areas is the *puteri*, or *main peteri*, a therapeutic dance-theater ritual performed in Malaysia and some parts of southern Thailand. In this ritual practice, healers dance to enter a trance and patients ultimately dance to bridge the human and spirit worlds. For the patient, the dance is curative, signaling health and a return to the community (Wright, 1980).

Tibetan Medical practice evolved from Tibet's indigenous and shamanic Bon spiritual tradition. Bon healing is ritual-based and has not vanished entirely from the culture, but has taken a backseat to current Buddhist traditions. In Tibetan Buddhist medical practice, art plays a primary, but very different, role. According to the Tibetan Buddhist tradition, the Buddha, Siddhartha

Guatama, established the foundation of the medical system through the creation of the Four Medical Tantras, or *Gyushi* (Baker, 1997). A series of paintings accompanies the written text. The 79 paintings, or *thangkas,* include nearly 8,000 images that offer insights into the system of health. The paintings are used for medical study by physicians and are also used by lay people. Sangye Gyamtso, painter of the original seventeenth-century paintings, noted that "art can convey truths that academic treatises only touch upon. The images within these paintings are keys to understanding the healing response within our own bodies and minds. They are potent examples of the Tibetan Buddhist concept of 'Liberation through sight'" (p. 15) as they transform ordinary perception into healing awareness. As the viewer contemplates the images, understanding arises and internal changes take place that can lead to both healing and spiritual growth. In this way, Tibetan Buddhist healing and spiritual traditions are deeply interconnected. While Tibetan Buddhism is today a primary spiritual practice in Tibet, the roots of Bon and its shamanic principles are still clearly present in the culture. Tibetan Buddhism is filled with ritualistic traditions including songs, dramas, and dances for healing, and even in the simple rituals of everyday life, such as the hanging of prayer flags, we see this rich history reflected.

## IMAGERY AND THE MIND

Each of these traditions has been practiced for thousands of years and can still be found today, illustrating the ways in which the arts facilitate healing rituals and healing itself. One of the primary foundations upon which these diverse healing rituals are based is the power of imagery, of the imagination, and of the mind. All of the references that can be found of the inclusion of the arts in healing practices involve one or more of the following components:

- an active use of the mind in developing or focusing on imagery
- the use of images as visual representation of an ideal or intention
- the use of the arts as a method for transcendence or altering one's level of consciousness
- the use of the arts as a symbol or manifestation of an intention

If we compare the use of the arts in healing 30,000 years ago with that of today we will see marked differences, but we can also find these essential traits present in both ancient and contemporary ways. The modern discipline of psychoneuroimmunology provides a scientific explanation for these animistic healing practices and for what humanity has known instinctively since the beginning of time—that imagery and the mind can trigger physical changes, including healing, in the body (see Pert, 1997). Psychoneuroimmunology explores the interactions between the mind, the nervous system (including the brain), and the immune system, and here may serve to broaden the reader's perception of these ancient animistic healing traditions.

It is important to consider that while the human species and our cultures have changed continuously over the course of our history, certain aspects of our being remain constant. Regardless of where or when we live, we generally strive to stay alive, avoid pain, seek comfort, joy, and love, and attempt to understand our existence and find meaning in it. We find consistent evidence of the use of the mind and imagination among humans to relate to both the natural and supernatural realms. The imagination lies at the center of much of this functioning, and consistently, we as human beings create to express the wonder of creation.

As we look now chronologically at the progress of healing traditions toward the development of Western medicine, we will see even more diverse, but consistently present, roles of the arts in healing practices. We'll start in Egypt.

## EGYPT: ANCIENT MEDICINE AND NARRATIVE

The oldest surviving medical book, dated 1550 B.C.E., derives from Thebes. Known as the Ebers papyrus, it documents a surprising level of medical sophistication and knowledge (Ebbell, 1937) and documents the diagnosis and treatment of a wide array of medical conditions. Approximately 1,500 pharmacological, herbal, and animal remedies are noted, as are numerous spells and incantations, suggesting that while medicine was developing as a physical science, beliefs related to the origin of illness and disease were still magical and supernatural in orientation. While spirit-based healing rituals were quite common in Egypt at this time, the roles of professional physicians were well developed and even specialized to include gynecology and surgery.

In ancient Egypt, there were three divisions of healers aside from physicians: the *swnu,* the Priests of Sekhmet, and the sorcerers. The Egyptians believed that good health was threatened by both earthly, or physical, forces and by supernatural forces such as evil spirits that could invade the body through orifices and consume an individual's vital substance (Porter, 1997). Spells and rituals were used to restore disruptions in balance between man and the spirit and ancestral realm. The gods were of such primary concern in daily life that it was only natural that they should be called upon for healing. Thoth, Egyptian god of writing, wisdom, music, and balance, was a central figure in Egyptian healing and was thought to be the most powerful magician in the world. Interestingly, he is credited with the invention of both medicine and writing.

Narrative incantations were commonly used in ritual form for sustaining or restoring good health. The following is the translated closing recitation from a Ramesside incantation to remove poison from a patient:

> Words spoken over an image of Atum Horus Hekenu, an image of Isis, an image of Horus, written on the hand of the bitten patient, to be licked off by the man, and drawn likewise on a strip of finest linen, placed at the neck of the bitten patient. The herbal remedy is the scorpion-herb, ground into beer or wine, to be drunk by the patient bitten by a scorpion. An item a million times effective. (Grajetzki, 2000, p. 1)

## GREECE: PLANTING THE SEEDS OF RATIONAL MEDICINE

In ancient Greece, illness was also explained in supernatural terms. As in many other aspects of culture, attitudes and traditions related to health and healing migrated from the Egyptians to the Greeks. Diseases were generally held to be caused either by malignant spirit demons or by the wrath of the gods (Loudon, 1997), who were mortals elevated to the position of gods. For example, in Homer's *The Iliad* (Seymour, 1990), the plague that decimates the Greek army attacking Troy is represented as supernatural in origin.

In general, the arrows of Apollo and his sister Artemis were believed by the Greeks of the Classical Era to be the bearers of sudden diseases sent by the gods. In addition to causing disease and death in this way, the gods were responsible for healing wounds and for curing diseases. Apollo and his son Asclepius were the most important of the healing gods, and Asclepius ultimately became the major god of healing in the fifth century B.C.E. Exquisite temples honoring Asclepius were erected throughout Greece, Italy, and Turkey, and it was there that the sick were tended to in an environment of art and beauty.

Within these temples, which often housed baths and theaters, dream therapy or "divine sleep" was a common treatment for difficult diseases. Within the ritual, a patient was prepared through fasting and music to enter a spiritual state in which he could best absorb divine communication from the dream state. This state, which occurred just before sleep and was accompanied by music, would bring Asclepius himself, appearing carrying a caduceus (the modern symbol of medicine). Asclepius would bring the patient either a cure or a recommendation for treatment. Greek physicians of the times were also known to commonly use the developing art of drama and Greek theater prescriptively. Greek tragedy was originally developed as a ritual of cleansing and atonement, and drama festivals in Athens were often preceded with ritual sacrifices (Figes, 1976). In the temples of Asclepius, comedy or satire was prescribed for depressive patients, and tragedy was prescribed for manic patients.

It was in these temples that Hippocrates, the father of modern medicine, is said to have studied the *iamata*, documents describing cures that were effected by the gods (Loudon, 1997). This study serves as the basis for one of the most important transitions in the history of healing: the invention of rational medicine, Hippocrates' new philosophy that attributed diseases not to gods or the spirit world, but to purely physical and natural causation. While Hippocrates is commonly credited with this invention, there also exists written evidence that credits the Egyptians with the establishment of medicine as a rational scientific discipline. This way of thinking correlated with the general tendency among philosophers of this era to explain the world in physical terms. Still, in this period we find references to medical practices that are not only spiritual, but very much involve creativity and the mind.

## THE MIDDLE AGES IN EUROPE: HEALING AND THE CHURCH

We'll leap ahead now to the Middle Ages, times of great illness and struggle, and also times of unprecedented conflict and transition in healing traditions in Europe. It is during this period that healing traditions were most challenged, and struggled to both maintain and depart from their roots. In Europe, Christianity was developing as both a formal religion and as a governmental power and affected healing practices to such a degree that some historians blame it for bringing about the darkest days in healthcare (Achterberg, 1985). The medical progress made by the Egyptians, Greeks, and Romans was halted during this time by the Christian denial of both animistic principles and principles of rational medicine, and healing became infused with religion.

By this point in time, all of the world's major religions had been well established, and are worth a bit of discussion as some had a tremendous influence on the medical practices of the times. Hinduism, Judaism, Buddhism, Christianity, and Islam each had well-defined and different perspectives on health and healing, but none had yet embraced solely rational ideas related to illness and disease. Judaism and Christianity shared Old Testament values that credited God and his wrath with the causation of disease and suffering, and credited faith, prayer, piety, repentance, and faith-based ritual with curing, making strong demarcations between the body and the soul. The soul was highly revered over the physical body, and during the Middle Ages in particular, the body was viewed as negative and sinful. These perspectives, and the rise of the Christian church as governmental power, led to the suppression of Western medical development during this time.

Numerous interesting references to the use of the arts for healing are found in Biblical scripture. In the Old Testament book of 1 Samuel (chapter 16, verses 14–16), David is summoned to play the harp to soothe the evil spirit from Saul:

The spirit of the Lord had departed from Saul, and he was tormented by an evil spirit sent by the Lord. So the servants of Saul said to him: "Please! An evil spirit from God is tormenting you. If your lordship will order it, we, your servants here in attendance on you, will look for a man skilled in playing the harp. When the evil spirit from God comes over you, he will play and you will feel better."

During the Middle Ages, plagues swept through Europe. The Black Death, one of numerous plagues, was credited with killing as many as 20 million people in its three-year reign. Church leaders were adamant that the plagues were God's wrath sent to punish mankind for his sins and that only piety, humility, repentance, and even suffering (reflecting the influence of Judaic values on Christianity) could bring an end to them. There was a pervasive belief in the church that "if God sends disease, then to try to cure it can be seen as interference with His will, and it is only He who should be asked to heal it; it may be visitation for sin, and then repentance and prayer are the proper therapy" (Loudon, 1997, p. 55). It was only after years of suffering and widespread death that the realization of the physical cause and spread of the disease was understood and the disease came under control.

Interestingly, the very ideals, and even some specific healing practices, upon which animism and paganism are based can be seen represented in Christianity during the Middle Ages in the context of a new vocabulary. Spirits and gods became saints; and diseases were termed to be caused by Satan rather than by spirits or gods. The divine sleep rituals of the Asclepian Temples could be seen in the church, but were now called the Divine Sleep of the Saints. Pilgrimages to holy places were popular and icons of saints were used to represent various virtues and healing qualities. While the language was different, the principles were nearly the same and still required faith, particular imagery, and ritualized practice on the part of healer and patient. Essentially, medicine still dwelled primarily in the realm of the imagination.

Also during this time, rational medicine was developing slowly in Greece and in the Middle East; and unbeknownst to many Westerners today, Islam was leading the way in the development of what would become Western medicine. In Europe, women healers and midwives, most notably Hildegard of Bingen and an Italian student of medicine known as Madame Trot, carried on the folk tradition derived from Greek and shamanic traditions, made tremendous advancements in the study and practice of herbal medicine, and contributed to the development of pharmacology and obstetrics (see Hildegard of Bingen, 1998).

The role of the arts was less central to the healing practices of the time, but could still be seen in both pagan and religious practices, including Christianity. Biblical accounts of miracle healing popularized belief in the healing power of relics and shrines; thus, pilgrimages to healing sites were quite popular and common. While the church denied and severely punished involvement in pagan healing rituals, the church itself encouraged faith-based healing. The word *pagan* derives from a Latin term meaning *countryside;* the term was used for the non-Christian belief system that was common in Europe and had essentially evolved from the earlier nature-based, or animistic, traditions (Molloy, 2002).

Scandinavian fire dances were pagan rituals performed to maintain health and to cleanse the body of illness. In this ritual, participants would dance all night to reach a state of transcendent spiritual ecstasy, then would repeatedly leap through a raging fire to burn off harboring diseases and help to restore and maintain health. Again, we see dance as a tangible action representing healing, thus engaging a belief system and the mind to effect physical change. Serlin (1993) notes the similarity of these fire dances and of Scandinavian ring dances with those performed by the Greek Orpheoteleste, who also danced around the sick for healing purposes in the fifth century b.c.e. Until the 1500s, rituals such as the fire dances continued to thrive in Europe. By this time, the persecution of the women healers had reduced their numbers, thus slowing the progress of rational healthcare severely.

## A SEGUE TO ISLAM: SCIENCE AND MYSTICISM

While Islam was leading the way in the development of scientific medical practices in the tenth, eleventh, and twelfth centuries, spiritual healing practices were also prevalent. In Islamic lands, medical care involved a rich mixture of religions and cultures—a coexistence of traditions that is unparalleled even in contemporary societies. Islamic physicians were developing the use of plant medicines that would become the foundation of Western pharmaceuticals, writing the texts that would become the foundations for Eastern medical practice and education in Europe, and establishing the first models of urban hospitals that would serve the sick exclusively (Loudon, 1997). At the same time, the Sufis were defining trance-based healing rituals reflective of indigenous practices.

Sufism, or Islamic mysticism, is a devotional movement that values deliberate simplicity and involvement of the emotions, and is sometimes referred to as "the heart of Islam" (Molloy, 2002). The practice of dancing or whirling is used to create a sustained state of ecstasy or altered consciousness in which one can experience God directly and effect change, including healing. In Sufi orders in the Asian subcontinent of India in the Sultanate period (the thirteenth through nineteenth centuries), *shatkhs* were the healers. The most common healing function that they performed was the writing of healing amulets. In this ritual, either the patient or the *shatkhs* would write the names of god or other healing words on a paper, which was placed in an amulet and worn around the patient's neck. It was believed that the power of the *shatkhs'* touch as well as the power of the words themselves were transferred to the paper and then to the patient as he wore the amulet.

The Sufi healer, who must train for 12 years before practicing, acts as a guide during some healing rituals, leading the patient to diagnose himself or herself in the state of ecstasy brought on through breathing techniques. In other rituals, the healer chants prayers over the patient and passes his hands over the patient's body (Lawrence, 1980). Interestingly, unlike other more orthodox faith healing practices, it is not necessary that the patient believes he will be healed. This structure represents an interesting departure from faith healing (although not from spirituality) and a belief in the healer's actions themselves as the cause of the healing.

## THE RENAISSANCE IN EUROPE: A NEW PARTNERSHIP FOR SCIENCE AND THE ARTS

Plagues dominated the lives of Europeans from 1348 until well into the seventeenth century. Syphilis and other diseases were also on the rise and the population in Europe was severely reduced. Medical care during the early Renaissance period was much the same as during the Middle Ages, with natural or rational medicine taking its place among magical and religious approaches. The coexistence of natural and divine healing is represented in the figures of Cosmas and Damian, the Catholic patron saints of medicine (Danilevicius, 1967) who, in keeping with the tradition of Asclepius, were reputed to have cured a patient in a dream. In the famous dream, the saints amputated the patient's ulcerated leg and replaced it with one from a recently dead Moor. When the patient awoke, he found a new healthy leg (although of a dramatically different skin coloration) in place of the old.

In the 1500s, the training of physicians moved formally into the university setting, and artists were found to be essential in both scientific discovery and in the teaching of medicine. Western medicine during this time was becoming professionalized through the development of hospitals for the sick and the increasing formalization of standards for professional medical practice. The role of the arts in the development of this Western medical system was changing but still quite important. At this time, achievements in the arts were as great as that of medical science. The level of visual detail that artists were capable of representing fell right into place in the medical system. Renaissance artists such as Lorenzo Ghilberti, Leon Batista Alberti, Leonardo da Vinci, and Michelangelo Buonarroti had begun to perform their own human dissections in order to study the human anatomy in detail. Physicians worked closely with these artists in order to understand the human form themselves and to produce visual models for experimentation and teaching (Loudon, 1997). Indeed, without the partnership of the arts, progress in medicine would have been far slower.

The arts also served another, shall we say, interesting purpose during the seventeenth century when, as the serious medical profession was evolving, so was the profession of quackery. Quacks were fringe healers who traveled from village to village pedaling cures and remedies. In order to bring attention to themselves and their products, these salesmen would set up in a busy marketplace and provide entertainment. Dancers, drummers, musicians, and actors were employed to draw the attention of a crowd and often to perform an enactment of the ailments at hand and the cures provided by the medicines for sale. A lofty period indeed for the arts in medicine!

## THE ENLIGHTENMENT: REDUCTIONISM IN EUROPE

Renaissance scientists and humanists aspired to return medicine to the purity of the Greek Era when tradition, faith, art, and rational thought collaborated in healing in a holistic manner. During the Reformation, as Luther broke from Rome, so medicine chose to depart from antiquity and the church and proceeded in a new purely scientific direction (Porter, 1997). However, some in the profession still recognized some of the basic principles of indigenous healing practices. The Swiss physician, Paracelsus (late fifteenth and early sixteenth centuries) wrote, "[T]he power of the imagination is a great factor in medicine. It may produce diseases…and it may cure them" (Gottlieb, 1995, p. 86).

During the eighteenth century, stunning developments were made in medicine including in the areas of surgery, pathological anatomy, chemistry, and pharmaceuticals. With the rise of literacy in the general public, demand for healthcare and healing of all sorts rose. Quackery still abounded, and the need for a medical system to oversee the profession arose, and so, standards and ethics for the profession began to be explored. The establishment of hospitals and the abundance of impoverished patients created an ideal environment for experimentation and clinical teaching (Loudon, 1997). It was here that the paradigm of the passive patient became commonplace. Hospitals became places designed for the facilitation of Western medical science and experimentation, rather than places where people could find respite and comfort in healing or in dying. Curing became the goal of the profession, as opposed to the broader concept of healing that centered in traditional healing perspectives, and could even include death as a positive outcome. Reductionist ideals pervaded medicine, marking a definite separation of the systems of body, mind, and spirit.

## THE NEW WORLD AND THE ARTS IN HEALTHCARE

At this point, we can turn our attention to America, where Europeans had, in the fifteenth century, begun settlement of the so-called New World. Tragically, Native American culture was decimated by the ensuing wars and the introduction of European diseases. Traditional Native American healing rituals persisted in reservations, but were replaced in the New World culture by European Western medicine. Imperialism was also taking Western medicine to many other parts of the world where indigenous practices had been relied upon for healing. Africa, Asia, and South America suffered the same losses of both cultural and healing traditions due to European imperialism.

One reference of the use of the arts in healthcare during this time involved Benjamin Franklin, one of America's founding fathers. In 1751, Benjamin Franklin, a scientist, writer, philanthropist, and publisher of the *Pennsylvania Gazette*, established Pennsylvania Hospital (Morgan, 2002). In keeping with Franklin's belief in the importance of activity and creativity, patients of the hospital were required to contribute works of writing to the hospital's "newspaper" publication.

During the eighteenth, nineteenth, and twentieth centuries, Western medical science made amazing progress and hospitals looked and functioned much as they do today. While gross experimentation had been curbed by a balance in medical progress and ethics, medical progress was stunning and disease survival rates as well as human life span increased significantly. Then, in the twentieth century, amidst this success, we saw the introduction of the arts therapies and arts in healthcare programs into hospitals, thus signaling, as my colleague John Graham-Pole asserts, the "second renaissance" in Western healthcare. This expansion of reductionist ideals to once again include consideration of a patient's emotional and spiritual systems as a part of the whole has begun to create a balance for the sterile, discomforting, and scientific environment of Western hospitals.

There is extensive representation in early literary works, including those of Egypt, Greece, and even the Bible, of the use of music in the treatment of illness. While anecdotal evidence such as this is present throughout history, it was not until the nineteenth century that controlled experimentation of music and healing was recorded. In the twentieth century, the field of music therapy was developed as a formal discipline. Drawing both from historical paradigms and present needs, music softened medical environments and nourished the spirit, mind, and body of patients.

The profession of music therapy was organized in the 1930s, "with attendant interest in accreditation, certification, dissemination of information, and coordination of research efforts" (Darrow, Gibbons, & Heller, 1985, p. 18). While the field of music therapy is often attributed to America, it actually originated in Britain. The oldest English text concerning music and medicine was written by Richard Browne, a physician, and printed in 1729. *Medicina Musica, or, A Mechanical Essay on the Effects of Singing, Musick, and Dancing on Human Bodies,* is the founding music-in-medicine text, making clear arguments for the usefulness of music in healing.

The twentieth century brought global warfare, which, due to unprecedented numbers of injuries and patients as well as crude makeshift medical facilities, provided a need to utilize alternative forms of treatment. Music was commonly used to effectively manage and comfort the sick and wounded on battlefields and in army medical facilities. Music was also prescribed as exercise for strengthening and retraining most of the joints and muscles of the body. The playing of musical instruments, singing, and the breathing required for both provided the means to exercise the lungs and the larynx. Music was also used as a direct anesthesia. It was observed that when phonographs were introduced into veteran's hospitals, the music not only entertained but also relaxed the patients. It was also found that patients could be anesthetized more easily and required less medication after surgery when music was playing in operating suites. Similar results were also observed in dentistry.

While all of the arts came to be organically utilized in healthcare throughout the twentieth century, the formal disciplines of the arts therapies and the arts in medicine were defined at different times. It should be noted that one of the primary designations between the arts therapies and the arts in medicine is that the arts therapies are primarily housed in, or stem from, the psychotherapies and psychiatric hospitals, while the arts in healthcare is primarily housed in physical medicine and in hospitals. While there are certainly overlapping foundational principles and similarities in practice, the two fields can also be differentiated in many practical ways.

Since the 1970s, there has been a movement toward rehumanizing formalized medical care. This trend follows the discoveries of structures and processes in the human brain linking perceived and imagined images and cerebral activity with somatic responses. Through the scientific studies of psychoneuroimmunology, both imagery and conditioning (including belief systems) are shown to have direct influence on body function. During the 1990s, 34 of the country's 125 medical schools included study of "alternative" healing practices, fostering a return to a more whole-person approach to healing and wellness (Wetzel et al., 1998). This attitude has rediscovered the potency of the arts in the healing process at a time when the mechanisms that make this phenomenon possible have been documented. A study conducted at the Tulane University School of Medicine in 2002 showed that 76 percent of the nation's 128 medical schools include arts and humanities activities in a planned way and 42 percent have arts and humanities courses offered as electives. As hospitals and healthcare organizations develop and expand arts programs for patients, future physicians are being educated in the roles of the arts and humanities in healing.

As the arts play a myriad of roles in healing practices once again, we see immense variety in programming and applications. Some are reviving ancient practices, some are developing new methods, but overall there is a growing cultural awareness worldwide of the importance of the arts for well-being. The renaissance of the arts and healing brings the arts back into the necessities of living, brings artists out of their studios and into hospitals where human beings face tremendous physical, emotional, and spiritual challenges, and brings deeper meaning and opportunity to the contemporary healthcare experience.

## TOOL KIT FOR CHANGE

### Role and Perspective of the Healthcare Professional

1. Knowledge and understanding of the many ways in which diverse cultures have approached health and healing throughout history can enhance a caregiver's ability to:
   a. empathize with a patient's perspective of his disease and healing
   b. think creatively about approaches to healing for an individual
   c. support the patient as a whole person
2. Understanding of the capacity of the arts to effect healing in a cultural, emotional, or spiritual context can broaden a healthcare professional's perspective of the range of approaches that can be employed in healing.
3. Consideration of the fundamental importance of a patient's belief system in healing and of the many ways in which diverse cultures approach healing can help the Western caregiver make meaningful and useful connections with patients.

### Role and Perspective of the Patient/Participant

1. The array of roles that the arts have played in health and healing can encourage patients to think creatively and intuitively about illness and healing.
2. Patients should take active roles in the healing process, including making choices about treatment and other support modalities such as the arts.
3. There is extensive and inspiring historical evidence of the usefulness of the arts and creative process in enhancing healing and well-being.

### Interconnection: The Global Perspective

1. While healing traditions are extraordinarily diverse throughout the world, there is a universality to the ways in which the arts have been and are still used to support health and healing.
2. In today's global society, it is more important than ever that diversity of belief systems and approaches to healing are respected.

## REFERENCES

Achterberg, J. (1985). *Imagery in healing: shamanism and modern medicine.* Boston: New Science Library.

Baker, I. (1997). *The Tibetan art of healing.* San Francisco: Chronicle Books.

Campbell, J. (1990). *Transformations of myth throughout time.* New York: Harper Perennial.

Csordas, T. J. (2002). *Body/meaning/healing.* New York: Palgrave MacMillan.

Danilevicius, Z. (1967). SS. Cosmas and Damian: The patron saints of medicine in art. *Journal of the American Medical Association, 201*(13), 1021–1025.

Darrow, A. A., Gibbons, A. C., & Heller, G. N. (1985, September/October). Music therapy past, present, and future. *The American Music Teacher,* 18–20.

Dissanayake, E. (1988). *What is art for?* Seattle: University of Washington Press.

Dissanayake, E. (2000). *Art and intimacy: How the arts began.* Seattle: University of Washington Press.

Ebbell, B. (1937). *The Ebers papyrus, the greatest Egyptian medical document.* Copenhagen: Levin and Munksgaard.

Eliade, M. (1964). *Shamanism: Archaic techniques of ecstasy.* New York: Pantheon.

Figes, E. (1976). *Tragedy and social evolution.* London: Calder.

Friedson, S. (1996). *Dancing prophets: The musical experience in Tambuka healing.* Chicago: University of Chicago Press.

Ghent, G. (1994). *African alchemy: Art for healing in African societies.* Moraga: Saint Mary's College of California.

Gottlieb, B. (1995). *New choices in natural healing.* Emmaus: Rodale Press.

Grajetzki, W. (2000). *Digital Egypt for universities.* University College London. Retrieved from http://www.digitalegypt.ucl.ac.uk/Welcome.html on July 20, 2005.

Homer. (1990). *The Iliad* (R. Fagles, Trans.). New York: Penguin.

Huang, C. K. & Williams, W. (1999). *The pharmacology of Chinese herbs* (2nd ed.). Boca Raton: CRC Press.

Hultkrantz, A. (1992). *Shamanic healing and ritual drama: Health and medicine in native North American religious traditions.* New York: Crossroad Publishing.

Kottak, P. (1998). *Anthropology: The exploration of human diversity.* New York: McGraw Hill.

Lawrence, B. (1980). *Healing rituals among North Indian Chisti saints of the Delhi sultanate period* (pp. 119–134). *Studies in History of Medicine.* 4(2):119–134.

Liberty, M. (1980). The sun dance. In W. R. Wood & M. Liberty (Eds.). *Anthropology on the Great Plains* (pp. 164–178). Lincoln: University of Nebraska Press.

Loudon, I. (1997). *Western medicine: An illustrated history.* Oxford, New York: Oxford University Press.

Molloy, M. (2002). *Experiencing the world's religions: Tradition, challenge and change.* Columbus: McGraw-Hill Higher Education.

Morgan, E. (2002). *Benjamin Franklin.* New Haven: Yale University Press.

Pert, C. (1997). *The molecules of emotion.* New York: Touchstone.

Porter, R. (10997). *The greatest benefit to mankind: A medical history of humanity.* New York: W. W. Norton.

Rinpoche, T. W. (1994). Shamanism in the native Bon tradition of Tibet. *Sacred Hoop Magazine, 7,* 1–2.

Razalý, S. M. (1999). Dissociative trance disorder: a case report. Department of Psychiatry, School of Medical Sciences, Universiti Sains Malaysia, Malaysia. *Eastern Journal of Medicine* 4(2): 83–84.

Sandner, D. (1977). *Navajo symbols of healing.* New York: Dover.

Serlin, I. A. (1993). Root images of healing in dance therapy. *American Journal of Dance Therapy, 15*(2), 65–76.

Seymour, T. (1891). *Homer's Iliad* (Books 1–3). Boston: Ginn and Company.

Smith, Huston. (1991). *The world's religions.* HarperSanFrancisco.

Wetzel, M. S., Eisenberg, D. M., Kaptchuk, T. J. (1998). Courses involving complementary and alternative medicine at US medical schools. *Journal of the American Medical Association, 280,* 784–787.

World Health Organization. (2005). Retrieved November 17, 2005, from http://www.who.int/en/

Wright, B. (1980). Dance is the cure: The arts as metaphor for healing in Kelantanese Malay spirit exorcisms. *Dance Research Journal , 12*(2), 3–10.

Chapter Three

# THE DEVELOPMENT OF THE CONTEMPORARY INTERNATIONAL ARTS IN HEALTHCARE FIELD

*Rusti Brandman, PhD*

At the end of a particularly wonderful dance concert by the David Parsons Dance Company, I heard another audience member exclaim, "I feel so much healthier now!" This was in the 1980s, long after Western thought had developed a schism between body, mind, and spirit, between science and art. This mode of thought had paved the way for the scientific method and the development of the contemporary medical model that uses primarily drugs and surgeries to cure the diagnosed condition. It was also long before I became aware of the "new" field of the arts in healthcare, which builds on an East/West, integrative contemporary yet ancient paradigm of healing.

Today, in the early twenty-first century, we see myriad applications of the arts to health, in addition to the creative arts therapies. We know that the transformative power of art has been intuited since the dawn of time and continued to play a major role in a majority of spiritual practices throughout the history of civilization. Though the concept of including paintings and sculpture in hospitals and other public buildings never completely died out, by the twentieth century, many considered spare functionality to be of greater importance, and art as a process was not even seen to be in the same universe as Western medicine (Haldane, 1999). But the twentieth century also saw a rebirth of the appreciation of the health benefits of participating in the arts on any level (audience or maker) that seemed to arise spontaneously from responses to traumatic situations or societal ills, personally meaningful experiences with art and healing, or intuitive sense by some visionary individuals. Due to this vision, the arts are now applied to the health of individuals, society, and environment; to recovery, prevention, or support of a multitude of conditions; and to general wellness of body, mind, and spirit (Haldane).

In contemporary society, intuition alone is not universally respected as a basis for establishing—and funding—programs in the healthcare and related fields. There now must be some demonstrable evidence of or objective explanation for this vision. This knowledge and evidence does exist. It came initially from study of the brain and nervous system, revealing the structures and functions that connect mental images with somatic response, and from clinical research undertaken primarily through the creative arts therapies. Leaders in the arts in healthcare fields are now calling upon this research to justify their past and current work, the expansion of existing programs, and the development of new programs.

## SCIENTIFIC SUPPORT

Definitive notions of brain mechanisms, based on the known characteristics of individual neurons, began to take shape in the 1940s. These constructs were inspired by two contemporaneous scientific developments: the rapid advances in computer technology, and a breakthrough in instrumentation that made it possible to observe the activity of single neurons in a functioning brain (Harth, 1995). Neurons were found to communicate with each other similarly to the on/off elements in a computer. This analogy led to the conceptualization of the neural net and pathways. Continued study brought knowledge of the roles that hormones and neurotransmitters play in creating somatic affects of mental imagery, such as that involved in making and observing art. This information was used as early as the World War I era by the creative arts therapies and then by the 1970s by healthcare professionals in the form of imagery applied to specific conditions and goals.

A strong base of academic research drawing information from science, medicine, and psychology is now supporting the behavioral medicine model. This model upholds the concept that behavior, both concrete external behaviors and internal attitudes, affects health (Achterberg, Dossey, & Kolkmeier, 1994). Since the 1970s, techniques in the realm of behavioral medicine have developed that use visualization, mental imagery, relaxation, and arts to positively affect pain and illness. Some of the specific scientific explanations of how art enhances health are discussed in the chapters by Evans and Graham-Pole. For hospital art programs seeking to provide evidence of the effectiveness of art in the healing process or of hospital arts programs, there are at least three compilations of research now available (Cooley, 2003; Ruiz, 2004; Staricoff, 2005).

## THE DEVELOPMENT OF CONTEMPORARY ARTS IN HEALTHCARE PROGRAMS

Following is a discussion of the contemporary developmental route to the integration of arts programs into the medical model for hospitals or other institutions. Because the field is relatively recent, this information was acquired primarily with Web-based research, and was strongly facilitated by membership in the Society for the Arts in Healthcare (SAH). SAH membership provided access to documents, membership databases, and personal contacts that were highly instrumental not only in amassing data, but in developing an understanding of influences and connections.

Data gathered in this way reveals that some arts in healthcare programs are housed in the hospitals themselves, and others are outside organizations offering arts programs to a number of healthcare institutions. There are at least four ways in which the arts impact healthcare today: "(a) by enhancing the environment, (b) by providing a therapeutic tool for patients, (c) by providing a therapeutic release for staff, (d) aiding the public understanding of health issues" (Rollins, 2004, p. vii). Discussions below will demonstrate how contemporary programs utilize these areas of influence in unique ways and even expand upon them. The concentration will be on programs that go beyond static exhibits or architectural features to include the presence of artists in the hospital in some role and will focus on programs that have exerted an overt impact on the development of the field.

### North America

The United States and Canada began developing arts programs in hospitals during the latter half of the twentieth century. In the United States, this began in the 1970s, followed by similar programs in Canada. In both cases, the movement was initiated by visionary individuals operating in relative isolation until networks were established to facilitate communication and dissemination of ideas. The earliest programs were concerned with art in the environment; only later did programs bring artists into the hospitals for interaction with patients, family, and staff. Discussion of the formative programs reveals the variety of structures and content found in hospital arts programs, as each program developed to fit the visions and resources of its unique situation (Dreschner, 2005).

The Society for the Arts in Healthcare (SAH) is a network of arts in healthcare professionals, students, and organizations from the United States and abroad. Founded by individuals from some of the earliest hospital arts programs in the United States in 1991 in order to provide an interface and mutual support, SAH now has nearly 2,000 members coming from many sides of the arts in healthcare community. The organization, in partnership with the Joint Commission on Accreditation of Healthcare Organizations (JCAHO) and Americans for the Arts, conducted a survey in 2004 to determine the prevalence of such programs, discovering that they exist in over 2,500 hospitals in the United States alone. The rationales include service to the patients for supporting mental, emotional, and physical recovery, creating a healing environment, supporting families, serving staff, and creating positive public relations (Wikoff, 2004). Discussion of the formative programs reveals the variety of structures and content found in hospital arts programs, as each program developed to fit the visions and resources of its unique situation.

The United States in the 1960s and 1970s was in the mood for change, and change in the direction of more inclusiveness in terms of diversity. Within this milieu, the National Endowment for the Arts (NEA) was established in 1965. By fostering artistic excellence, encouraging arts education, and "improving access to the arts for all citizens, the agency strengthens American democracy to the core" (Ivey, 2000). During the following decade, several independent organizations that were to be influential to the development of arts in healthcare were established. These agencies reflected the spirit of inclusion both in the sense of accessibility to diverse audiences and in terms of embracing nonmainstream modes of medical treatment. Two such organizations were Hospital Audiences, Inc. (HAI) and VSA Arts. HAI was founded in 1969 by Michael Jon Spencer to bring arts experiences to populations in New York that are isolated from such events, thus mainstreaming these individuals (Hospital Audiences, Inc., 2006). Jean Kennedy Smith founded VSA Arts, which became an affiliate of the John F. Kennedy Center for the Performing Arts in 1974, and the U.S. Congress designated the organization as the coordinating agency of arts programming for people with disabilities (VSA Arts, 2006). Originally called Very Special Arts, this international nonprofit agency now has affiliates in most states and in at least 60 countries worldwide. Today VSA stands for: "Vision of an inclusive community; Strength through shared resources; and Artistic expression that unites us all" (VSA Arts, 2006). Its goal is inclusiveness of educational opportunities and experiences rather than healing per se, yet the spirit of the organization, and often its funding, have been quite influential to arts in healthcare programs.

These agencies served as precursors to the development of seminal arts in healthcare programs in the 1970s. Duke University's exemplary Cultural Services Program, renamed the Health Arts Network in 2003, began through the interest and efforts of physicians Dr. James Semans and Dr. Wayne Rundles (Dreschner, 2005). These doctors, recognizing the importance of the arts to their own lives, considered the possibilities that the arts could provide "healthy distraction" for patients and their families (Palmer, 2001). A visit to HAI in 1975 prompted the initiation of monthly performances in the hospital cafeteria, a way of enhancing the healthcare environment. The Cultural Services Program was firmly established in 1978 with a grant from the NEA, and a director and program assistant were hired. Over the years, Duke has initiated programs in all the performing arts, visual arts, literary arts, video, medical education, arts medicine and science, employee programs, and network building on local and national/international levels. (Palmer, 1991). Duke has influenced the further development of the field through its Hospital Arts Handbook, and was one of the instrumental players in the creation of the Society for the Arts in Healthcare, hosting the first National Hospital Arts Programs Convocation on the year of their tenth anniversary (Palmer, 1991).

In 1976, the University of Iowa Hospitals and Clinics, through interest from the hospital architect and physicians, embarked on a project to humanize the hospital environment. They began by exhibiting carefully selected prints in various public areas. Project Art, with Joyce Summerwill as coordinator, took on a formal organization in 1978 and is credited by some with being the "first hospital arts program of its kind" (Lohr, 2004). Initially, the program consisted of monthly visual art exhibits. A performing arts component, a traveling art cart with framed prints and posters, and art studio workshops were added during the next several years, and by 1984 Summerwill began a program of consultations for other hospitals interested in beginning their own art programs (University of Iowa Healthcare, 2006).

Gifts of Art at the University of Michigan, another early comprehensive hospital arts program, was officially established for the opening of a new system hospital in 1986 (Dreschner, 2005). The planning came from the facilities area by interior design personnel and an art committee of both hospital and university art personnel. Iowa's Summerwill was an influential consultant, so that in its earliest manifestation, Gifts of Art placed a similar emphasis on artworks in the environment, particularly on exhibits. While the Iowa program emphasized permanent collections, UM emphasized changing exhibits (Dreschner). Part of the University of Michigan Health Systems, Gifts of Art includes art on the walls, performances in hospital spaces, a meditation garden, and music at the bedside (University of Michigan Health System, 2006). The goals of this program, like the original goals of the Iowa and Duke programs, were to provide an enriched and comforting environment for patients and staff and to promote healing. Under its first director, Gary Smith, the program was able to establish a somewhat stable funding structure (Dreschner) and the program is now funded by Friends of the University of Michigan Hospitals and Health Centers as well as through grants, gifts, and proceeds from art sales (University of Michigan Health System).

Duke, Iowa, and Michigan each hosted national convocations that led to the establishment of SAH, thus creating a high level of influence on the field in the United States. Another influence on the arts in healthcare movement during the 1980s came from the world of circus, the Big Apple Circus specifically. Director Michael Christensen founded the Clown Care Unit in 1986 in response to a hospital's request for the circus performers to see some of the pediatric patients. Noticing how clowns transformed the environment positively, he developed a training system that has helped establish Clown Care units worldwide, with at least 17 in the United States (Big Apple Circus, 2006).

In 1991, with the establishment of both SAH and another network, Art as a Healing Force, the field in the United States began to assume an identity. SAH's founding and influence has already been discussed. The latter was created in order to facilitate establishing "art and healing as a recognized field in both art and in medicine" (Art as a Healing Force, 2006).

Shands Arts in Medicine at the University of Florida, unlike the programs previously discussed, began a participatory artist-in-residence program early on. The program resulted from the visions of two individuals. Both were familiar with the medical model and had experienced the power of the arts in their lives. John Graham-Pole was seeking to strengthen arts and humanities in medical education and Mary Rockwood Lane began envisioning artists working in the hospital (Samuels, 1998). Through meeting with and studying other programs, like the University of Iowa's, they formulated the idea of an artist-in-residence program at the hospital. Over the years, the program has evolved a two-part model of both building aesthetics and bedside art making (Shands Arts in Medicine, 2006). The Shands Healthcare system now has artist-in-residence programs at eight of its locations.

This program has created several structures and events that have influenced further development of the arts in healthcare field, such as hosting national symposia in 1995 and 1997, establishing a structure for consultations for other institutions through site visits (Dreschner, 2005, p. 5), and seeding 11 additional programs in Florida through partnerships with VSA Florida, the Florida Fine Arts Council, and the Department of Education.

An additional influence stems from AIM's partnership with an interdisciplinary center of the College of Fine Arts at the University of Florida. The Center for the Arts in Healthcare Research and Education (CAHRE) was officially established in 1999, and augments the Arts in Medicine program's clinical emphasis with training for future artists-in-residence, programs for caregivers, interdisciplinary theoretical courses, supportive research, and national and international outreach programs This program marks a first, providing education and training in the field, beginning with the first course in 1996 and implementing a comprehensive international training program in 2002 (Center for the Arts in Healthcare Research and Education, 2006).

Founded in 1993 in New York City by Adrienne Assail and Geraldine Herbert, the Creative Center is a community of artists, cancer patients, and survivors. As a social worker in a bone marrow transplant unit, Herbert had used arts activities with her patients and had observed the high degree of absorption that accompanied this creative work (Dreschner, 2005). Her observations prompted her to initiate this program to nurture patients, families, and survivors through the arts. The Creative Center is an independent organization supplying artists to a number of area hospitals.

Starting in 2002, the organization added education and training of artists-in-residence to its goals and programs, offering its first week-long training program (The Creative Center, 2006).

Another training program is offered by the North Carolina Arts for Health Network. This network was developed by representatives of arts in healthcare programs across the state at the 1996 SAH conference hosted by Duke, and was funded in 2000. The group established an annual conference-style training institute in 2001 (North Carolina Arts for Health Network, 2006).

The continuing maturation of the field in the United States has been greatly influenced by the NEA, SAH, and the arts-in-education programs of some states' arts councils, as well as by partnerships among these and other agencies. For example, the NEA has made the arts in healthcare a national initiative, funding SAH's Consultant Services program and partnering with the organization for a national interagency symposium in 2003 (Brenner, Palmer, & Leniart, 2003). Another partnership providing great impetus and support to the growth of the field is between SAH and Johnson & Johnson, providing grants to exemplary healing arts projects (Society for the Arts in Healthcare, Johnson & Johnson Grants, 2006). The arts councils of some states are now encouraging artists to go not only into the schools, but also into hospitals, and very recently there has been growth in the use of arts for disease-specific projects and for such health-related areas as aging and palliative care (G. Hanna, personal communication, December 28, 2006). With the existing supports and new networking organizations yet to develop, the field of the arts in healthcare in the United States will undoubtedly continue to develop new programs and models.

Although at present Canada has no overarching organizational network for arts in healthcare programs, the country "has many programs equally as old and as large, as successful, and as mature as many programs in the US" (S. Pointe, personal communication, June, 16, 2006). Initially Canadian programs were, as in the United States, grassroots developments by local personnel working in relative isolation from other programs until about 2001. At about that time, some had found SAH, and in 2005, Friends of the University of Alberta Hospitals hosted that organization's annual conference. This facilitated Canadian programs in locating each other (Pointe). Also in 2005, the British Columbia Arts Council sponsored the Canadian Forum on Arts and Health to provide an opportunity for people who are active at the intersection of health and the arts to network, share their research and programs, and discuss issues of importance to the field (British Columbia Arts Council, 2006). In preparation for the forum, coordinator Nancy Cooley prepared a paper citing research in the field and compiled a listing of those involved with arts in healthcare practice (N. Cooley, personal communication, June 28, 2006). Her report of forum discussions revealed that Canada was in the "gathering momentum" stage of the adoption curve and that it was the consensus of the participants that a national network is a priority for the field (Cooley, 2005).

There is a network in British Columbia, and following the 2005 SAH conference in Edmonton, the provincial government of Alberta appropriated resources toward establishing an arts in healthcare network there. That is presently in process, as are efforts to create a national organization. So although Canadian arts in healthcare is not sufficiently networked to have an overriding sense of its own history on a national level, it is making progress in that direction and is certainly in an active state (S. Pointe, personal communication, June 16, 2006). Cooley's *Canadian Catalogue of People and Activities: Arts and Health* (2005) and the SAH membership list (Society for the Arts in Healthcare, 2006) indicate that the hubs of networked arts in healthcare programming are presently in the western provinces of British Columbia, Alberta, Manitoba, and in the eastern province of Ontario, especially around Toronto and Ottawa.

According to Pointe, Canadian, American, British, and European hospitals had been housing art on the walls for many years before their programs began including interactive arts activities (S. Pointe, personal communication, June 16, 2006). For example, Toronto's present Bloorview MacMillan Children's Centre Creative Arts program represents a fusion of the older MacMillan Spiral Gardens, founded in 1984 ("Bloorview MacMillan Children's Creative Arts Centre," 2006), with Bloorview Hospital. The 1996 merger resulted in the 1997 development of an arts program called the Cosmic Bird Feeder, which provides an artful environment and an extensive array of arts activities to resident and community children ("Bloorview MacMillan Creative Arts," 2006).

In 1984, the University of Alberta Hospital was undergoing renovations for which hospital board member and renovation committee chair Bill McMullen mandated the creation of an art gallery. The McMullen Art Gallery opened in 1986 to embody the committee's philosophy that art in a hospital environment could help ease pain and promote healing. At that time, the hospital developed the position of Art Advisor, funded through Friends of University Hospitals, to offer professional guidance for its collections and exhibitions (Dreschner, 2005). In 1999, Susan Pointe took the position and soon became involved in SAH, thus allowing her to become acquainted with the concept of bedside arts activities (Dreschner). Modeled after Shands Arts in Medicine's artist-in-residence program, Artists on the Wards was established in 1999 (Dreschner). This program provides free bedside activities including visual arts, writing, and music, to alleviate boredom, ease pain, and reduce emotional stress. (University of Alberta Hospitals and Health Facilities, 2006).

Art à la Carte (based in Calgary, Alberta), Artswell in Ottawa, Ontario, and Manitoba Artists in Healthcare, Inc., are all programs inspired by personal experiences with the healing power of the arts. Art à La Carte is a tribute to Patti Hronek, who had visited cancer patients as Provincial Coordinator for the Canadian Cancer Society's CanSurmount volunteer program while living herself with a rare form of bone cancer. When she herself became bedridden, another CanSurmount volunteer, Debbie Baylin, brought posters and photographs to the bleak hospital room. In 1994, Baylin founded Art à la Carte with a selection of donated posters and later the organization established galleries as part of its mission to bring comfort, "beauty and the privilege of choice to the sterile hospital environment" (Art à la Carte, 2006). The program has served as a prototype for the development of eight additional programs.

The Perley and Rideau Veterans' Health Centre, in Ottawa, Ontario, has offered "exceptional art and recreational programs to seniors with physical limitations and/or dementia" (Perley and Rideau Veteran's Health Centre, 2006). Since 1995, Mary Pfaff had served as a social worker there observing the transformative power of the arts as she facilitated painting, sculpture, ceramics, and gardening programs (Artswell, 2006c). Her belief that the arts positively affect all who experience them inspired her to found Artswell in 2002. Artswell is a nonprofit organization based in the city of Ottawa that focuses on promoting the relationships among the arts, healthcare, and medicine with the goal of offering empowerment through creativity (Artswell, 2006a). The organization's Arts in Health service develops and delivers programs to hospitals, palliative care, support and special needs groups, long-term care facilities, and schools, primarily in Ottawa and surrounding areas. Some Artswell programs work within the model of creating an aesthetically healthy environment, such as providing an art cart; others work with the concept of one-on-one creative activities that are therapeutic for patients; and still others instruct patients and staff in the use of arts materials. (Artswell website, 2006b). Committed to research and education supporting the value of the arts to health, Artswell supports linkages to academic and other organizations worldwide to foster awareness of the transformative powers of the arts, particularly in relation to health (Artswell, 2006a).

Manitoba Artists in Healthcare, Inc., was incorporated as a charitable organization in 2001 (Manitoba Artists in Healthcare, 2006b). MAH's mission is to develop and deliver programs and services to promote mental, emotional, spiritual, and physical health for healthcare communities throughout Manitoba (Manitoba Artists in Healthcare, 2006a). MAH has used information on best practices and evidence-based research to design programs tailored to the community. "Our vision is to improve individual and community health through engagement with the arts and artists using the international language of art" (Manitoba Artists in Healthcare, 2006b). It now supplies a variety of programs, like *Music to My Ears*, that brings live music to soothe the stressful environment of medical areas, for several area hospitals (Manitoba Artists in Healthcare, 2006c).

SAH and MAH, and a perceived need for arts and health programming within the province, inspired and influenced the formation of the British Columbia Artists in Healthcare Society, which became a nonprofit organization based in Port Coquitlam, British Columbia, in 2003 (British Columbia Artists in Healthcare Society, 2006a). The goals of the society encompass promotion of the role of the arts in healthcare and healing, providing artistic services to healthcare facilities, and establishing artist-in-residence programs in healthcare institutions and palliative care centers in British Columbia (British Columbia Artists in Healthcare Society website, 2006b). During its first year, the society initiated ArtCare, offering community and hospice participatory arts activities and special public community events. ArtCare trains volunteers in delivering art opportunities without agenda, and participates in an interprovincial partnership with Manitoba Artists in Healthcare, Inc. (British Columbia Artists in Healthcare Society, 2006c).

## Europe

Countries in Western Europe have a long tradition of public art, and often hospitals are seen as public buildings. Artful environments for hospitals are far more prevalent than participatory art programs. In Europe, arts in healthcare often deals even more with preventive community health programs and education, and there is more governmental support for arts programs of all kinds, including those in healthcare. Participatory programs are the last types to develop, but are now gradually emerging in hospitals, as well as the community venues.

The National Network for Arts and Health (NNAH) is the British parallel to SAH. It disperses information and facilitates links among its membership and responds to the needs of the field in general through developing products and services that may often be tailored to the specific interests of each member. NNAH is very effective at advocating for the field, aiding in mainstreaming the concept locally, regionally, and nationally (National Network for Arts and Health, 2006). NNAH now has about 500 members drawn equally from the arts and the healthcare sectors. Much as in the United States, the beginnings of the arts in healthcare movement in Britain could be described as a grassroots process. There are now many different threads in the fabric of British arts in health: primary care, hospitals, mental health, and community health. According to Mike White, Director of Projects at the Centre for

Arts and Humanities in Health and Medicine (CAHHM) at the University of Durham, it is the temperament and vision of the individual that drives this work (M. White, personal communication, April 28, 2006). Probably the first hospital arts program in Great Britain was started when Peter Senior became an artist in residence at St. Mary's Hospital in Manchester in 1973 (Senior, 1997). He built a team of artists who painted murals on the hospitals' walls, leading to Hospital Arts, Britain's oldest group of artists serving the healthcare field (Senior). By the 1980s, the idea of artworks in hospitals was well established, and new hospitals included arts programs. It was during this same era that White helped establish an arts program in a primary practice and the National Network for Arts in Health was founded. Also in the 1980s, there was a movement in which derelict industrial spaces were converted into art studios. This was done in conjunction with local mental health services that referred patients recovering from a variety of mental issues to come to the studios to work with professional artists. There is now a national network of arts in mental health studios (M. White, personal communication, April 28, 2006).

By the 1990s, arts programs were emerging in hospitals, primary care, mental health, and community health settings, and this diversity of practices began to be represented at conferences. The arts in hospital environments have been supported through a government initiative to build or significantly refurbish 70 new hospitals around the country. Many of these new hospitals have arts commissioning as integral parts of the building budgets (M. White, personal communication, April 28, 2006).

In primary care and community health during the last five years, there have been two major initiatives supportive of the arts: Health Action Zones, and Healthy Living Centres. Though that funding is presently declining without a replacement plan, art is now being considered in the building programs of these healthcare sectors and is part of the budget (M. White, personal communication, April 28, 2006).

Participatory arts programs in hospitals have developed much more slowly than arts in the environment. However, more and more hospitals are using their atrium spaces for performances and there are a growing number of hospital artists in residence. Such programs may represent the next step in the development of arts in healthcare. Increased artist-in-residence programs would be a powerful way for healthcare to continue the relationship with the arts, as the artists can open up a dialogue between the healthcare and patient communities (M. White, personal communication, April 28, 2006). What White finds encouraging is that there seems to be a growing number of health professionals who "get it, who want it, and who will champion it" (White).

CAHHM, founded in 2000, is a research center in Durham University's multidisciplinary School of Health that focuses upon interdisciplinary research and educational initiatives, developing the relationships between humanities, the arts, and medical and healthcare practice. CAHHM's activities encompass three sorts of relationships: medical humanities, arts and health, and healthcare environments. Therefore, projects may use the arts therapeutically, deal with beautifying the environment or otherwise improving healthcare staff working conditions, or focus on disseminating health information using the arts as agents to do so (Center for Arts and Humanities in Health and Medicine, 2006a). CAHHM is primarily interested in research that is directly applicable to healthcare practice. The organization has developed some influential links internationally and the staff has been invited to share expertise in Australia, New Zealand, and South Africa (Center for the Arts and Humanities in Health and Medicine, 2006b).

Dr. Michael Ertl describes challenges, both met and unmet, of visual art in the environment in two hospitals in Vienna. The Vienna General Hospital, the Allemeine Krankenhaus (AKH), was 30 years in the building and it includes some very high-quality and valuable art pieces (Ertl, 1999). While at the building's entrance the pieces are presented in exhibition style, elsewhere in the building pieces seem to be displayed in a haphazard fashion, diminishing their value in terms of creating an artful environment (Ertl).

The Donausptial (Danube Hospital) or Sozialmedizinisches Zentrum (Ost) (SMZ-Ost), on the other hand, involved planners, architects, and artists for a more integrated approach. Some of the art is thematic of the positive side of hospital functions or provides an interactive environment, such as in some waiting areas and outdoor spaces. The hospital also arranges for the artists to be present and available to talk with visitors (Ertl, 1999).

Viennese psychiatric hospitals now also have departments called Art and Creativity that offer creative experiences to their patients (Ertl, 1999). The hospitals find that patients engaged in creative activity are more interested in participating in their prescribed therapies and have a more positive outlook. These programs generally involve movement, dance, music, and visual arts including interaction with artists (Ertl). Since the Art and Creativity programs are not considered part of the prescribed treatment, they do not fall into the realm of the arts therapies, but rather are seen as part of the process of returning the patients to nonhospitalized life (Ertl).

Since its inception in the 1980s, the French Ministry of Culture has embraced a goal of facilitating exposure to the arts for underserved populations, forming partnerships with other ministries. In 1999, the Ministries of Culture and Health defined a national policy for making cultural programs part of hospitals, consolidating the agreement in 2006. This policy supports the creation of positions for hospital cultural program directors (French Ministry of Culture and Health, 2006a). The ministry's Web site gives practical information for those who wish to practice arts in hospitals. The relatively codified system of government oversight includes legal definitions of the artist, artistic competencies, and conditions for artistic "interventions." The site gives examples of types of works that are created in such interventions, and defines legal issues of artistic copyright, artists' wages, and artists' taxes. It provides a useful list of print and web resources (French Ministry of Culture and Health website, 2006b).

European participatory arts programs are slowly appearing. Such a program is being developed in Hildesheim, Germany, through the research of graduate student Anna Lisa Meckel (A. Meckel, personal communication, July 26, 2006), and the Arts and Health program at Adelaide and Meath Hospital in Dublin includes a writer-in-residence program as well as music performances in the atrium and music therapy (H. Moss, personal communication, July 19, 2006).

## Australia

Sally Clifford and Joanne Kaspari founded the Australian Network for Arts and Health (ANAH) in 1997 to fill a need for supporting artists working in healthcare settings through networking, advocacy, lobbying, research, and evaluation (Clifford, 2001). At the onset, most of the related activity was in community art and cultural development. At that time, the major issue facing artists in healthcare was that of professional isolation and the accompanying challenges to securing continuous support from administrators to sustain such programs.

The founders discovered that the programs existing at the time had been initiated by a doctor or other healthcare professional committed to the role of the arts to health and had been delivered by hired short-term artists. Once either the artist or the healthcare connection had left the facility, others were not necessarily as interested in putting effort into the arts programs (Clifford, 2001). Nevertheless, there had been quite successful programs in operation in Australia for many years, notably hospital programs at Westmead established in the early 1980s and the Toowoomba Base Hospital Artist-in-Residence program dating from 1988. In addition, numerous community health centers had been hosting arts projects using creative process to investigate health-related issues. The term "arts in health industry" had been used in Australia since the late 1980s, and there were some key artists who focused their work in that area (Clifford).

The Australian Arts and Health field is extremely diverse, encompassing participatory community cultural development, public art, curated collections, architecture and design, art for healing, art for health promotion and education, and art therapy. By including all these fields, the possibilities for communication among practitioners are increased and facilitated. The field is also diverse in terms of geography and outcomes (Clifford, 2001).

## South America

One example of how the concept of arts and health is practiced in Brazil is *Doutores da Alegria—Arte, Formação e Desenvolvimento* (Doctors of Happiness—Art, Education and Development). Brazilian citizen Wellington Nogueira performed with the Big Apple Circus, Clown Care Unit in New York from 1988 to 1991. Upon returning to Brazil, he formed a similar troupe, as other Clown Care Unit alumni had in France (*Le Rire Médecin*) and Germany (*Die Klown Doktoren).* In 1991, Nogueira's Doutores da Alegria (Doctors of Happiness) began its program in the *Hospital Nossa Senhora de Lourdes,* in São Paulo (currently called Hospital da Criança, Children's Hospital) with a duo of clowns. The mission of *Doutores da Alegria* is to bring happiness to hospitalized children, their families, and their caregivers through the art of clowning. The *Doutores* find that the traumas of loss of control over bodies and lives suffered by hospitalized children can be eased through the art of "besteirologia" (silliness), aiding in the development of positive and healing attitudes. *Doutores da Alegria* now provides programs for hospitals in São Paulo, Rio de Janeiro, and Recife (Doutores da Alegria, 2006).

## Asia

Though steeped in rich cultural health traditions and practices, many Asian nations have adopted the Western medical model in hospitals. Some are also using the contemporary ideas of arts in hospitals as practiced in the West. Since the 1990s, Japan has been one of the most economically and technologically advanced nations in the world. However, "A nation of full employment until recently, but with no weekends, Japan is a country where people literally work themselves to death..." (Cooper, 1999). According to Graham Cooper, chairman of art and architecture and an environmental artist and design consultant from Britain, Japanese hospitals must be built to use land efficiently, and yet provide artful environments for healing (1999). Newer hospitals have left the traditional Japanese architectural styles, influenced from the contemplative tea house, but rather have developed from a more Western influence (Cooper). However these hospitals have been artfully conceived to integrate architecture, light, gardens, and art to create a relaxing, beautiful, and healing atmosphere. Some hospitals have also acquired artworks that create a sense of familiarity for patients (Cooper).

In 1997, Japan's Tanpopo-No-Ye Foundation sponsored a Conference on Art in Healthcare that covered topics ranging from arts in the hospital environment through hospital artist-in-residence activities. Rationales cited for holding the conference note that modern technology has brought material abundance, but also a sense of isolation. Particularly with the development of a greater demographic of elders, it is necessary to help people find self-realization in order to promote a healthy society. Art is seen as a potential tool for promoting positive attitudes, and the Arts in Healthcare movement in Europe supplied a model. The purpose of the conference was to provide information, communications, and 32 networking possibilities, and to form a national Society for the Arts in Healthcare (Tanpopo-No-Ye, 2006).

Hong Kong's Art in Hospital was founded in 1994 from the inspiration of a young artist who had survived cancer. After diagnosis and admission to a typically sterile hospital, he felt his condition had worsened due to the bleakness of his surroundings. He made a commitment to beautify the hospital environment after his recovery, sensing that doing so would bring comfort to other patients who, like himself, were fighting grave illnesses (Art in Hospital, 2006a). The initial project for this new program was a mural at the Radiotherapy Unit at Prince of Wales Hospital. Upon successful completion of this project, Art in Hospital was officially established with the mission to use the arts to create favorable healing environments for patients and to provide patients with opportunities to actively explore their artistic potentials as a potent way to express and share their feelings to support healing. In addition, the program's goals involve the larger healthcare, artistic, and general communities (Art in Hospital, 2006b). Recently, AIH has been investigating additional hospital art options, including the promotion of these ideas to other Asian locales. To date, the program has initiated projects in Beijing, India, and Cambodia, thus influencing the use of the arts in healthcare in these countries (Art in Hospital, 2006c).

## Emerging Programs

U.S. consultants are presently helping to establish hospital arts programs in Siberia and Kenya. These represent the very few instances in the development of the contemporary arts in healthcare movement in which program initiation was instigated from outside the local community. Having previously visited Siberian villages in 2003, Naj Wikoff, former president of SAH, earned a Fulbright Scholarship for 2005–2006 to help develop hospital arts programs there. He made presentations on the use of the arts in healthcare in at least four cities in Siberia and worked in four children's hospitals in the town of Ulan Ude and a hospital in Orlik (*Letters Home*, 2006).

These hospitals face challenges very similar to those faced by hospitals in the United States and other Western countries: staff burnout, the need to enhance community relations, the desire to create more welcoming and healing environments for patients and families, and efforts to lift spirits, give patients a break from pain, relieve staff stress, and deal with an aging population. The hospitals in Siberia are particularly bleak in design. Wikoff suggests that the presence and use of the arts would make vast improvements in these hospital situations (*Letters Home*, 2006).

Wikoff began working within the concept of enhancing the aesthetic appeal of the hospital environments. In all the hospitals, he used input from patients and staff in order to ensure that local cultural values were reflected in the hospital environments and to achieve a sense of ownership on the part of the hospital personnel. He also called upon additional consultations, when appropriate, to establish designs. For example, the Buryat History Museum provided information helpful for keeping the design consistent with Buryat culture, and colleagues from the United States gave helpful suggestions for meeting a challenge provided by a neonatal unit: how to make the space more uplifting for staff and families while maintaining a dim and quiet atmosphere for the patients. Paula Most, from Lifespan; Hasbro Children's Hospital; and Annette Ridenour of Aesthetics, Inc., gave recommendations, using music of 60 beats or less (to mimic maternal heartbeat), painted borders with natural imagery in muted colors, and carefully focused directional lighting *(Letters Home*, 2006). Although the majority of work was concerned with visual art in the environment, music was also introduced, and there are plans to develop a music performance component. Besides the improved conditions of the specific hospitals, the project showed the potential for individuals and aesthetics to make differences in lives (*Letters Home*, 2006).

A new arts in medicine program is presently being established in Kenya due to the efforts of a Kenyan native, David Akombo, and the CAHRE Center. In Kenya, Akombo had witnessed a dichotomy concerning the confluence of the arts and healing. Though music and the arts were the primary means of healthcare in rural villages, Western-style hospitals prevailed in the urban centers with virtually no artists working to bring hope and inspiration to the patients (D. Akombo, personal communication, May 10, 2006). While studying for his doctorate in music education at the University of Florida, Akombo sought direct experience in the practice of the arts in the contemporary healthcare model through participating in Shands AIM and CAHRE's Arts in Healthcare Summer Intensive. After seeing how seriously the discipline of the arts in healthcare is taken in Western cultures, he collected information, including clinical studies and data on the effectiveness of existing Western programs, to present to Kenyan hospitals (D. Akombo, personal communication, May 10, 2006).

The Mater Hospital in Nairobi, as with all the hospitals approached, has embraced the Western medical model and wanted evidence that arts in healthcare works and is now accepted in mainstream Western institutions (D. Akombo, personal communication, May 10, 2006). As a privately run hospital, owned by the Sisters of Mercy and serving the public, the Mater is a good environment for arts due to its staff retention issues and its founding principles of compassion and affordability. It is committed to providing quality training for staff, but is challenged in terms of staff retention because the other privately funded hospitals offer much higher salaries, and often Mater-trained staff will leave to assume these higher-paying jobs. Although located on the edge of a depressed industrial district, the Mater Hospital is rated as one of the top four hospitals in Kenya and is rated first in patient care (K. Ayoti and M. Dolan, personal communication, April 20, 2006). It is in the realms of patient care and staff retention that the CEO, Kennedy Ayoti, sees the arts fitting into their setting. He would like the Mater Hospital to be the first hospital in Kenya to have an arts in medicine program. (K. Ayoti and M. Dolan, personal communication, April 20, 2006) Through visits to Shands Arts in Medicine and participation in the CAHRE Centers Arts in Healthcare Summer Intensive, the Kenyan artists and hospital personnel familiarized themselves with the possibilities of an arts program to meet their needs in terms of patient and staff satisfaction. CAHRE personnel were on site at the Mater in October 2006 to facilitate implementation of the new program.

## SUMMARY AND CONCLUSIONS

The programs discussed above are just a sampling of the varied and exciting work being done worldwide today with intersections of the arts with health. From this discussion, it is apparent that scientific evidence notwithstanding, the initial founding of the majority of the programs was inspired by personal experiences rather than objective reference to the evidence itself. The visionaries have come from several sectors of the arts and health communities: artists, health caregivers, administrators, and facilities personnel. Having a supporter within the local healthcare system has been helpful to the initiation of the majority of programs.

The earliest programs began in 1970s in Britain and the United States, with precursors starting in the late 1960s. Additional programs developed gradually during the 1980s and then, beginning in the early 1990s, a small explosion occurred in additional programs and networks. There was no international fanfare when the first programs developed to spur others to start. In fact, program founders and directors were too busy developing their programs to initiate connections at the onset (S. Pointe, personal communication, June 16, 2006). Programs developed as favorable conditions appeared in their local scenes, and for the most part, the field has come into existence with grassroots initiatives. In fact, with very few exceptions, such as the French Ministry of Culture, these programs have resulted from local initiatives rather than mandates or requests coming from an outside source. Even government policy in Great Britain that health buildings should be beautiful as well as functional came into being after the Hospital Arts program developed in St. Mary's Hospital in Manchester. The umbrella associations, too, grew to meet the networking needs of the grassroots programs rather than the other way around. And these umbrella organizations, in turn, fostered continued proliferation through their abilities to provide networking opportunities, disseminate information, and offer support.

While there does not appear to be one linear developmental thread within the growth of the field, there does seem to be somewhat of a network of influences among the programs discussed. For example, the Duke program was directly influenced by Hospital Audiences and helped influence others through founding the Society for the Arts in Healthcare and writing informational materials. Iowa's program directly influenced the University of Michigan and Shands Arts in Medicine, which in turn influenced numerous artist-in-residence programs, including the University of Alberta. Ideas are indeed carried from place to place, but are always made creatively unique to the situation for programs to flourish.

The earliest programs were begun by bringing arts into the environment for visual arts exhibitions and/or performances. Some programs that began with arts in the environment added participatory components; and a few programs, like Shands AIM, began with participatory arts for patients delivered to the bedside. Besides these types of programs, the arts in hospitals have also been used for way-finding, and to help illustrate and emphasize educational health information. Arts techniques are even taught in the hospital setting, and some hospital arts programs help deliver arts education to medical students. There is also a great variety in the way the arts programs are structurally aligned with hospitals, from being an integral part of the hospital to being an independent organization offering programs to a number of hospitals.

Since the late 1990s, the field seems to be growing exponentially, or at least, knowledge of programs is eminently more accessible due to the umbrella organizations and the Internet. Anyone wishing to locate hospital arts programs need only consult the Web sites of the various national networking organizations. In the early twenty-first century for the first time there is some purposeful arts in health migration, with international consultants being called in, or proposing programs to hospitals outside of the consultants' countries. And arts in health models are perhaps equally present in venues outside of hospitals to aid in recovering health on a physical, mental/emotional, and /or spiritual level from a plethora of challenges: substance abuse, disaster relief, preventive programs, arts for disabilities, support for those living with life-limiting or life-altering conditions, and probably new applications being developed at this instant.

The field is also accumulating an ever-growing body of respectable research on the beneficial effect of the arts on health in addition to research in the creative arts therapies. At least three documents compiling such results are available on the Internet, and SAH in conjunction with CAHRE has posted a searchable database of studies. Some of the findings show that:

Participation in arts activities or being placed in a well-designed environment can result in:

- Reduced stress levels
- Improvement in mood
- Distraction from medical problem
- Reduction in medication
- Quicker recovery rates
- Reduction in patients suffering depression
- Less visits to the primary care physician
- Improved communication skills in those with special needs
- Development of new skills by careers and increased confidence
- Managers being aware of the benefits of creativity in a hospital-based setting
- Development of interpersonal skills, new friendships and increased involvement by those participating in the activity, leading to an enhanced sense of well-being. (Ruiz, 2004, p. 61)

The availability of this sort of evidence-based information is very helpful to new programs seeking support from institutions, as well as to existing programs called upon to present rationales for continuing and upgrading support. This research also can provide impetus and support to additional ideas for incorporating the arts into our concept of healthcare and indeed for new research initiatives. As the field has matured, the need for studies and evaluation has grown, as has the motivation to undertake such projects. Most programs seem to invite innovation. The field is fed by the very creativity that it values—it is kept healthy by the way it strives to keep its clients healthy—artfully.

## TOOL KIT FOR CHANGE

### Role and Perspective of the Healthcare Professional

1. For those interested in practicing the arts in healthcare, there are educational programs and consultancies available to train practitioners and foster program development as well as resources available from national networking organizations:

   Society for the Arts in Healthcare (USA): http://thesah.org/
   National Network for Arts and Health (UK): http://www.nnah.co.uk/work.html
   Australian Network for Arts and Health: http://www.anah.org.au/

French Ministries of Culture and Health: www.culture.gouv.fr/culture/
politique-culturelle/hopital/
Tanpopo-No-Ye Foundation (Japan): http://popo.or.jp/english/artinhealthcare.
html

2. Practitioners are now engaged by more than 2,500 hospital arts programs in the
United States alone for providing arts in the environment, artists in residence,
and/or arts activities for staff. These practitioners may be artists, health caregivers,
or therapists acting in the capacity of artists in residence.

### Role and Perspective of the Participant

1. There is evidence that being in an artful environment and/or participating in
creativity is beneficial to returning to and maintaining health. Patients can seek
out arts programs and/or find ways to enhance their environments for healing
through personally significant and pleasing décor.
2. Patients wishing to reap these benefits may find arts programming present in
an increasing number of healthcare facilities, generally offered through volunteer services, child life, pastoral services, patient services, or other administrative
structures.
3. In some cases, arts programs in hospitals were founded by former patients or were
influenced by patients' positive experiences with arts or adverse affects of the lack
thereof.

### Interconnection: The Global Perspective

1. Hospital programs exits on all continents. Each develops uniquely to suit its
situation.
2. Most programs were started by an individual local to the community with a commitment to the benefits of the arts to health.
3. There now is scientific evidence of the effectiveness of the arts in integrating
body, mind, and spirit for health as well as numerous model programs to reference
for promoting the establishment, maintenance, and development of hospital arts
programs.

## REFERENCES

Achterberg, J. Dossey, B. & Kolkmeier, L. (1994). *Rituals of healing: Using imagery for health
and wellness.* New York: Bantam Books.
Art à la Carte. *Mission statement.* (2006). Retrieved March 30, 2006, from http://www.
artalacarte.org/old/.
Art as a Healing Force. (2006). *Art as a healing force, the organization.* Retrieved March 16,
2006, from http://www.artashealing.org/ahfworg.htm.
Art in Hospital. (2006a). *Introduction* (English). Retrieved April 30, 2006, from http://aih.
org.hk/e/e_intro.htm.
Art in Hospital. (2006b). *Mission statements.* (English). Retrieved April 30, 2006, from
http://aih.org.hk/e/e_mission.htm.
Art in Hospital. (2006c). *Services* (English). Retrieved April 30, 2006, from http://aih.org.
hk/e/e_services.htm.
Artswell. (2006a). *Homepage.* Retrieved April 30, 2006, from http://www.artswell.ca/
homepage.htm.

Artswell. (2006b). *Programs.* Retrieved April 30, 2006, from http://www.artswell.ca/Programs.htm.

Artswell. (2006c). *Bios.* Retrieved April 30, 2006, from http://www.artswell.ca/Bio.htm.

Big Apple Circus. (2006). *Community programs: Clown care.* Retrieved April 15, 2006, from http://www.bigapplecircus.org/CommunityPrograms/ClownCare/.

"Bloorview MacMillan Children's Creative Arts Centre Spiral Gardens." (2006). Retrieved May 10, 2006, from http://www.bloorviewmacmillan.on.ca/Spiral/sub/about.html.

"Bloorview MacMillan Creative Arts." (2006). Retrieved May 10, 2006, from http://www.bloorviewmacmillan.on.ca/creativearts/.

Brenner, S., with Palmer, J. & Leniart, K. (Eds.). (2003). *Report on the Arts in Healthcare Symposium.* Washington, DC: National Endowment for the Arts and Society for the Arts in Healthcare, March 19–20, 2003. Retrieved December 29, 2006, from http://thesah.org/doc/NEASymposiumReport.doc.

British Columbia Artists in Healthcare Society. (2006a). *Homepage.* Retrieved April 30, 2006, from http://www.bcartistsinhealthcare.org.

British Artists in Healthcare Society. (2006b). *About us.* Retrieved April 30, 2006, from http://www.bcartistsinhealthcare.org/about.php.

British Columbia Artists in Healthcare Society. (2006c). *Art care programs.* Retrieved April 30, 2006, from http://www.bcartistsinhealthcare.org/artcart.php.

British Columbia Arts Council. (2006). *Canadian Forum on Arts and Health.* Retrieved May 30, 2006, from http://www.bcartscouncil.ca/healthcanadaforum/.

Center for Arts and Humanities in Health and Medicine. (2006a). *Home.* Retrieved April 30, 2006, from http://www.dur.ac.uk/cahhm/.

Center for the Arts and Humanities in Health and Medicine. (2006b). *Arts and health.* Retrieved April 30, 2006, from http://www.dur.ac.uk/cahhm/reports/artsinhealth/.

Center for the Arts in Healthcare Research and Education. (2006). Retrieved March 30, 2006, from www.arts.ful.edu/cahre.history.asp.

Clifford, S. (2001). *In response: The Australian arts and health industry.* The Australian Network for Arts and Health. Presented at the Sixth National Rural Health Conference, Canberra, Australia, March 4–7, 2001.

Cooley, N. (2003). *Arts and culture in medicine and health: A survey research paper.* Cooley and Associates: Embracing Change Creatively.

Cooley, N. (2005). *Canadian catalogue of people and activities: Arts in health.* Canadian Forum on Arts and Health, British Columbia Arts Council.

Cooley, N. (2005). *Canadian Forum on Arts and Health 2005: Forum summary report.* Retrieved from http://www.bcartscouncil.ca/healthcanadaforum/program/.

Cooper, G. (1999). "Art in Japanese hospitals." In D. Haldane & S. Loppert (Eds.), *The arts in healthcare: Learning from experience.* London: King's Fund in association with Lulham Art Publications, Roehampton Institute.

The Creative Center. (2006). *History.* Retrieved March 30, 2006, from http://thecreativecenter.org/History/.

Doutores da Alegria. (2007). *Informações históricas.* Retrieved May 27, 2006, from http://www.doutoresdaalegria.com.br.

Dreschner, J. W. (2005). *Arts in healthcare: Programs and practitioners. Sampling the spectrum in the US and Canada.* White Paper No. 1. New York: Center Colloquium Group.

Ertl, M. (1999). *Art in Vienna's hospitals—decoration or challenge?* In D. Haldane & S. Loppert (Eds.), *The arts in healthcare: Learning from experience* (pp. 47–55). London: King's Fund in association with Lulham Art Publications, Roehampton Institute.

French Ministry of Culture and Health. (2006a). *Culture à l'hôpital* Retrieved June 16, 2006, from http://www.culture.gouv.fr/culture/politique-culturelle/hopital/.

French Ministry of Culture and Health. 2006b. *Hospital interventions.* Retrieved June 16, 2006, from http://www.culture.gouv.fr/culture/politiqueculturelle/hopital/interventions.htm.

Gottlieb, B., ed. (1995). *New choices in natural healing.* Emmaus, PA: Rodale Press.

Graham-Pole, J. (2000). *Illness and the art of creative self-expression.* Oakland, CA: New Harbinger Publications, Inc.

Haldane, D., & Loppert, S. (1999). *The arts in healthcare: Learning from experience.* London: King's Fund in association with Lulham Art Publications, Roehampton Institute.

Harth, E. (1995). *The creative loop: How the brain makes a mind.* Reading, MA: Addison-Wesley.

Hospital Audiences, Inc. *Homepage.* Retrieved August 10, 2006, from http://www.hospaud.org/hai/index.htm).

Ivey, B. (2000). Introduction. In B. Koostra (Ed.), *National Endowment for the Arts 1965—2000: A brief chronology of federal support for the arts* (p. 5). Washington, DC: Office of Communications.

*Letters home: Naj Wikoff in Ulan Ude, Russia.* (2006). Retrieved April 30, 2006, from http://www.northcountrypublicradio.org/news/naj/.

Lohr, G. O. (2004, Fall). Where art and healing meet. *Surface Design Journal,* 19–23.

Manitoba Artists in Healthcare. (2006a). *Home page.* Retrieved April 30, 2006, from http://www.mahmanitoba.ca/home.htm.

Manitoba Artists in Healthcare. (2006b). *About.* Retrieved April 30, 2006, from http://www.mahmanitoba.ca/about.htm.

Manitoba Artists in Healthcare (2006c). *Programs.* Retrieved April 30, 2006, from http://www.mahmanitoba.ca/programs.htm.

National Network for Arts and Health. (2006). *Homepage.* Retrieved March 30, 2006, from http://www.nnah.co.uk/work.html.

North Carolina Arts for Health Network. (2006). *About NCAH.* Retrieved March 30, 2006, http://www.ncartsforhealth.org/about.htm.

Palmer, J. (2001). *An introduction to the arts-for-health movement, or how the arts sneaked in on the medical model.* Community Arts Network Reading Room. Retrieved March 30, 2006, from http://www.communityarts.net/readingroom/archivefiles/2001/11/introduction_to.php.

Palmer, J., and Florence, N. (1991). *The hospital arts handbook.* Durham, NC: Duke University Medical Center.

Perley and Rideau Veteran's Health Centre. (2006). *Homepage.* Retrieved June 16, 2006, from http://www.prvhc. com/homepage.htm.

Rollins, J. (2004). *Art activities for children at the bedside.* Washington, DC: WVSA Arts Connection.

Ruiz, J. (2004). *A literature review of the evidence base for culture, the arts and sport policy.* Social Research, Research and Economic Unit, Scottish Executive Education Department.

Samuels, M., and Lane, M. (1998). *Creative healing.* San Francisco: HarperSanFrancisco.

Senior, P. (1997). The arts in health movement. In T. Kaye (Ed.), *The arts in health-care: A palette of possibilities* (pp. 20–25). London and Bristol, PA: Jessica Kingsley Publishers.

Shands Arts in Medicine. (2006). *Homepage.* Retrieved March 30, 2006, from http://www.shands.org/aim/.

Society for the Arts in Healthcare. *Homepage.* Retrieved June 15, 2006, from http://thesah.org/.

Society for the Arts in Healthcare(2006). *Johnson & Johnson Grants.* Retrieved December 29, 2006, from http://thesah.org/template/page.cfm?page_id=15.

Staricoff, D. R. (2005). *Arts in health: A review of medical literature.* (Arts Council England Report No. 36).

Tanpopo-No-Ye. (1997). *Arts in healthcare conference.* (English.) Retrieved May 1, 2006, from http://popo.or.jp/english/artinhealthcare.html.

University of Alberta Hospitals and Health Facilities: *Artists on the wards.* Retrieved April 15, 2006, from http://www.capitalhealth.ca/HospitalsandHealthFacilities/Hospitals/UniversityofAlbertaHospital/AboutUs/Artists_on_the_Wards.htm.

University of Florida News. Retrieved June 12, 2006, from http://news.ufl.edu/2006/06/12/performing-arts-in-medicine/.

University of Iowa Healthcare. Retrieved March 15, 2006, from http://www.uihealthcare.com.

University of Michigan Health System. *Gifts of Art Program.* Retrieved March 30, 2006, from http://www.med.umich.edu/goa/.

VSA Arts. (2006). *About.* Retrieved March 20, 2006 from http://www.vsarts.org/x16.xmlWikoff, N. (2004, November). *Cultures of care: A study of arts programs in U.S. hospitals.* Washington, DC: Americans for the Arts.

Chapter Four

# THE HOSPITAL ARTIST IN RESIDENCE PROGRAMS: NARRATIVES OF HEALING

*Jill Sonke-Henderson, BA, and Rusti Brandman, PhD*

## CREATIVITY AND THE ROLE OF THE ARTIST IN THE HEALTHCARE SETTING

Our Western hospitals may look quite different from indigenous healing sites, but they are nonetheless places of transcendence. When we enter a hospital to receive care, we leave behind much of what we consider to be our identity—our job, home, clothing, hairstyle, all of our belongings—and we find ourselves in the same situation as anyone who has experienced illness at any point in history, that of facing our own mortality. This is a very essential space. In this space, one's search for life's meaning is often urgently intensified (Johnson, 2005), and people instinctively respond to opportunities for expression, insight, and connection that the arts can provide.

Although the specific roles of the arts in the realm of healing have changed over the course of our human history, art and healing have never been entirely separated. The mind and one's belief systems still lie at the heart of our relationship to medical treatment and the recovery from illness, or the healing journey into either life or death in a more holistic sense.

The arts can provide an adaptive mechanism (Dissanayake, 2000) to the uncertainty that comes with illness. In situations of uncertainly and anxiety, which many hospital patients experience, the sympathetic nervous system's release of glucocortoids and adrenaline inclines one toward action at a very primal level ("fight or flight"). Unfortunately, the limitations of the hospital environment and of illness itself inhibit this response. Thus, the arts as they have been adapted for facilitation within the context of the healthcare environment provide an important mechanism for this natural inclination. Watson and Clark (1994) have shown that in this situation, activity (doing, rather than thinking) and social interaction are positive adaptive mechanisms. The former enhances immune function and cognition, while the latter has a positive effect on mood.

Today, many hospital patients have the opportunity to experience the arts. Since the 1970s, arts in healthcare, also referred to as arts in medicine, programs have been established at over 2,500 hospitals in the United States (Wikof, 2004). As discussed in chapter 3, the majority of these programs focus on the aesthetics of the healthcare environment, while many also include the performing arts and interactive arts programs for patients, family members, caregivers, and visitors. Typically, these programs are funded by the hospital administration and/or grants and private funds, and do not involve third-party or direct patient billing for services. This is an important distinction in the role of the arts and artists in the healthcare setting.

Within the context of many arts in healthcare programs, artists in residence work with patients to facilitate creativity as a way of enhancing healing, well-being, and the overall experience of healthcare. Arts in healthcare programs have become important components of our healthcare system that provide basic humanistic elements of care and contribute significantly to holism in Western healthcare. Hospital artists and arts programs attend to a vast array of patient needs that often go unmet by the healthcare system. These programs are extremely cost-effective, and provide patients with a broader range of attention, care, and control. This chapter will highlight numerous examples of the types of care that artists provide for patients.

## Artists in Residence

Artists in the healthcare setting are facilitators. They share with patients their expertise in accessing what we will refer to as the "creative state": a state of consciousness resembling meditation or prayer, and transporting the person to a different level of reality—from objective to subjective, from left brain to right brain, from corporal to spiritual. Dr. Jean Shinoda Bolen (1999) describes this state using the Greek term *kairos*, or participatory time. One becomes so absorbed in the moment that there is often no perception of time passing.

Access to this state draws upon physical, emotional, mental, and spiritual factors in varying degrees for individual artists. There are many ways to reach it. Sometimes it is an actual physical space. Sometimes it is a temporal space. For Henry Thoreau, being in the physical space he developed at Walden Pond was key to his creative process in writing. The choreographer Twyla Tharp also relies on a physical space, her "white box" of an empty studio (Tharp, 2003), to access her optimal creative state. While many artists rely on an optimal physical space to access a creative state, many can create art under any physical circumstances, and some have discovered an optimal creative state in hospitals and other unusual places. Frida Khalo, Toulouse-Lautrec, Edvard Munch, and Herni Matisse are among the many accomplished visual artists whose creative processes were discovered or heightened during illness (Herrera, 1983; Lucie-Smith, 1983; Wong, 2001).

Mary Dean Atwood's (1991) discussion of Native American rituals cites many instances using sensory deprivation of some sort (going without food, going into an isolated area, etc.), to facilitate reaching a receptive state, and calls this process shifting from left to right brain mode. The hospital experience deprives patients of many of the typical references of everyday life. Without all the markers of one's "normal" identity, one may develop a very essential state of being, a state that brings the most primary aspects of living to the fore, opening possibilities for new experiences and for the imagination to take flight. The essence of a creative state is not physical, but one in which the mind, emotions, spirit, and body are altered and allow one's creativity and expression to flow. It is a state of deep concentration. It is similar to the internal focus that athletes access in order to perform at their best, and the space that meditation practitioners find when the mind is quieted. It is the state that all artists, including the great ones, strive to access.

Artists often recall a certain degree of relaxation as necessary to reaching their creative state. Mozart remarked, "When I am, as it were, completely myself, entirely alone, and of good cheer—say traveling in a carriage or walking after a good meal—it is on such occasions that my ideas flow best and most abundantly" (Myers, 1999, p. 1). It is in this creative space that deeply personal truths and insights can be found and where the individual's unique voice and vision originate. It is a state wherein the mind can be deeply unified with the spirit and the body, and where expression can be unedited and uninhibited by the intellect. It is the same universal state that has been sought throughout time by artists and healers alike. Hospital artists in residence are familiar with this state and become adept at facilitating it for patients.

## The Artist's Relationship to the Healthcare Setting

Artists in residence are not shamans or healers or therapists. They are accomplished, professional artists who are also skilled facilitators and have personal experience with the transcendent nature of the arts. They are employed or contracted by hospitals to bring the arts to patients, visitors, caregivers, and the physical environment as a way of humanizing and enhancing the healthcare experience. As noted above, many hospitals have implemented artist-in-residence programs for this purpose. These programs, while unique to each setting, utilize artists to create visual and auditory enhancements for the physical environment and to bring opportunities for creative engagement to patients at the bedside and in groups. These activities are generally geared toward patients, family members, visitors, caregivers, and other hospital staff.

Hospital artists are professional practicing artists who receive specialized training for working in the clinical setting. This differs from the preparation of other clinical professionals, including arts therapists whose goals and relationships to the clinical environment differ slightly. Many hospital artists have training or credentials in the arts therapies or in nursing, and while these are extremely useful backgrounds for this work, they are not required for employment in most situations. While artists are often a part of the clinical care team, in that they meet with medical staff to discuss patient care issues and plans, they do not have clinical privileges and typically do not enter notes into patient records or provide services that are directly billable. As a result, artists enjoy a uniquely nonclinical relationship with patients.

Over the past 40 years, the Western healthcare system has come to recognize the importance and usefulness of artists in residence in providing important components of care. Awareness that the arts can be a positive element in the hospital environment of care and can help to meet the psychosocial needs of patients has been embraced by hospitals as well as by healthcare oversight organizations such as the Joint Commission on Accreditation of Healthcare Organizations (JCAHO).

The importance of these values is reflected in the experience of a woman who lived for many months in the hospital while she waited for a heart transplant. During this time, she transitioned from being a reluctant participant in arts activities to becoming a performer in the hospital's theater troupe:

Anne had been fascinated when she attended her first Reflections show a few months earlier. Raised in the country, she had never attended a live theater performance. Bored by the tedium of a long hospitalization while she awaited a heart transplant, she had participated in a variety of art and writing activities. After quietly watching her first playback theater performance, she shyly asked if the troupe would be willing to come to her room sometime. In the privacy of her own room over the course of the following weeks, Anne began to tell her own stories. The troupe played them back to her as theater pieces, and over time became aware that she was learning the playback forms.

The director of the troupe invited Anne to join them as an actor. On the day of her premiere, Anne's usual pajamas were replaced by the black clothing worn by the other actors; and at the end of the performance, she was surrounded by the enthusiastic congratulations of her fellow patients and caregivers. She was beaming and related to her friends, "I have received so much while I have been a patient here. But today, in being a playback actor, I finally had the opportunity to give back. I feel great!"

Opportunities such as this provide patients with a way to feel more whole; to participate in a generative process, to interact, and to give to others. In times of illness, life can seem to screech to a grinding halt, and feeling productive can significantly enhance a patient's sense of wellness and well-being.

The artist also serves as a model and a reminder for hospital caregivers of the role of the arts as tools for professional longevity. The arts provide a superb mechanism for expressing both the agonizingly painful and immensely meaningful experiences that caregivers accumulate in their stressful jobs. John Graham-Pole (2002), in the introduction to his collection of poems entitled *Quick,* notes that "Medicine is a bottomless well of poems." This certainly applies to the other arts as well. The experience of healthcare is rife with life's richness, hints as to its meaning, and enough emotional intensity to inspire a lifetime of creative expression. Hospital artists lead workshops for caregivers in and out of the hospital setting, and through their work with patients serve as a reminder of this important and accessible resource.

Inverse and symbiotic to the caregiver's attraction to the arts is the artist's attraction to the healthcare environment as a source for deepening life experience and artistic inspiration. Hospital artists find fuel for their creative process in their experiences, which helps them find a deeper sense of meaning in their work. In the early 1990s in her book *The Reenchantment of Art,* Suzy Gablick (1992) challenged artists to come out of the seclusion of the studio art world and to engage in community. Where in the past several decades, there has been a movement in healthcare toward humanism that has significantly embraced the arts as a means, so over the past decade has there been a parallel movement within the fine and performing arts toward deeper meaning and human connection. The arts are fulfilling a basic human need within healthcare; and the link between healthcare and the arts is also fulfilling that same need within the fine and performing arts.

## The Artist's Relationship to the Patient/Participant

Hospital artists work with patients in a caring and supportive way. They enter each patient's room not with a particular agenda, but simply with an intention to provide attention and support through art if it is useful to the patient. Artists offer opportunities that are as simple (and significant) as distraction from pain and worry or as meaningful and life-altering as insight and direction. Just as professional or accomplished artists become adept at accessing their creativity (great painters paint *more* great paintings, and faster), patients also learn to use and rely on the arts for a variety of purposes. Some seek transcendence, some empowerment, some insight; some seek to gain a sense of control, and some to manifest joy and connection. People in the hospital may often learn and deepen these skills as fast as or faster than students of the arts. The sense of urgency that often accompanies illness shapes the patient's creative process and redefines the art form they engage in, using it to suite their needs. The artist in residence simply encourages and supports the patient, and then has the incredible honor of witnessing and sharing in the depths of creativity that ensue.

The artist in residence's relationship with a patient is not clinical in the medical sense. The artists do not access a patient's medical and personal information, yet they have the unique opportunity to form a meaningful relationship with the patient. The autonomy of the role of the hospital artist allows him to spend as little or as much time as is appropriate and needed with a patient. This is a rare luxury in the healthcare setting. In subsequent sections, we will discuss at length the importance and functionality of the relationship formed between the artist and patient.

## The Artist's Relationship to Medical Staff

Artists in residence sometimes work in partnership with clinical caregivers. In some settings, such as on the Adult Heart Transplant, or "Status One," service at Shands Hospital at the University of Florida, artists are a part of the clinical care team and meet with physicians, nurses, social workers, and other care providers on a regular basis to design the most comprehensive plan of care for patients, including the arts. In most programs, artists in residence respond to referrals or orders from clinical staff to bring creative activities to patients. Requests are made based on physical, emotional, social, and spiritual needs of patients. Many clinical caregivers rely on artists to provide aspects of care, such as unlimited attention and listening, that their own time constraints do not allow. Many artists in residence respond to referrals throughout the hospital, while others are assigned to a specific unit or units.

Artists often work most closely with nursing and social work staff in the hospital. These clinicians tend to know their patients well and can identify unique needs that extend beyond the traditional range of physical and even psychological medical care. Clinicians refer patients to an artist in residence, for example, when a patient has difficulty in complying and needs creative motivation to reengage with her treatment. The most common reasons stated for artist referrals are loneliness, boredom, noncompliance, long-term admission, chronic pain, lack of activity/engagement and depression, and a need for distraction; or inversely, that the patient is very outgoing and interested in art and activity. Creative activities often provide a point of engagement for patients that other therapies lack. For instance, a patient who is struggling with and achieving little result from physical therapy exercises may find that painting is enjoyable and can provide a level of engagement and even physical distraction that can facilitate the prescribed movement more easily than a focused exercise. In this way, clinical staff members utilize artists in residence as partners in providing care, recognizing that the arts can assist them in accomplishing important outcomes in patient care.

## FACILITATING CREATIVITY IN THE HEALTHCARE SETTING

### Engaging the Patient in a Creative Process

We will now look now at the "how" of facilitating the arts at the patient bedside. In this regard, the authors have, over the past 13 years of clinical practice within the Shands Arts in Medicine Program at the University of Florida, developed a helpful metaphor for the facilitation of the arts at the bedside. It is important to note that what follows is not a method to be applied, but is simply an observation of the progression of what often occurs in this process. This metaphor, which we call the "Four Bridges," is very similar to other systems that have been developed to map the stages of creativity or the stages of ritual. Mellick (1996) describes four stages through which creativity undertaken for the sake of the soul must evolve as "intentional departure from ordinary awareness; inner journey into the imagination; return to ordinary awareness, and reflection on the journey" (p. 17). Achterberg, Dossey, & Kolkmeier (1994) describe the three stages of rituals for healing as separation, transition, and return. A similar process is described here from the perspective of an artist facilitating the arts at the bedside. We will begin with a discussion of the artist-patient relationship and will then describe the Four Bridges with the assistance of narratives that illustrate the roles of the arts in healthcare today. Both authors use dance as a primary artistic medium in their work with patients; thus, we will begin with a brief discussion of dance in healthcare and will use a number of examples of patients who have explored dance as a creative medium.

The physical nature of dance makes its application in the medical setting quite powerful. Patients often describe feeling betrayed by their bodies (Finlay, 2003; Montgomery & Graham-Pole, 1997; Wendell, 1996). This feeling, as well as the pain and discomfort associated with illness and treatment, can cause a sense of separation from the body; and sometimes patients describe feeling angry with their bodies. Through dancing, a patient can have a positive, joyful physical experience and begin to bridge that separation. Levels of cortisol and other hormones rise, causing a physical sensation of pleasure that is also associated with feelings of success and control (Flinn et al., 1996). Patients discover meaningful personal knowledge, or insight, that they otherwise might not obtain. JoAnn provides a wonderful example of how a patient gains important insight through a creative process:

---

JoAnn was immediately attracted to the idea of moving when she was introduced to the Dancer in Residence at Shands Hospital. She had moved only between bed, chair, and bathroom for more than a week since being admitted to her isolation room on the bone marrow transplant unit. She told the artist that she lived near and loved the beach, and so the session was begun with movement in which the arms cross an imaginary horizon, followed by a scooping up of water from the ocean and a movement that tossed it overhead to shower gently down. The artist invited JoAnn to repeat the same movement sequence for a few minutes with her eyes closed.

After a few moments, she took in a deep breath and then let out a sigh. "Now I know I'm going to be alright," she said. "All of the seashells just turned to jewels." The image she had discovered inside her movement was a clear indication to her that she was going to live. This insight gave her tremendous confidence and meant more to her than her prognoses or the statistics she had been given for her survival. For the first time, she really knew that she was going to live (Sonke-Henderson, 1996).

---

Some people describe this knowing as coming from deep within them; some describe it as seeming to come from beyond them or through them. Nonetheless, this type of insight is a fruit of creativity; it is much the same for the untrained artist as the trained artist. Each individual redefines dance, reinvents the art form. The essential nature of the healthcare experience assists the patient in approaching creativity as a tool for healing.

JoAnn's experience, although short in duration, beautifully exemplifies a patient's journey across the Four Bridges. The artist spent time getting to know the patient, invited her to participate in movement, and led movement based on the patient's interests and experience. The patient then moved into a state of deepened concentration and discovered a very personal and meaningful insight. She then found closure by sharing and celebrating her experience verbally with the artist. In the following sections, we will discuss each of the Four Bridges and will present other patient stories as illustrations.

## The First Bridge: Moving into Relationship

Relationship is the absolute basis upon which a hospital artist in residence facilitates a creative process for patients. While our societal values and the pace of our lives today do not allow for much emphasis on the art of conversation, this is an extremely important skill for an artist in residence. Indeed, it is one of the great pleasures of the role. In the hospital environment, efficiency of communication is highly valued, and while it may be important for caregivers, it can be highly depersonalizing and alienating for patients. Hospitals are rife with high-speed, highly condensed, and highly impersonal dialogue. Artists have the unique opportunity to talk with patients and, even more importantly, to listen.

Hospitalized patients often struggle with frustrations regarding communication with caregivers, and a patient's perception of caregiver empathy have been shown to affect emotional health, symptom resolution, and health outcomes (Kaplan, 1989; Reid-Ponte, 1992; Stewart, 1995). Patients often describe a feeling of not being heard by their caregivers, as was the case with a woman on an oncology unit at Shands Hospital that the poet John Fox met during a residency with Shands Arts in Medicine. The patient was very weak and had great difficulty in speaking with any significant volume. She was also, due to her critical condition, in the throes of decision making. After listening to her frustrations, Fox asked her if she would like help in writing a poem describing her feelings. After Fox read a poem to her that he had written about listening (see chapter 9), she poured out a series of words and images describing how she would like to be listened to:

### When Someone Deeply Listens To Me

When someone deeply listens to me
I feel like a baby bird
Being held for the first time.

Secure. Like nothing could
Break the security blanket
That's wrapped around me.

When someone deeply listens to me
I feel HEARD, not just
Responded to.

When people don't listen to me
I feel angry, frustrated. It's like
Tense eyes. No one is hearing
What I am saying, they hear
What they want me to say—
Not what I am saying.

It's cloudy in there when
No one is listening to me.
Cloudy in my head.

The frustration is overwhelming and
I have to self-protect
And get into this mode of fogginess.

When someone deeply listens to me
It's nice, comforting.
When I say I'm scared and they
Really listen and they say:
I'm scared too.
That's really listening.

Instead of trying to talk
Me out of
Being scared.

Fox hung the poem over the sink in the entryway of the patient's room so that her caregivers, while they stood to wash their hands, might read it and understand better how she wanted to be listened to. Over the next few weeks as she moved from room to room and the poem went with her, she happily reported a significant change in the way her caregivers related and attended to her.

There is no way to overstate the importance of listening and of making a relationship with a patient as a basis for facilitating creativity. Not only is it functionally useful, but it is one of the richest parts of the work of a hospital artist. Artists receive the benefit of hearing about vast human experiences and this informs their work with patients. They come to better understand the amazing diversity of people, and glean powerful wisdom and insight from those who are in a very essential state of being. This level of communication is a tremendous honor and the basis for the artist's work, and simply engaging in conversation and being listened to can be extremely comforting and nourishing for a patient. Although an artist is available for further creative interaction, it does not make the process any more or less successful. Whatever is useful and meaningful for the patient defines a successful artist/patient interaction.

The establishment of relationship as described above is the foundation of facilitating the arts at the bedside. The confidence for the patient to create is most often cultivated through a rapport with the artist. Sometimes patients are familiar and comfortable with their creative process, particularly if they already consider themselves to be artistic, but most often the work of the artist includes building a relationship that will provide the patient with the comfort and security to move into a creative process. The process often begins with conversation or storytelling. It can occur quickly or over an extended period of time, but should never be rushed. An artist is typically observant of what the patient displays (or does not display) in her room—what was brought along, what was sent, and so forth. These are effective conversation starters. What is most important in this stage is the artist's capacity for attentive and compassionate listening. While listening, the artist may take note of parts of the conversation or stories that seem to stir the patient's energy, the moments when the patient lights up, when his eyes widen, or when he sits a little taller or beams proudly. These memories and images can be used as a starting point for a creative activity.

Engagement in an arts activity can also be an excellent basis for building a relationship. For some people, focusing on an activity can take the pressure off the relationship building. Sometimes an artist will simply ask the patient if she can sit with him while she works on her artwork. This takes the pressure off the conversation and it can be very relaxing for patients to watch a piece of art emerge.

An artist in residence who works in an emergency room waiting area during the wee hours of the morning related the following experience one day at an Artists Rounds meeting at Shands Hospital:

> A man came in to the emergency room waiting area having a panic attack. He was advised that the wait would be long and he was very anxious. After a short time, the painter asked him if he would like to have his portrait painted while he waited. At first, he was confused and slightly irritated by the question, but with the apparent realization that he had nothing else to do, consented. He sat quietly for a long time as the artist painted, but eventually began to tell her about his life. She listened as she painted, and when she finally handed him his finished portrait, he stood up and thanked her, adding, "I don't need to see a doctor any more, I feel fine." He embraced her with gratitude and a sense of connection as he left.

It is important to note that some people don't want to do anything creative. It is not for everyone. One of the greatest skills of the hospital artist is to know how to be encouraging and supportive without being pushy or coercive. A useful hospital artists' credo is to "go into a patient's room with an intention (to support the patient through creativity), but without an agenda (to get him to make art)." This skill takes time to develop and can be observed in the seasoned hospital artist who views every patient's room as personal and sacred space.

## The Second Bridge: Moving into Creativity

The rapport and trust established between the artist and patient within the first bridge allows the patient to comfortably give him- or herself permission to be creative. Adults in particular are likely to respond to an invitation to make art with, "Oh, no, I can't draw" or "I would feel silly." But once the rapport has been established, the patient will often cross the second bridge into creativity with relative comfort. At this point, when the patient is ready to begin a creative activity, the artists generally guides the process. This is the "Hey, I've got an idea, follow me…" part of the process.

Using the memories, images, and even the physical gestures provided by the patient in the first bridge's conversation, the artist can lead with ideas that have personal meaning to the patient. This part of the process can be extremely therapeutic in itself. Dancing, singing, reading poetry together, or painting, even without creating something uniquely personal or metaphorical, can be extremely joyful, physically invigorating, and inspiring. Sometimes the second bridge is as far as the journey goes within the sequence of the bridges, but can be continued or maintained over time. Jamie is a good example of a patient whose creative process was extremely important, but not metaphorical or symbolic:

---

The Dancer in Residence was referred to Jamie by her physician. The 12-year-old girl was experiencing a relapse of cancer after several years of good health. Her previous treatment for a brain tumor had left her blind, but she had mentioned to her doctor that she wanted to learn to dance. She asked the dancer to teach her ballet, jazz, modern dance, swing dance, and hip hop. The dancer worked with her each day. Despite her lack of sight, she learned quickly and even began creating original swing steps. She loved it when her family, nurses, and doctors would come and watch her dance. She effectively used dancing to define her environment and to affirm her orientation toward life. Her room was filled with music and dancing, and whoever came in was invited, usually expected, to dance with her.

---

Another child, a four-year-old boy who spent three days per week coping with the cramping and fatigue associated with his dialysis treatments, described his experience of painting with a visual artist in residence in the following conversation with his nurse:

---

"Sean, you seemed to have an easier time with your dialysis today," the nurse observed.

"It's the medithine," he said with his endearing lisp.

"But you didn't have any medicine. Nothing was any different, sweetie," she pointed out.

"It's the medithine!" he insisted.

The nurse looked at him, perplexed. "What medicine?"

"It's the Arts in Medithine!!" he said in a tone that indicated that grownups just don't know anything.

## Third Bridge: Moving into the Patients' Creative Process

Some patients may begin directing the creative experience immediately, but most will expect or need the artist to be a definitive leader in the beginning. The third bridge represents the transition in leadership of the creative process from the artist to the patient. There is often a visible shift in the patient that the artist can recognize that signals this transition. Within a movement activity, the patient may alter her gaze from outward (following the artist's lead) to inward (following her internal imagery or impulse), or might initiate this shift by sharing images, memories, or feelings that arise from the movement. The artist may take a variety of approaches to support the patient in developing her creative process. In dance, this could include gently mirroring or echoing the patient's movement, physically supporting the patient, or improvising from the patient's images or movement motifs in a way that helps that patient to not be distracted from her focus.

The insights discovered during this stage of the creative journey can range from interesting to life-altering. It is also highly empowering to the patient to have his or her work affirmed by another. In the hospital, artists have the honor of witnessing some of the most profound and meaningful creativity from patients. The artistic expression may not be trained or polished, but it is powerful and it often exemplifies extraordinary creative mastery. Beatrice is a 17-year-old patient who has used dance in the hospital and at home to control her sickle cell disease pain for over a decade:

When Beatrice was 14 years old, she came into the hospital in a terrible pain crisis. Because her medical record noted that she had a long history of using dance as an effective distraction for her pain, the Dancer in Residence was called. Through her excruciating pain and her tears, she told the dancer that she could try to move and requested Chopin for accompaniment. She sat up on the side of the bed, her limbs swollen

*(Continues)*

*(Continued)*

and only minimally mobile. The dancer began the movement by holding her hands and moving her arms slowly. Beatrice closed her eyes and
relaxed in the movement. After a while, Beatrice lifted her hands from
the dancer's and began to lead the movement. She lost herself fully in
the music and moved into a state of intensely deep concentration. Her
range of motion rapidly increased and her face was visibly relaxed.

This session began a new stage in Beatrice's creative process and in her pain
management strategies. She has continued to use Chopin to accompany her
movement and to facilitate her transition into the deep level of concentration
she uses to transcend her pain. No music moves her like Chopin, and this
recognition provides her with a consistently effective tool for managing her
pain. When asked by clinical staff about what happens to her pain when she
is dancing, Beatrice responds that the pain is still there, but she feels so good
overall that she can coexist with it.

Hospital artists do not attempt to interpret or assign meaning to a patient's
images or creative process. If a patient chooses to explore the meaning within
his work, the artist listens and honors his thoughts. Artists support the patient
in his or her creative journey, knowing that the process itself has therapeutic
value and that it may also yield important discoveries, but does not guide
the patient toward interpretation, therapeutic exploration, or catharsis. If this
occurs, the artist supports as any fellow human being might, and if additional
psychological support is needed, garners the assistance of mental health staff.

The artist may notice that the ritualized creative practices that patients
develop are indeed representational or metaphorical of their current situation
or desires. These metaphorical rituals can become powerful affirmations for the
patient (Texter & Mariscotti, 1994) and can also allow the patient control and
the ability to assert his own will. Natasha's story illustrates this experience:

Natasha, a beautiful, soft-spoken five-year-old, was about to undergo a
bone marrow transplant. Over the first few days that she worked with the
Dancer in Residence, Natasha created a beautiful movement sequence
that would become her daily ritual. In her dance, she and the dancer flew
up into the sky and gathered all of the stars into their baskets. Natasha
would then [literally] give herself and the dancer an alcohol swab and
a gauze pad. They sat down and cleaned each star meticulously, front
and back, until she felt that they were all clean. Sometimes she would
even count the stars to make sure they had them all. When they were all

clean, they would dance again and toss all of the stars back up into the sky. This was an extraordinary metaphor for a bone marrow transplant. In Natasha's case, with no matching donor, her own bone marrow had been harvested, cleaned of cancer cells, and transplanted back into her body as a basis for a new immune system.

Natasha did this each day, including the day of her transplant, and for about a week after. As it happened, on this day Natasha's new bone marrow cells were beginning to grow and her white blood cell counts were going up, signaling that her transplant was working successfully. Instinctively, she changed her ritual; her dances shifted to a focus of being at the beach, swimming, and doing all of the things she wanted to do when she left the hospital.

Natasha demonstrated that even a child of five years, who could not consciously create a metaphorical ritual for healing, can embody a stunning example of the functional capacity of the arts in the healthcare setting. In her ritual, Natasha asserted each day that that her bone marrow was clean and that she would return to her normal child's life.

This third stage of the journey can be experienced directly, as when the patient makes the art him or herself; or can be experienced in what might appear to be an indirect manner. Some patients may be reluctant or unable to provide much physical input; others may have very limited capacities, both mentally and physically; and others may simply prefer to be somewhat passive in the process. Artists may paint an image for a patient, dance a patient's dance, theatrically act or musically sing out a patient's story, or write it for him. Although the role of the patient may seem passive in these instances, it is indeed a very engaging and meaningful experience. It is akin to what we can experience as audience members at performances, or to what we experience when we view art in a museum or gallery. These experiences, although often considered to be passive, are indeed active, engaging, and often transformative.

In this way, artists can become the instrument of expression for patients who may be too ill to actively participate, but are nonetheless determined to express their experiences, ideas, and hopes. For example:

Gloria was a strong and independent woman who had raised six children herself after her husband had died of a heart attack while in his 40s. In her present condition, she was unable to speak above a whisper, and

*(Continues)*

*(Continued)*

was despondent and subdued. She told the visiting artist that violet was her favorite color and as they talked, the artist made violet paper flowers for her. She told the artist about her life as a girl in New England where she loved walking in the woods and picking blueberries in the bogs. She brightened up when the artist asked if she would like her to create a dance from her imagery. Delighted, Gloria selected music from the artist's collection, and watched eagerly as the dancer improvised for her. The dance ended with the artist symbolically presenting her with a basket of freshly picked blueberries, to which Gloria declared "Muffins!" After more conversation, which now was animated, the dancer created a movement motif that Gloria might be able to do herself. It was just a slight flick of the foot with some shaking as if she were trying to get her wading boots off. Gloria smiled and relayed with enthusiasm as she shook her foot, "That's exactly what you do."

## The Fourth Bridge: Moving toward Closure

Closure is the transition from the creative space back to a focus on the present. This is analogous to the return phase of ritual and, much like the *denouement* in classical comedy, provides closure to the experience and a way of bringing the transformation back into the present physical world. Mellnick (1996) suggests that when one is ready to leave the inner realm, he should carefully allow the experience to come to a close and then reenter normal awareness.

Sometimes, particularly with children, closure can be very challenging. Children often will not want to stop dancing, singing, or drawing, and have difficulty with the artist's leaving. In this case, closure must be facilitated by the artist. This can require tremendous creativity in itself, particularly with young children. Typically, it is a considerable respite for the patient to be engaged in an imaginary place "out of" the hospital, and if the artist were to say, "Okay, I have to go now; we have to go back to the hospital," it would leave the patient with a feeling of disappointment rather than with a sense of lingering happiness and fulfillment. So, we find a playful way to get back to the room and leave the patient with a project, such as drawing or writing, which keeps him connected to his creative space.

Even for adults, return can be difficult, particularly given the bleakness of a hospital environment. It can be very helpful to talk about the creative experience and to orient it toward continuation. Talking, journaling, writing a poem, creating a visual representation of the experience are all good ways to externalize the process and to provide some lasting symbols for the powerful process that has just occurred. This not only brings the process out of the self, but also solidifies the sense of completion. The following story illustrates an exceptionally important experience of closure:

Violet, who was in the hospital awaiting a lung transplant, explained to the visiting artist in residence that she had a dream of what she would do after she received her lung. She was determined to dance across a bridge spanning the intercoastal waterway near her home to the sea. During the many visits the artist made to her room, Violet would provide imagery—usually involving water—and ask the artist to dance it for her. It was during these moments that the medical staff would notice significant increases in her blood oxygen saturation levels, and an increased level of overall relaxation.

Over the months that Violet waited for her lung, her imagery never involved crossing the bridge; she often approached it, but never crossed it. After she received her lung however, on the day before she was to return home, she finally joined the dancer physically in her dance, ritually crossing the bridge and "rehearsing" her further recovery. When they reached the top of the bridge in their dance, Violet looked out over the ocean, she cried out triumphantly, "I'm alive…and I can breathe!" Several months later, on the Fourth of July, Violet called the artist to report that she had indeed walked across the bridge as she had envisioned, and did indeed do a dance on the top!

For some artists, leaving the patient's room can be as difficult as the initial entrance. Having something to leave with the patient for the future makes the exit seem more appropriate. Visual arts or crafts often provide a natural product for the patient to keep. While it is the process itself that is transformative for the patient, when there is such a product, it serves as a symbol for the process and as a means of honoring the experience. Since dance is so ephemeral, dancers in residence often give the patient the gift of a small movement motif, preferably something that the patient is physically able to do himself, which comes from the session's shared experience. This type of offering, as well as a suggestion to continue with "prescribed" visual art or writing exercises, can help to provide a sense of both closure and continuance for the patient.

## CONCLUSION

The outcomes of patients' creative processes vary greatly. For some patients, the opportunity to engage in a creative process can be a pleasant diversion from the current hospital experience. This, while seemingly very simple, can be extremely useful and patients are often very grateful for the distraction. The effects of laughter, fun, and joy on well-being cannot be overstated. Distraction itself has been shown to have positive effects on pain and anxiety, and even on the need for medication (Eccleston, 1995; McCaul & Malott, 1984; Vessey, Carlson, & McGill, 1994).

Engaging in a creative activity can bring physical relief from pain or discomfort, can increase range of motion, lung capacity, and physical energy, and can significantly alter mood and outlook (see Staricoff, 2004). Physicians, physical therapists, and nurses often refer patients to Arts in Medicine for these reasons. It has become apparent through the presence of artists in the hospital setting that patients often respond favorably to creative inspiration and motivation as opposed to physiological directives. For example, a patient recovering from a mastectomy who dreads the painful range of motion exercises mandated in her physical therapy might happily achieve the same range through dancing or painting.

The arts provide opportunities for people to express themselves, to be supported, and to be honored. These experiences can often be transformative. Within them, people discover deeply personal insights that can guide decision making, interactions with family and caregivers, and their outlook toward healing, living, or dying. The arts also provide people with opportunities to create something tangible that can represent or serve as a legacy to a significant time of life, or can serve as a memorial to a deceased family member. Hospitals today are filled with ceramic tile wall installations, ceiling tile installations, and murals that honor the experiences, including life and death, of patients and caregivers. The major theme of these works of art is hope. And what better place for the arts—humanity's medium for exploring and reflecting the human experience—than in hospitals, where we face some of life's greatest challenges.

## TOOL KIT FOR CHANGE

### Role and Perspective of the Healthcare Professional

1. The hospital artist in residence is a facilitator for the patient's creative process and uses his artistic sensibilities to help the patient find her own creative voice.
2. The artist in residence must take care to not take on the role of clinician or therapist. The uniquely nonhierarchical artist/patient relationship serves as an effective basis for facilitating a meaningful creative experience.
3. The artist in residence enters each patient's room with a clear intention for supporting healing, but without a rigid agenda.
4. The artist in residence should provide the patient with a sense of self-sufficiency in his creative process so that it can continue without dependency on the artist.

## Role and Perspective of the Participant

1. A patient can use a creative process for distraction, enjoyment, expression, communication, connection, physical movement, insight, and inspiration.
2. Creative exploration and expression complement medical care by assisting the patient with the integration of the physical, emotional, and spiritual aspects of healing.

## Interconnection: The Global Perspective

1. Artist-in-residence programs throughout the world create unique ways of facilitating the arts at the bedside. Practices fit with local cultural paradigms and "reinvent" each art form on a continuing basis.
2. Artists in residence from healthcare settings throughout the world meet annually at the Society for the Arts in Healthcare conference in various locations in the United States and Canada. See www.thesah.org for more information. There are similar umbrella organizations in Great Britain, Australia, and Japan.

## REFERENCES

Achterberg, J., Dossey, B., & Kolkmeier, L. (1994). *Rituals of healing: Using imagery for health and wellness.* New York: Bantam Books.

Atwood, M. D. (1991). *Spirit healing: Native American magic and medicine.* New York: Sterling Publishing Co.

Bolen, J. (1999). "*The creative encounter,*" *the soul of creativity: Insights into the creative process.* Novato, CA: New World Library.

Dissanayake, E. (2000). *Art and intimacy: How the arts began.* Seattle: University of Washington Press.

Eccleston, C. (1995). Chronic pain and distraction: an experimental investigation into the role of sustained and shifting attention in the processing of chronic persistent pain. *Behaviour Research and Therapy, 33,* 391–405.

Finlay, L. (2003) The intertwining of body, self, and world: A phenomenological study of living with recently-diagnosed multiple sclerosis. *Journal of Phenomenological Psychology, 34*(2), 157–178.

Flinn, M. V., Quinlan, R., Turner, M., Decker, S. A., & Engladn, B. G. (1996). Male-female differences in effects of parental absence on glucocorticoid stress response. *Human Nature, 7*(2): 125–162.

Gablick, S. (1992). *The reenchantment of art.* London: Thames & Hudson.

Graham-Pole, J. (2002). *Quick.* San Jose: Writer's Club Press.

Halley, F. M. (1991). Self-regulation of the immune system through biobehavioral strategies. *Biofeedback and Self Regulation., 16*(1), 55–74.

Herrera, H. (1983). *Frida: A Biography of Frida Kahlo.* San Francisco: Harper & Row.

Johnson, T. (2005). Intensive spiritual care: A case study. *Critical Care Nurse, 25,* 20–26.

Kaplan, S. H., Greenfield, S., & Ware, J. E. (1989). Assessing the effects of physician-patient interactions on the outcomes of chronic disease. *Medical Care, 27,* S110–S127.

Lucie-Smith, E. (1983). *Toulouse-Lautrec.* Oxford: Phaidon Press. McCaul, K., & Malott, J. (1984). Distraction and coping with pain. *Psychological Bulletin, 95,* 516–533.

Mellick, J. (1996). *The natural artistry of dreams: Creative ways to bring the wisdom of dreams to waking life.* Berkeley: Conari Press.

Montgomery, J., & Graham-Pole, J. (1997). A conversation: Humanizing the encounter between physician and patient through journalized poetry. *Journal of Poetry Therapy*, *11*(2),103–111.

Myers, T. P. (1999). *The soul of creativity: Insights into the creative process.* Novato, CA: New World Library.

Reid-Ponte, P. (1992). Distress in cancer patients and primary nurses' empathy skills. *Cancer Nursing, 15,* 283–292.

Sonke-Henderson, J. (1996). Healing through art. *Women's Health Digest, 2*(4), 330–331.

Staricoff, R. L. (2004). *Arts in health: A review of the medical literature.* London: Arts Council England.

Stewart, M. A. (1995). Effective physician-patient communication and health outcomes: A review. *Cancer Medical Association Journal, 152,* 1423–1433.

Texter, L., & Mariscotti, J. (1994). From chaos to new life: Ritual enactment in the passage from illness to health. *Journal of Religion and Health, 33*(4), 325–332.

Tharp, T. (2003). *The creative habit.* New York: Simon and Schuster.

Vessey, J. A., Carlson, K. L., & McGill, J. (1994). Use of distraction with children during an acute pain experience. *Nursing Research, 43,* 369–372.

Watson, D., & Clark, L. (1994). The vicissitudes of mood: A schematic model. In P. Ekman and R. J. Davidson (Eds.), *The Nature of Emotion: Fundamental Questions* (pp. 400–405). New York: Oxford University Press.

Wendell, S. (1996). *The rejected body: Feminist philosophical reflections on disability.* New York: Routledge.

Wikof, N. (2004). *Cultures of care: A study of arts programs in U.S. hospitals.* Washington, DC: Joint Commission on Accreditation of Healthcare Organizations.

Wong, C. (2001) Great artists, their medical conditions, and how their work was affected. *studentBMJ, 9,* 443–486.

Chapter Five

# THE SCIENCE OF CREATIVITY AND HEALTH

*Jeffrey E. Evans, PhD*

I have several times applied to the work of art the metaphor of a mode of nourishment.

—Susan Sontag (1965)

When, at the end, the artist was willing to rest his case on what his eyes and hands had arrived at, he had been able to see what he meant.

—Rudolf Arnheim (1962)

The purpose of this chapter is to discuss concepts from behavioral and biological science that explore how creative activities can promote health and well-being. We will show that creative activities promote harmony or *coherence* between person and world; that creative activities build *abilities*, or *competencies*, that promote *self-efficacy* and defeat boredom and depression; that enhanced engagement and mood can improve immune system functioning and other markers of physical as well as mental health, signaling a concordance, in the creative process, between mind, brain, and behavior. We will first define creativity in the context of arts in healthcare (AIH), then present a model of the creative process that explores the competencies involved—what people actually do when they create. Next we explore connections between creativity, self-efficacy and health, and between mind, brain, and behavior in the creative process.

## WHAT IS CREATIVITY FOR ARTS IN HEALTHCARE?

Creativity is a complex concept whose definition depends upon context, including the motivations and interests of those using the term. *In AIH practice the principal interest is in the capacity of creative activity to reduce human suffering and its potential to promote health.* This implies that our concept of creativity is not limited to those with special talent, nor is it defined by criteria external to the person. Rather, it is *inclusive,* applying to anyone who presents as a patient, and it is *personal.* That is, we regard people in general as having creative potential and, furthermore, that creativity is a process with component abilities that can be developed.

## THE CREATIVE PROCESS

Creativity is also complex in the sense that it is a process composed of many parts. Specifically, like growth and development, the creative process can be divided into stages or *moments* traversed on the way to maturity. And those moments can be further divided into cognitive, perceptual, physical, and affective abilities, many of which can be developed. For example, your creativity may involve facility with a particular medium—words, or clay—or in especially acute visual perception, powers of concentration, or perseverance. It may involve collaborating productively with other people. It may involve sensitivity to certain forms in the environment or to contradictions or ironies in society. In short, creative activity can be grounded in any number of skills and sensibilities that motivate and help you work.

In the section below we outline moments in the creative process and briefly describe each one in terms of component skills and abilities. For practitioners of AIH, such analysis can help define a client's "creative style" (Evans, 1992) and therefore identify natural strengths on which to build.

### Moments of the Creative Process as Problem Solving

Historically, the creative process has been conceived as a series of stages in the solving of problems, principally in science and mathematics (Hadamard, 1954 (1945); Wallas, 1926). We use the term *moments,* rather than *stages,* to minimize the impression of lock-step inevitability. Moments rarely occur singly, in order, or in their entirety. That is, in any given creative activity a particular moment may be brief or extended, it may repeat, it may alternate, and it may overlap with other moments. Defining such moments retains useful distinctions between categories of behavior but suggests a more realistic complexity than implied by ordered stages.

Wallas's original model proposed four stages, which we expand to six, to apply to artistic activities as well as to science and mathematics. An expanded model of the creative process is as follows:

Inspiration
Preparation
Incubation
Insight
Execution
Evaluation

In expanding Wallas's model we are also applying problem solving to the realm of art. The idea of art as problem solving should be clear if you consider the obvious difficulty of capturing complex feelings and perceptions in media. Anyone who has tried to put thoughts and feelings into words with any degree of precision or artistry knows that there is a huge problem of *translation* (Reddy, 2001) from the internal medium of the senses, including feelings and emotions, to the external medium of written language.

Second, problem solving recognizes that behavior is motivated. All animals do things, art included, for a reason: to accomplish something, to set things right, to move from point A to point B, to achieve greater satisfaction. And motivated activity implies a problem to be solved. This expanded view of problem solving—from math, to art, to life problems—implies that creativity has much in common with other complex behaviors, including resolving psychological conflicts and making complex judgments and decisions. Further, the concept of problem solving forms the connection between creativity and health, because implicit in problem solving is tension reduction, learning, and novelty, all of which have been shown to promote healthy brain development as well as mental well-being. We will develop this further in part 3. At this point we will describe each moment of the model with reference to component processes.

### Inspiration

Creativity requires cognitive and affective engagement. Inspiration is the spark of interest that launches us to make something new. In AIH, clients are often under stress, have strong feelings, and may be encouraged to translate those feelings and emotions into tangible form. Such translation can serve to organize the person and reduce tension. Inspiration in that context can result from the relationship with an AIH practitioner or simply from the availability of materials and the time and space to employ them.

### Preparation

Like the growth of a plant, for the creative process to result in something new and useful the ground is prepared in a way that makes that emergence more likely. Following are categories of activity that make up preparatory moments typical in AIH practice.

1. Setting the stage. In AIH, clients are *invited,* and often encouraged, to enter into creative activity. The ready availability of materials and a place to work are basic. This is not just true for patients in the hospital. For anyone interested in self-expression, arranging a place and time of day conducive to work facilitates release into creative activity.
2. *Relationship building.* Working with an AIH practitioner, mentor, or teacher can help one simply *to begin,* through introducing media, and through conversation or other shared experience.
3. *Psyching up.* It is helpful to achieve a mental or emotional set that facilitates creative activity, especially the basic belief that one is capable of being creative. It is important to feel assured that in creative or productive activity it is natural to make mistakes and that revision is part of the process.
4. *Use of ritual.* Ritual in AIH practice can involve scheduling regular times to create, so that it becomes an expected part of daily routine. Finding a ritual that works can help jump-start creative activity. In *The Creative Habit,* the choreographer Twyla Tharp describes how ritual helps start her day (Tharp, 2003).
5. *Skill building.* People can prepare for creative activity by consciously developing a skill, procedure, or technique such as watercolor or calculus. AIH clients can use their time to try something new or to revisit an old interest, developing skill and gaining confidence.
6. *Cognitive Structuring.* Having a client articulate his style of creating can help focus his efforts and consciously develop his own version of the creative process.
7. *Sketching* is a special form of preparation that minimizes conscious control of the outcome and therefore encourages unconscious self-organizing. Sketching, in other words, is an act of intentional playing with and within a medium to see what turns up. Sketching can suggest possible outcomes that may later become part of the final product. And while the unconscious automatically organizes the mind, the medium exerts its own influence. The medium is like a third party that literally *mediates* between the person and the developing work. That is, it facilitates the artist's effort, but also sets limits. Imagine the contrast between the limits of watercolor to a painter and granite to a sculptor.

Sketching also highlights the overlap of moments in the creative process: it can be part of preparation, like calisthenics that loosen you up. It can also be an element of execution and therefore be itself a finished product.

### Incubation

The emergence of a creative product—an insight, for example—benefits from not-doing as well as from doing. Incubation is a break or time-out that involves thinking about or doing something else. It can be as simple as taking a short walk in which attention is free-floating or directed at a simple, repetitive activity. It can involve rest or relaxation of attention, such as dreaming, daydreaming, or meditating. The advice "sleep on it" recognizes the value of removing attention from a problem or task and allowing the mind to process autonomously.

Incubation can occur at any time and can overlap with other moments. It can be several seconds of relaxed reverie during effortful preparation, after which you return to directed thought. Learning that incubation is a recognized and helpful part of the creative process can result in confidence that relaxation of effort can be productive. Knowing the benefits of incubation can also remind us to keep track of ideas that come to mind during off times, as unconscious mental processes automatically organize our many impressions. For example, students and others interested in creative endeavors are typically encouraged to carry a small notebook to keep track of ideas that occur when they aren't consciously working.

Incubation, therefore, refers to spans of mental idling when our impressions undergo a largely unconscious process of self-organizing with the result that ideas simply "come to mind." When such ideas have particular significance we often refer to having an insight.

### Insight

Insight is arguably the most dramatic moment of the creative process. It includes the well-known "Aha!" experience, a moment of sudden understanding or clarity when thoughts fall into place with a special feeling of resolution. The intensity of the "Aha!" experience varies from a bolt from the blue to a less dramatic feeling of *resonance*. Bolts from the blue are hard to miss; resonance can be subtle and fleeting. Learning to be receptive to these subtler forms of insight can take the form of cultivating an attitude of relaxed attention—for example, of alertness to potentially useful ideas during periods of incubation.

Insight can also appear as the very first moment of the creative process and therefore overlaps with inspiration. For example, you might by chance notice (have insight into) a juxtaposition of forms that inspires a piece of visual art. Such ongoing mental processing adds strands and color to the fabric of experience and, if we are receptive, can infuse everyday life with aesthetic experiences and creative ideas.

The interplay of conscious and unconscious thought that occurs during mental self-organizing and insight undoubtedly involves brain areas for more and less controlled mental processing; therefore as self-organizing occurs in the mind, so it occurs in the brain. Another way to conceive of self-organizing is the development of *coherence* between, for example, perception and action, as we see below.

### Execution

We might "execute" in a medium in order to transform an idea into a work of art. Execution can also transform the ideas themselves as the unique properties of the medium speak back reflexively to us and modify or produce fresh ideas. The execution of a sketch can be conscious preparation for later execution of the formal work.

A unique document in the creativity literature is Rudolf Arnheim's chronicle of Pablo Picasso's preliminary studies for his monumental painting *Guernica* (Arnheim, 1962/2006). With the eye of an art historian and a Gestalt psychologist, Arnheim reveals Picasso's creative process from his legacy of numbered and dated drawings: the starts and stops, progress and regress, and the moments of slowing down for a problem posed by the state of the painting at the time. Arnheim demonstrates that the work is reflexive: it slowly yet finally succeeds in revealing the artist's meaning to himself.

### Evaluation

When insight is gained in problem solving and the work is seemingly complete, evaluation is a moment of stepping back and assuming a critical distance. This is a skill in itself. In science and math it means checking the validity of a solution. In both art and science it can mean asking yourself: "Does this work?" "Am I satisfied?" "Does something need to be added or changed?"

## Moments Progress Organically

As progress is made on a work of art, moments occur, recur, and cycle back upon themselves. As in psychological development, the image of a spiral represents recurrence yet steady progression toward greater maturity. While it is possible to isolate each moment for the purpose of definition, in practice moments are not separate. They overlap, feed into each other, and often appear to just happen. You are working for the college newspaper and become inspired, perhaps by empathy or a chance encounter, to write an article about local homelessness. You gather information, perhaps do an interview, and so make preparations for writing. Along the way you have other things to do, or simply tire of the work and take a break: you incubate by choice or by necessity. At some point you execute a rough draft. You look back over your draft, asking yourself if it "sounds right," perhaps referring back to what inspired you, in order to recapture the spirit of your original intent. Perhaps you need an additional bit of information or decide to sleep on it before again revising the draft: the process cycles back, moments recur, your piece grows (see also Arnheim, 1962, part 4; Elbow, 1973, chap. 2).

## Moments Are Composed of Cognitive and Affective Abilities

In order to get closer to what can occur in AIH practice, it is important to define further what people actually *do* during moments of the creative process. We call such "doing" the exercise of *abilities* that can be as simple as defining and sticking to a ritual that assists in preparation; the ability to write a sentence needed for expository writing; perceptual acuity or empathy that begets inspiration; an objective attitude needed to evaluate one's work. All these component abilities and more can be learned. Even incubation, seemingly a time of mental idling, comes more naturally to some, and for the "incubation-challenged," it can be learned (see Adams, 1974/2001, chap. 3; Seifert, Meyer, Davidson, Patalano, & Yaniv, 1995). Sternberg (2005) calls such component abilities *developing competencies,* to emphasize their dynamic nature.

As with creativity itself, with component abilities we avoid external criteria and summary judgments. That is, abilities are personal and are judged only insofar as they assist in self-expression and problem resolution.

## THE CREATIVE PROCESS AND HEALTH

The creative process is composed of moments and abilities that solve the problem of translating inner thoughts and feelings into an external medium, that is, of articulating meaning. Success at articulating meaning is an exercise in *self-efficacy* (Bandura, 1996; cited in Sternberg, 2005) and cognitive *control,* called by Wegner, *perceived control* (Wegner, 2002). In self-efficacy and perceived control is the potential for enhancement of mood and of health in general (Haidt & Rodin, 1999; for reviews see Skinner, 1995, cited in Wegner, 2002). How is self-efficacy healthy for us? That is, what is the organic component of the satisfaction that arises when we have been effective? There are two concepts that are useful to us in this regard: the *relaxation response* and *flow.*

### The Relaxation Response

The common sigh of relief when we succeed in adequate self-expression is akin to what Benson (1975) has called the "relaxation response" and is a physiological sign of psychological resolution. The relaxation response suggests a release of tension, and it is a response that can be learned and repeated. In clinical practice it is taught through psychophysiological techniques such as biofeedback, or through "integrative" methods, such as meditation (e.g., see Segal, Williams, & Teasdale, 2002). Dialogue in counseling or psychotherapy also promotes the relaxation response through insight into oneself and being understood by the therapist. These experiences, though, are not limited to clinical situations. The relaxation response can also result from everyday instances of understanding and being understood, of aesthetic appreciation and problem resolution, and from finding the right way to express a thought, feeling, or perception.

### Flow

Motivations to understand and to be understood involve novelty and learning, and they engage physical as well as mental activity—*flow,* the sheer pleasure of *doing.* Flow (Czikszentmihalyi, 1990) is a state of unselfconscious involvement in which the self is brought into interaction with features of the world—ideas, media, one's own body—for expression, enjoyment, and play. More than 40 years of evidence confirm a correlation between similar active involvement and brain development. Data from laboratory rats has shown that brains were more highly developed in animals exposed to "enriched environments" of toys, tunnels, and exercise wheels (e.g., Krech, Rosenzweig, & Bennett, 1962) or to social compared to isolated environments (Diamond, 1978). More recent evidence shows that neurogenesis, the birth of new brain cells, is promoted by environmental complexity and learning. This has been shown in older as well as younger animals and in primates as well as rats (see Gross, 2000). Conversely, chronic stress decreases the amount of neurogenesis (see Gross, 2000). Furthermore, in humans, the health effects of active engagement and play apparently slows development of amyloid plaques associated with Alzheimer's disease and other dementias (e.g., Marx, 2005).

The absence of engagement can result in boredom and depression (Czikszentmihalyi, 1990); stress can result in anxiety. Both depression and anxiety are linked to a poverty of connections among brain cells, as shown in imaging studies of major depression and posttraumatic stress disorder (PTSD). Specifically, major depression results in reduced grey matter volume in the prefrontal cortex and the hippocampus (cited in Castren, 2005), and PTSD results in shrinking of the hippocampus. Grey matter is made up of brain cells (neurons), and its volume and organizational complexity is an index of health. It may be significant that the prefrontal cortex and hippocampus, which are associated with higher mental and emotional functioning, are particularly affected by the presence or absence of active engagement.

Flow and the relaxation response, then, are two components of solving a tension-producing problem. But what is the problem that is solved? What is held in common between being understood by another person, finding the right words or image to express a thought, working out a math problem, or deciding where to go to college? They differ in the details and implications, of course, but when the problem is solved, all have established *coherence* between the person and some aspect of the world. Coherence reduces tension and results in euthymia (literally "good mood," the opposite of dysthymia and depression). *That is, in the creative process, self-expression is responsible for creating coherence between the person and some aspect of his or her experience.*

The creative process as an insight-seeking, problem-solving activity provides many occasions for flow and the relaxation response. But does creative engagement really reduce stress and enhance health?

## Creativity and Health: Empirical Studies

It has been a central tenet of psychotherapy since Freud that self-expression is important for mental and emotional health. Founding humanistic psychologists

Abraham Maslow and Carl Rogers concluded that creative self-expression may be a uniquely human need tantamount to self-actualization (Runco, 2005). More recently the equating of creative self-expression with health has been subjected to experimental scrutiny, and it has been found in some contexts that creative self-expression promotes mental health, and possibly physical health as well. The medium in which this has been most extensively studied is *narrative writing*.

James Pennebaker has pioneered research on the effect on health of narrative writing about traumatic experiences. In a descriptive review of over two dozen studies, Pennebaker and Seagal (1999) found "positive health and behavioral effects" reported across different populations, including arthritis and chronic pain sufferers, postpartum women, college students, distressed crime victims, maximum-security prisoners, and men laid off from their jobs. They found writing associated with lower pain medication use, higher college grades, lower levels of depression and faster reemployment. Not unexpectedly, other results show comparable effects of writing and *talking* about traumatic experiences. Apparently the important feature is not writing per se, but the process of putting thoughts and feelings into words. It has also been found that a variety of writing topics produce comparable health benefits. The critical feature for the effect on health is that people explore their thoughts and feelings on topics that are meaningful to them. The authors also report from four different laboratories that "writing produces positive effects on blood markers of immune function" (p. 1245).

In a statistically rigorous meta-analytic review of 13 studies, Smyth (1998) found that several types of superior health outcomes were reported one month postwriting: "reported health (including health center visits), psychological well-being (including happiness, adjustment), physiological functioning (including immune function), and general functioning (including school grades, absenteeism)" (p. 180). How might translating thoughts and feelings into words promote health through the immune system?

In a recent meta-analytic review of 30 years of research on stress and the immune system, Segerstrom and Miller (2004) show that the relationship is not simple; that is, studies define various forms of acute and chronic stress and reveal differing effects of stress on the immune system. Principally important for our purposes, acute stress tends to increase rapidly responding "natural immunity." For example, during fight or flight the body is protected by an increase in the number of natural killer cells and large granular lymphocytes in peripheral blood. This can happen on a moment's notice when there is a threat to the body of physical injury and immune cells are required close to the body's surface to fight potential injury and infection. However, under conditions of chronic stress, such as living with a disability, or caring for a chronically ill spouse—or, we might imagine, the stress of hospitalization—almost all immune system functions are suppressed, including natural killer cell cytotoxicity and proliferation of lymphocytes.

The jury is still out, however, on whether the critical psychological mechanism linking stressors with the immune system involves emotion, motivational states, cognitive appraisal, or behavior, although an emphasis on behavior (e.g., physical activity and behavioral habits) has proven useful in studies of clinically depressed patients (Segerstrom & Miller, 2004).

Outside of the arts therapies (e.g. music, painting, dance) the value of other expressive media to health has not been extensively studied. Pennebaker and Seagal (1999) briefly describe an experiment in their laboratory in which students were asked to express a traumatic experience either through dance alone or through dance followed by writing. Control subjects were asked to exercise in a prescribed way for 10 minutes per day over three days. Only the movement plus writing group showed improvements in physical health and grade point average, although both "movement expression groups (dance alone and dance plus writing) reported that they felt happier and mentally healthier in the months after the study" (p. 1247–1248). Thus, nonverbal means alone seem to produce health benefits, although apparently two modalities are better than one.

In sum, translating experience into multiple modalities of expression results in increased coherence between self and world. That is, in the above example of writing and dance, not only does the verbal modality encode the experience, but so do somatosensory and kinesthetic modalities. And in the brain, each modality has its basis in specific, though overlapping, large-scale distributed neural networks (e.g., see Mesulam, 1985). Furthermore, each modality is a "language" with its own specialized neural code for experience (e.g., Pribram, 1977). The fact that we recognize the external world each time we open our eyes, are familiar with the feel of the world as we move through it, and recognize objects by their names attests to massive neural encoding of multiple overlapping aspects of the world. To reproduce that impression through the creative process is an act of re-creation of that which has been given us by nature and by experience. Again, creative self-expression *organizes the person* with reference to the world of experience and creates coherence between the person and the world.

## WHY WE CREATE: THE QUEST FOR RESONANCE AND COHERENCE

We have reviewed evidence that the creative process can benefit emotional and even physical health. We also introduced the idea of the relaxation response and flow as likely physiological mediators between creative self-expression and health. In flow, the person experiences unimpeded cognitive and emotional flexibility and is therefore capable of drawing on the resources of the past, the present, and the future to express her experience of the world. Similarly, the relaxation response often follows relatively subtle events, such as translating an idea into words. With translation comes a felt correspondence, or *resonance,* between internal and external structures—for example, between feeling and written language. That is, when the words work, a rather profound thing has happened: mind and brain have made a choice from within the vast lexicon, grammar, and tone of the English language. That choice is a group of words that translates meaning—a formerly mute cognitive and affective structure—into a medium that communicates. And as I feel resonance between my words, sketch, or music and my experience, *coherence* (Thagard, 2000) develops between myself and the world. How the mind and brain work together in the quest for resonance and coherence is the subject of this section.

## Coherence, Mental Flexibility, and Mental Control

In the creative process resonance is felt and coherence develops through translation between modalities, such as the language of visual perception and the language of words. Resonance, then, is a feeling that signals coherence between myself and the world I am writing about. The development of coherence implies growing understanding of myself and my experience; that is, with coherence, learning has occurred. In a complex and changing world, achieving coherence requires access to modalities of perception and of expression, and the mental flexibility to shift back and forth between those modalities and between the levels of control they represent.

*Mental control* waxes and wanes. Flexibly shifting among moments and component abilities of the creative process, from visual perception to imagination and memory, from prose writing to logic and empathy, weaves coherence between the person and the world. Sometimes such flexibility involves a high degree of control and sometimes less. When an artist switches between, say, observing a landscape and beginning to paint it, he may feel a high degree of control: the shift from observation, to mixing a color, to applying it may appear to him a series of conscious decisions. At other times shifts may seem to happen automatically, without conscious direction. For example, when I emerge from reverie and generate words that I mentally "heard" while daydreaming the switch may seem automatic, not controlled or willed.

Most important for our purposes is the *perception* of mental control and the feeling of effort involved in such *perceived control* (Wegner, 2002). Perception of control allows us to have a clear sense of *authorship* of ideas and actions. The sense of authorship of our efforts enhances the sense of self (Wegner, 2002), that when our efforts work, *we have been effective.*

The concept of *mental flexibility* arose in the neuropsychological assessment of brain-injured persons, where it is typically defined as the shifting of mental sets, also called task switching in cognitive psychology (e.g., Gilbert & Shallice, 2002; Rubinstein, Meyer, & Evans, 2001). The inability to shift set has been studied extensively and is characterized by concrete, unimaginative, perseverative thinking (Goldstein, 1944; cited in Walsh, 1994). Many forms of brain injury blunt mental flexibility and interfere with everyday functioning, especially with executive mental functions unique to humans.

Considering brain injury helps us further understand the concept of *coherence*. In many cases people with brain injuries have great difficulty perceiving, comprehending, and behaving in ways appropriate to the current context (e.g., see Damasio, 1994). This is a problem with coherence more basic than stunted creativity; it involves difficulty shifting attention among features of the world, between the self and what is outside the body, and between levels of control or of abstraction. There is a difficulty *reading* the world, so responses are awkward at best, resulting in lack of coherence between the self and the social world and its requirements. Awkward or inappropriate responses lead to unsatisfying responses from others, eroding feelings of self-efficacy.

For healthy people in relatively unchallenging circumstances, coherence between person and world may seem effortless. When we are thus fortunate, we shift sets and read the world adequately, we understand what is going on, and we fit in well enough to meet our needs. The creative process can provide opportunities for finer-grained, more complex coherence that adds new insights to what we may be conscious of at any given moment. The creative process articulates in words, paint, or other media, what was formerly inarticulate, yet what formed part of our *felt relationship*, or embeddedness in the world. To the extent that relationship is problematic or conflictual, the creative process has the potential to reduce stress and enhance coherence. For hospital patients creating can provide a welcome opportunity to reflect and to achieve a greater measure of peace with their circumstances.

## Coherence and the Brain

The whole brain is involved in developing and maintaining coherence. Nonetheless, just as our ongoing experience can be discussed in terms of separable functions—verbal memory, visual attention, and so on—some areas and networks of the brain are more involved in the processing of one function than another. Our lived experience is based on communication between those brain areas and a blending of those functions. *Structure-function relationships* are correlations between those features of anatomy and those functions of the mind, and they serve as handy guides to help us understand how the brain contributes to subjective states, including creativity. In this section we will consider three broad relationships between structure and function:

1. the anterior (front) versus posterior (back) of the cerebrum, which corresponds broadly to action versus perception
2. cortical versus subcortical brain regions, which corresponds to more versus less conscious control of mental processing
3. the right versus left cerebral hemispheres, which corresponds to a wider versus narrower focus of attention

### Anterior Versus Posterior Cerebrum

Broadly construed, the anterior third of the cerebrum (which contains the frontal lobes) specializes in action, and the region posterior to the frontal lobes, in perception. Perceptual processes—visual, auditory, tactile, and somatosensory perception, for example—are relatively receptive rather than active mental states. The primary brain areas for perceptual processing are all located "behind" the frontal lobes in the temporal, parietal, and occipital lobes. In addition, multisensory processing is also located posteriorly. An example is spatial processing that combines other senses to form perception of ourselves in relation to objects in the environment, and of objects in relation to each other. These perceptual, receptive functions also imply less obvious mental control (although unconscious control operates to maintain stability of perception; Powers, 1973). Of course there are close connections between posterior and anterior brain areas, supporting functional connections between perception and action, which is a continuous part of our waking experience.

By action we mean a wide range of functions united by the fact that they act on the world. Some actions affect the world directly, some indirectly, and their degree of directness also correlates with cerebral locations. Direct actions involve the precentral gyrus, the posterior-most strip of the frontal lobes that runs from the apex of the head to just in front of the top of the ears. An example of a direct action is hitting a tennis ball. It directly affects the ball itself, the space through which the ball moves, and anything in its way. Indirect actions involve prefrontal regions of the frontal lobes, which are anterior to the precentral gyrus. Indirect actions involve preparation for direct action—getting ready to hit the ball—but also what we know and how we interpret the world. For example, knowing that it may be advantageous to hit to an opponent's backhand is an abstract, preparatory form of action that guides placement of the shot. In addition to direct and indirect action on the world outside the body, the frontal lobes are also involved in controlling our own mental functioning. Think of the control and flexibility involved in shifting attention, for example, between the ball, the net, the position of the opponent's racquet, his posture, and so forth. The past 20 years has seen an explosion of interest in the frontal lobes, as researchers have employed increasingly sophisticated experimental designs and imaging technologies (e.g., Stuss & Knight, 2002).

### Cortical versus Subcortical Brain Regions

Until you become good enough at tennis for attention to become more global and action more automatic, massive mental control and widespread frontal *cortical* activation accompanies the action of simply getting the ball over the net. The cerebral *cortex* is the so-called grey matter, the outermost "skin" of the cerebrum that contains many billions of brain cells, or *neurons,* that communicate with each other and with neurons in other parts of the brain and spinal cord. As one gains expertise, and mental control is more unconscious, brain activation becomes increasingly *subcortical,* that is neurons deep within the brain, below the cortex, become more active. With recruitment of subcortical neurons, you get the ball over the net with less effort, almost without thinking. That is, with increasing expertise much preparation for action happens outside the focus of attention, including planning, coordinating, sequencing, and abstracting. So, mental control also varies from the brain's surface to its depths—from the grey matter of the cerebral cortex to subcortical nuclei, such as the basal ganglia, that automatically generate patterns of movement.

Shifting from moments of thought that are active to receptive, less controlled to more controlled and back again is central to the creative process. The creative process is thus a weaving together of the objective with the subjective. To accomplish this blend requires shifts of attention, joining of impressions, and monitoring of results as well as relaxed receptivity to what is given in the environment and what comes to mind from past impressions. Awareness of this mix of functions, and what it feels like to shift between them, increases control of the creative process and of opportunities for self-expression. For hospital patients, by putting creativity on the agenda, AIH practice does more than create a temporary diversion from the patient's problems. It also has the potential to develop lasting mental flexibility and self-awareness, and improved coping and adjustment.

### Left versus Right Cerebral Hemispheres

Like variations in action and in mental control, the creative process has moments that vary in how wide or narrow the *focus of attention* might be. For example, the artist is concerned with both the features of a face, painted at close range with a fine brush, and with the overall pattern of the face—how it appears when she steps back to evaluate the effect of the last brushstroke. She is also concerned with the face as a detail of the overall canvas: perhaps the face is part of a crowded scene; perhaps there are other faces. Furthermore, a group of faces can be seen as a detail of the painting as a whole, and also as a whole unto itself. Switching back and forth between narrower and broader perceptions of the work is fundamental to execution and evaluation (e.g., Arnheim, 1962/2006). And, of course, analogies can be drawn to other visual and plastic arts, to music, writing, and even to problem solving in math or science.

Wider focus correlates with activation of the right cerebral hemisphere, and narrower focus with the left. In neuropsychology this is termed "hemispheric specialization," with the left hemisphere specialized in the perception and manipulation of details and the right specialized in perception of patterns and a "feel for the big picture."

Since the 1960s and 1970s, the popular view of hemispheric specialization held that the left cerebral hemisphere was responsible for logical, analytic thinking while creativity was a function of the right hemisphere (e.g., Ornstein, 1972). Although an overgeneralization, this view was supported by a century of progress in clinical neurology and neuropsychology in which cases of stroke and brain trauma consistently demonstrated, in most people, left hemisphere dominance for speech, language, and arithmetic operations. The right hemisphere was for many years considered silent, both in the sense of nonverbal and of mysterious. Studies showing right hemisphere dominance for nonverbal visual, spatial, and musical functions added to its mystery and to its association with creativity and artistic endeavors.

While the left brain/right brain dichotomy devolved into a popular overgeneralization, in clinical science a distinction was made between *local* (left) versus *global* (right) mental processing (e.g., Delis, Kiefner, & Fridlund,1988; Lezak, Howeison, & Loring, 2004). A similarly useful dichotomy is crystallized versus fluid intelligence (Goldstein, 1944), and, more recently, established versus novel patterns of thought (Goldberg, 2005). That is, the left hemisphere with its verbal specialization can be said to represent more established, crystallized thinking insofar as established patterns of thought—information that has been learned, thoughts that have been thought before—tend to be verbally encoded. More novel juxtapositions of words—in poetry, for example—tend to recruit the right hemisphere. Presumably, the breadth of connotation and association in poetry involves right hemisphere processing, as the left is involved in the more concrete denotational function of language. The right hemisphere, with its global processing, puts the focus on fluidity and on context, in which a small shift in detail can change everything.

Hemispheric specialization involves the emotions as well as cognition. Specifically, the frontal region of the left hemisphere is specialized for emotions resulting in approach, and the right, withdrawal (Davidson, 1995). Approach and withdrawal is a basic rhythm in all of biology, from plants and paramecia to primates. In people it may be related to disordered global versus local cognitive processing seen in depression and anxiety. Global versus local processing is also a basic rhythm in perception. When the hemispheres are working together, rhythms of emotion, perception, and action contribute to coherence across the brain and between person and world.

### Insight as a Special Moment of Reduced Control and Global/Local Integration

Insight is a special case of receptivity and reduced control, with its own pattern of activation involving the hippocampus and the right hemisphere (Jung-Beeman, 2004; Luo & Niki, 2003). When insight occurs in the process of creation, often two or more ideas are connected or associated. This involves the context-oriented functioning of the right hemisphere, discussed above, and also of the hippocampus. The context orientation of the hippocampus can be seen in its specific functions. First, it is a part of the limbic network, which processes emotions and the overall "feel" of things. Second, along with the posterior right hemisphere it is involved in spatial orientation. Finally, it is central to the creation of new memories and therefore to the processing of novelty (e.g., Goldberg, 2005). When novel elements are introduced, global and local are integrated, and coherence develops. This happens in insight, for example, when a new detail is the missing piece that causes many details to coalesce into a meaningful whole.

## COHERENCE, RELAXATION, AND FLOW: ELEMENTS OF CREATIVE ENGAGEMENT

The goal of AIH practice is to reduce suffering and to promote health. But how does engagement in creative activity approach that goal? Can it be of lasting value or is it simply distracting in the moment? First of all, distraction can itself be valuable, if nothing else as relief from harsh reality, pain, or uncertainty. However, a foundation of creative activities, as we have shown, is exercise of one's abilities, development of competencies, and self-efficacy; self-efficacy promotes euthymia, which can last beyond the moment. Much as success makes an athlete feel "pumped" for the next round of play, working out a problem can prime you for the next challenge; it can even "make your day." For a hospital patient, effective self-expression can distract, can counteract loss of autonomy and challenges to identity inherent in the patient role, and can enhance coping and adjustment. But beyond the satisfaction of personal effectiveness, and even beyond euthymia, engaging in creative activities is shown to have positive effects on the brain and on health. This has been discussed for three elements of creative engagement: the relaxation response, flow, and the development of coherence.

Sometimes we create to work something out, sometimes simply to relax. But in any creative endeavor the underlying goal is to solve a problem of coherence between what we know, perceive, or feel, and what we write, paint, sing, or otherwise create. And what we create comes back to us as better understanding of the world and of ourselves. In other words, the goal of the creative process is translation from the inner to the outer world, and is what is served by developing our creative abilities. To the extent that euthymia and enhanced immune functioning result, the creative process has had a positive effect on mental and physical health.

Coherence between self and world has neuropsychological correlates in the harmonizing of action and perception, of controlled and automatic processing, and of global and local attention. Furthermore, achieving coherence, "getting it right," implies expectancy, that there is something one is looking for, that one has an internalized sense of what might be right or coherent. This search, and the intimation of an answer even before the answer is found, may account for absorption in a work both as audience and as creator (Hagendoorn, 2004).

The purpose of arts in healthcare is not to teach expertise in art. However, for persons united in their concern with illness, pain, and recovery, AIH provides a focus on creative abilities that can enhance mood, and promote coping and health.

## TOOL KIT FOR CHANGE

### Role and Perspective of the Healthcare Professional

1. The healthcare professional is a guide within the creative process, to the subjective states participants may experience. The professional's role, first and foremost, is to establish rapport with participants.
2. Next, the professional's role is to introduce participants to *moments* of the creative process, so they may begin to identify those moments in their own creative activity: that is, moments of inspiration, preparation, incubation, insight, execution, and evaluation.
3. The professional's role is also to facilitate participants developing cognitive and affective *abilities,* or *competencies* that are involved in moments of the creative process and that fulfill both expressive and problem-solving functions of creativity.
4. Finally, the professional introduces participants to the *relaxation response* and *flow* as psychophysiological indicators of creative engagement, and helps to identify as a goal of the creative process, development of harmony, or *coherence,* between person and world.

### Role and Perspective of the Participant

1. To engage with the healthcare professional in developing means of self-reflection and self-expression.
2. To be receptive to thinking about one's own creative process and to engaging in creative activities.

### Interconnection: the Global Perspective

1. This perspective seeks to reduce the mystery of the creative process by placing it in the realm of ordinary cognitive and affective abilities that are available to anyone.
2. However, this perspective seeks to honor the mystery inherent in the notion of harmony or coherence between person and world, which may be experienced and interpreted in languages of mind, body or spirit.

## REFERENCES

Adams, J. L. (1974/2001). *Conceptual blockbusting.* Cambridge, MA: Perseus Publishing.

Arnheim, R. (1962/2006). *The genesis of a painting: Picasso's Guernica.* Berkeley, CA: University of California Press.

Bandura, A. (1996). *Self-efficacy: The exercise of control.* New York: Freeman.

Benson, H. (1975). *The relaxation response* (Avon Books ed.). New York: William Morrow.

Castren, E. (2005). Is mood chemistry? *Nature Reviews Neuroscience, 6*(3), 241–246.

Czikszentmihalyi, M. (1990). *Flow: The psychology of optimal experience.* New York: HarperCollins Publishers.

Damasio, A. R. (1994). *Descartes' error.* New York: Avon Books.

Davidson, R. J. (1995). Cerebral asymmetry, emotion and affective style. In R. J. Davidson & K. Hugdahl (Eds.), *Brain asymmetry.* Cambridge, MA: MIT Press.

Delis, D. C., Kiefner, M. G., & Fridlund, A. J. (1988). Visuospatial dysfunction following unilateral brain damage: Dissociation in hierarchical and hemispatial analysis. *Journal of Clinical Neuropsychology, 10,* 421–431.

Diamond, M. C. (1978). The aging brain: some enlightening and optimistic results. *American Scientist, 66,* 66–71.

Elbow, P. (1973). *Writing without teachers.* New York: Oxford University Press.

Evans, J. E. (1992). Language and the body: communication and identity formation in choreography. In G. C. Rosenwald & R. L. Ochberg (Eds.), *Storied lives* (pp. 95–107). New Haven, CT: Yale University Press.

Gilbert, S. J., & Shallice, T. (2002). Task switching: a PDP model. *Cognitive Psychology, 44,* 297–337.

Goldberg, E. (2005). *The wisdom paradox.* New York: Gotham Books.

Goldstein, K. (1944). Mental changes due to frontal lobe damage. *Journal of Psychology, 17,* 187–208.

Gross, C. G. (2000). Neurogenesis and the adult brain: death of a dogma. *Nature Reviews Neuroscience, 1,* 67–73.

Hadamard, J. (1945/1954). *The psychology of invention in the mathematical field.* New York: Dover.

Hagendoorn, I. (2004). Some speculative hypotheses about the nature and perception of dance and choreography. *Journal of Consciousness Studies, 11*(3/4), 79–110.

Haidt, J., & Rodin, J. (1999). Control and efficacy as interdisciplinary bridges. *Review of General Psychology, 3,* 317–337.

Krech, D., Rosenzweig, M. R., & Bennett, E. L. (1962). Relations between brain chemistry and problem solving among rats raised in enriched and impoverished environments. *Journal of Comparative and Physiological Psychology, 55,* 801–807.

Lezak, M. D., Howieson, D. B., & Loring, D. W. (2004). *Neuropsychological assessment* (4th ed.). New York: Oxford University Press.

Luo, J., & Niki, K. (2003). Function of hippocampus in "insight" of problem solving. *Hippocampus, 13,* 316–323.

Marx, J. (2005). Preventing Alzheimer's: A lifelong commitment? *Science, 309,* 864–866.

Mesulam, M.-M. (1985). *Principles of behavioral neurology.* Philadelphia: F. A. Davis.

Ornstein, R. (1972). *The psychology of consciousness.* San Francisco, CA: W. H. Freeman.

Pennebaker, J. W., & Beall, S. K. (1986). Confronting a traumatic event: Toward an understanding of inhibition and disease. *Journal of Abnormal Psychology, 95,* 274–281.

Pennebaker, J. W., & Seagal, J. D. (1999). Forming a story: The health benefits of narrative. *Journal of Clinical Psychology, 55*(10), 1243–1254.

Powers, W. T. (1973). *Behavior: The control of perception.* Chicago: Aldine.

Pribram, K. H. (1977). *Languages of the brain.* Monterey, CA: Brooks/Cole.

Reddy, W. M. (2001). *The navigation of feeling: A framework for the history of emotions.* New York: Cambridge University Press.

Rubinstein, J., Meyer, D. E., & Evans, J. E. (2001). Executive control of cognitive processes in task switching. *Journal of Experimental Psychology: Human Perception and Performance, 27,* 763–797.

Runco, M. A. (2005). Motivation, competence, and creativity. In A. J. Elliot & C. S. Dweck (Ed.), *Handbook of Competence and Motivation* (pp. 609–623). New York: The Guilford Press.

Segal, Z. V., Williams, J. M. G., & Teasdale, J. D. (2002). *Mindfulness-based cognitive therapy for depression.* New York: Guilford Press.

Segerstrom, S. C., & Miller, G. E. (2004). Psychological stress and the human immune system: a meta-analytic study of 30 years of inquiry. *Psychological Bulletin, 130*(4), 601–630.

Seifert, C. M., Meyer, D. E., Davidson, N., Patalano, A. L., & Yaniv, I. (1995). Demystification of cognitive insight: Opportunistic assimilation and the prepared-mind perspective. In R. J. Sternberg, & J. E. Davidson (Eds.), *The nature of insight* (pp. 65–124). Cambridge, MA: MIT Press.

Skinner, B. F. (1995). *Perceived control, motivation and coping.* Thousand Oaks, CA: Sage.

Smyth, J. M. (1998). Written emotional expression: Effect sizes, outcome types, and moderating variables. *Journal of Consulting and Clinical Psychology, 66*(1), 174–184.

Sontag, S. (1965). On style. In *Against interpretation and other essays* (Picador USA ed., pp. 15–36). New York: Farrar, Straus and Giroux.

Sternberg, R. J. (2005). Intelligence, competence, and expertise. In A. J. Elliot & C. S. Dweck (Eds.), *Handbook of competence and motivation* (pp. 15–30). New York: Guilford Press.

Stuss, D. T., & Knight, R. T. (Eds.). (2002). *Principles of frontal lobe function.* New York: Oxford University Press.

Thagard, P. (2000). *Coherence in thought and action.* Cambridge, MA: MIT Press.

Tharp, T. (2003). *The creative habit.* New York: Simon & Schuster.

Wallas, G. (1926). *The art of thought.* New York: Harcourt, Brace.

Walsh, K. (1994). *Neuropsychology: A clinical approach.* New York: Churchill Livingstone.

Wegner, D. M. (2002). *The illusion of conscious will.* Cambridge, MA: The MIT Press.

Chapter Six

# THEORY AND PRACTICES OF ART THERAPIES: WHOLE PERSON INTEGRATIVE APPROACHES TO HEALTHCARE

*Ilene A. Serlin, PhD, ADTR*

This chapter introduces the creative and expressive arts therapies from an existential perspective that sees the creative act as a courageous affirmation of life in face of the void or death. From this affirmation of life comes the healing medicine of creation. The need to create, communicate, create coherence, and symbolize is a basic human need.

> Thus the artists—in which term I hereafter include the poets, musicians, dramatists, plastic artists, well as saints—are a "dew" line, to use McLuhan's phrase; they give us a "distinct early warning" of what is happening to our culture....The artists thus express the spiritual meaning of their culture.
>
> —May (1975, p. 17)

In a reflection on "The Place of Beauty in Therapy and the Arts," Swiss expressive arts therapist Paolo Knill (1995) reminds us that creative acts or works of art "touch the depth of soul, evoke imagination, engage emotions and serene thought." Art is crucial for the healing journey because it touches and also expresses the whole complex human person, including levels of mind, body, and spirit. In Jung's (1966) essay "On the Relation of Analytical Psychology to Poetry," Jung proposed that the origin of a work of art lies not in the personal unconscious of the artist, but in the collective unconscious, which is the "common heritage of mankind" (p. 80). The humanities connect people across different cultures and traditions to common challenges of the human condition.

The arts heal in a number of important ways. First, the arts can provide a diagnostic image of culture and the individual, and provide healing for mental and physical health. Aristotle observed that there are two instincts basic to human nature: (1) imitation; and (2) harmony and rhythm, and "even dancing imitates character, emotion, and action, by rhythmical movement" (Aristotle, 1961, p. 50). Traditional healers were artists, and many contemporary healing practices draw on aspects of the arts. Studies show that the artistic endeavor may reduce stress and health complaints, improve immune function, provide both physical and psychological benefits, and even help people live longer (Kiecolt-Glaser et al., 2002; Pennebaker, 1990).

Art also provides access to multiple modes of intelligence (Gardner, 1993), thinking, communicating, and problem solving. Arts expand psychological horizons. Clinical studies with mood disorders and creativity indicate how different cognitive styles, modes of representation, and even processes considered in some contexts to be deviant can open us up to new creative possibilities and untapped powers of the human spirit. For example, outsider art, a collector's item, is the expression of those who have been diagnosed as mentally or emotionally ill and who are often on the outside of society.

Art connects us to the imagination (McNiff, 1992), and bridges the conscious and the unconscious. It takes us into expanded states of consciousness, helping us understand our waking reality, mindfulness, altered states, and dreamtime. And, in many cultures, art takes us to the sacred.

- *Arts promote health.* Traditional healers were artists, and contemporary healing practices draw on the arts. Studies show that the artistic endeavor may reduce stress and health complaints, improve immune function, provide both physical and psychological benefits, and even help people live longer. Work by Pennebaker, Kiecolt-Glaser, and others support the many healthy functions of emotional disclosure and the relationship of different modes of expression to brain function.

- *Art provides access to multiple modes of intelligence* (Gardner, 1982): thinking, communicating, and problem-solving. Aesthetic inquiry is a way of knowing through images, similar in structure to philosophical, psychological, or spiritual inquiry. Art is also a form of expression, and both verbal and nonverbal communication express outwardly the indwelling of images. It is holistic, drawing on multiple modes of inquiry and learning (Arnheim, 1969), and research (McNiff, 1998).

- *Arts expand psychological horizons.* Work with mood disorders and creativity indicate how different cognitive styles, modes of representation, and even processes that are considered to be deviant in some contexts can open us up to new creative possibilities and untapped powers of the human spirit.

- *Art expands consciousness.* Art takes us into expanded states of consciousness, helping us understand our waking reality, mindfulness, altered states, and dreamtime (Schlitz, Amorok, & Micozzi, 2005).

- *Art is social.* It reflects cultural differences, and it creates community. It reflects social change, and it effects social change. Art is political, and can be used in conflict resolution and in community rituals (Imber/Black, 1992).

## THE EXPRESSIVE AND CREATIVE ARTS THERAPIES

In this section, we will define the arts therapies and take a look at some of the professions created around the arts in therapy. Should you want additional information, please contact one of the listed organizations for follow-up.

The expressive and the creative arts therapies have healing as their primary objective, while the arts are the modality of healing. Expressive and creative arts therapies have both general organizations and theoretical approaches, and the specific modalities of art, music, dance, poetry, drama, and psychodrama each have their own associations and practices. Some expressive arts therapists believe that the expressive therapist should be trained in all modalities and that effective therapy requires an ability to use a variety of modalities to follow and deepen psychological images (see Knill, Barbra, & Fuchs, 1995; Robbins, 1994), while other arts therapists believe that each art form is a discipline that has its own knowledge base and requires years of practice. The earliest organizations and training programs represented one discipline, such as the Art Therapy Association. Graduates of these programs and members of these associations are called "art therapists" and they are certified in art therapy. Other organizations, such as the International Expressive Arts Therapy Association (IAETA), combine all the arts together. Graduates of this program are called "expressive arts therapists" and they are certified by the IAETA.

The creative arts therapies also come in a variety of theoretical and philosophical perspectives, and those will be represented in this volume. For example, a psychodynamic model for the creative arts therapies is outlined by David Read Johnson (1998) as a combination of psychoanalytic theory, developmental psychology, and object relations theory. In this model, inner states are externalized through the arts media; conflicts are transformed creatively and then reintegrated into the client's experience. Some arts therapists' decisions about how to practice are based on clinical and theoretical considerations, while others' decisions are based on political considerations (for example, the creative arts therapists work together in some states to lobby for hospital-based positions; see the National Coalition of Creative Arts Therapies Associations, 2004b). While all traditions have merit, the clinician learning about the expressive and creative arts therapies should be familiar with the broad spectrum of theoretical perspectives and be able to situate each art approach within that spectrum.

In *Expressive Therapies,* Malchiodi (2005) estimates that 30,000 individuals in the United States have been formally trained at the graduate level in expressive therapies. She defines "expressive therapies" as the "therapeutic use of the arts and play with children, adolescents, adults, families, and groups" (p. xiv). Noting that individuals have different expressive styles such as visual or auditory, Malchiodi suggests that therapists' communication can be enhanced by reaching these clients with an expanded repertoire of different styles and with a combination of verbal and nonverbal expression. Although research in the expressive arts therapies is needed, there is already a body of literature on the use of expressive therapies for assessment of individuals, capacities, and psychological, psychosocial, and cognitive skills (Feder & Feder, 1998). In addition, the arts therapies are generating their own forms of research that work specifically with imagery and the creative process (Hervey, 2000; McNiff, 1998). The use of the arts in a therapeutic context has roots in the early 1900s as music therapy reached veterans of World War I, and Moreno (1923) used enactment to work through their emotional issues. Art was also used to understand children's drawings (Goodenough, 1926) and in sand trays (Lowenfeld, 1969). After World War II, the arts began to be used with patients who had severe mental illness in psychiatric hospitals like the Menninger Clinic and St. Elizabeth's Hospital. Professional organizations were established with training guidelines, standards, and ethics. Recently, the expressive arts have also been used successfully with people with primarily medical issues. Other organizations called *arts medicine* (Pratt & Tokuda, 1997) focus on an international application of the arts in medicine, while some bring the arts into the community (Kaye & Blee, 1997), and others bring artists from the community to patients' bedsides (Graham-Pole, 2000). Finally, a recent trend shows other expressive arts therapists working within the new field of alternative and complementary medicine, bringing the arts into integrative healthcare (Goodill, 2005; Serlin, Classen, Frances, & Angell, 2000).

## Art Therapy

One of the earliest art therapists in the United States was Margaret Naumburg (1966), who brought a psychoanalytic perspective to use art as a way of making unconscious imagery and symbols conscious. Most art therapists believe that art is a "form of visual language through which people can express thoughts and feelings that they cannot put into words," and "a way to communicate experiences that are difficult to verbalize, such as physical or sexual abuse, trauma, grief, and other complex emotional experiences" (Malchiodi, 2005, p. 17). Various theoretical approaches to art therapy include psychoanalytic, archetypal, object relations, humanistic, cognitive-behavioral, and developmental, while the American Art Therapy Association's recent survey showed that most art therapists consider themselves to be psychoanalytic (Elkins & Stovall, 2000). Theorists of *psychoanalytic art therapy* include:

1. Naumburg (1966), who believed that spontaneous drawings represent and project unconscious thoughts and feelings.
2. Kramer (2001), who proposes that art expressions sublimate anger and negative emotions.
3. Levick (1969), who suggested that art expressions identify individual defense mechanisms.
4. Arthur Robbins (1989), who brings a psychoaesthetic experience approach to depth-oriented treatment.

Other eminent art therapists are Landgarten (1991), Liebman (1990), McNiff (1981, 1986, 1988, 1992), and Wadeson (1980). Citations to their work can be found in the references section.

- *Humanistic art therapy* relies less on interpretation than on the experiential process of art making and its power as a transformative and self-actualizing force (Betensky, 1995; Garai, 2001; Silverstone, 1997). Gestalt art therapy is an action-oriented approach, and includes theorists Zinker (1978) and Rhyne (1995).
- A *developmental approach to art therapy* is used especially among those art therapists who work with children, and includes psychosexual, psychosocial, and object relations approaches, as well as stages of normal artistic development.
- A *soul perspective on art therapy* understands psyche in the classical sense to be an expression of soul. As such, it has its own language that is more closely related to art than to science. Its therapeutic assumptions are that the soul has powers of self-healing, which art can unleash (McNiff, 1992, p. 3).

Finally, art therapy is used with *children, adults, groups, and families.* As an "action-oriented modality" (Malchiodo, 2005, p. 42), art therapy provides "facilitation of individual's discovery of personal meaning for their art expressions" and "a variety of avenues for children, adults, families and groups to overcome emotional distress, reframe problems, resolve conflicts, achieve insights, change behaviors, and increase an overall sense of well-being" (Malchiodo, 2005, pp. 42–43).

## Music Therapy

Music therapy is defined as: "the prescribed use of music by a qualified person to effect positive change in psychological, physical, cognitive, or social functioning of individuals with health or educational problems" (Forinash, 2005, p. 46). It has ancient and global roots: Joseph Moreno shows how what he calls "ethnomusic therapy" has been an important part of the practices of traditional healers. Successful with post–World War II veterans, music therapy's first training program began in 1944, and in 1950 the American Music Therapy Association (AMTA) was founded. There are estimated to be 15,000 music therapists around the world (Grocke, 2002). They practice in approximately six major areas, including education, medical, healing, psychotherapeutic, recreational, and ecological (Bruscia, 1998). Their approaches range through psychodynamic (Benenzon music therapy), behavioral, biomedical, humanistic, and transpersonal (Nordoff-Robbins music therapy and Bonny method). Their methods include improvisation, recreative experiences, composition experiences, and receptive experiences, and they can practice as auxiliary therapists, or augmentative, intensive, and primary therapists (Alvin, 1975; Bruscia, 1998; Hodges, 1996; Levin, 1969). Major schools of music therapy are:

- *Behavioral music therapy*—uses music to change behavior, using positive and differential reinforcement.
- *Developmental music therapy*—uses music to reach blocked developmental goals.
- *Music psychotherapy*—music to facilitate self-awareness, emotional expression, and healing.
- *Medical music therapy*—is used in medical settings to help patients work with the emotional issues that accompany medical treatment (Adridge, 1992, 1998; Spintge & Droh, 1996).
- *Humanistic music therapy*—uses music to bring self-actualization and personal meaning (Campbell, 1991).

## Dance/Movement Therapy

The American Dance Therapy Association defines dance therapy as: "the psychotherapeutic use of movement as a process which furthers the emotional, cognitive, physical, and social integration of the individual" (Lomen, p. 68). Dance therapists work in a variety of settings with individuals and groups to help their clients express themselves; dance therapy "encourages new behaviors and symbolically communicates hidden emotions, releases anxiety, and serves as a vehicle to integrate body, mind, and spirit" (p. 68).

Dance therapy has roots in ancient healing practices (Serlin, 1993). It became a profession in the United States through the work of a number of creative dancers who found that they could reach patients others could not by communicating nonverbally with them. Marian Chace is described as "key to the successful beginnings and development of dance therapy as a recognized and validated form of psychotherapy" (Thomas, 1994, p. 128) and her students founded the American Dance Therapy Association (Chaiklin, 1969; Dyrud, 1970; Sandel, Chaiklin, & Lohn, 1993). Early pioneers who give depth to the theory include: Trudy Schoop (Schoop, 1974), Blanche Evans (1991), Janet Adler (1996), Valerie Hunt, Judith Kestenberg (1975), Mary Whitehouse

(1986), Liljan Espenak (Espenak, 1969), Elizabeth Polk (Ederer-Schwartz, 1991), Alma Hawkins (Hawkins, 1991), and Irmgard Bartenieff and Anna Halprin (Serlin, 1996). Isadora Duncan as the archetype and "creative source of dance therapy" is discussed by Miriam Berger (Berger, 1992), and a history of the founding and development of the American Dance Therapy Association is given by Beth Kalish (1973) and Elissa White (1973). What all these approaches share is a fundamental belief that (1) health comes from an integration of mind, body, and spirit, (2) psychological and/or physical illness comes from a problem with this integration, and (3) change can come through a movement intervention.

The following are the major approaches:

- *Chace approach* (Chace, 1993): uses rhythmic bodily action to mirror clients' actions and establish a relationship.
- *Depth approach:* either Freudian or Jungian based, uses movement to reach unconscious symbols carried in the body. Modalities include: psychoanalytic (Siegel, 1995), Jungian (Chodorow, 1991), authentic movement (Adler, 2002; Whitehouse, 1986), and depth/existential (Serlin, 1977, 2000).
- *Developmental approach:* works with developmental stages in movement and helps clients work through blocks (Loman, 1998).
- *Medical Dance/Movement Therapy:* uses movement to work with people with physical or life-threatening illnesses that have a psychological component (Goodill, 2005).

Dance/movement therapy has its own assessment tools, used to interpret nonverbal behaviors. These include Laban Movement Analysis, Kestenberg's Movement Profile, Espenak's movement diagnostic tests, Davis's Movement Psychodiagnostic Inventory (see Rothstein, 1970), and Kalish-Weiss's Body Movement Scale for Autistic and Other Atypical Children. Major principles in dance therapy include: nonverbal mirroring and attunement, containment, developmental sequencing, and reexperiencing and working through of bodily held blocks and issues. Because dance/movement therapy is action-oriented and spontaneous, it is creative and works with mind, body, and spirit.

## Drama Therapy and Psychodrama

Drama therapy and psychodrama rely on an innate human sense of story, narrative, and the ability to create one's life. Drama as healing was also used in early shamanic healing practices, but it has been used as a psychotherapeutic modality in the twentieth century. The founder of psychodrama was Jacob Moreno (1889–1974), a Viennese psychiatrist who used dramatic enactment to replay problematic incidents in his patients' lives in the context of a supportive group (Moreno, 1946). Current leaders of psychodrama include Renee

Emunah (1994), David Read Johnson (1998), and Robert Landy (2005). While psychodrama therapy and drama therapy are similar, they differ in that drama therapists may work with fictional narratives and are closer to theater, while psychodrama uses the personal experiences of the protagonist as narrative. In psychodrama, the protagonists may play roles that include the psychosomatic, psychodramatic, social, and cultural. Techniques include doubling and role reversal. Finally, psychodrama and drama therapy have been very effective with children, and with victims of natural and man-made disasters (Gersie, 1997; Jennings, 1992).

## Poetry Therapy

Poetry therapy uses the language of poetry to evoke central images of the clients' existence. According to the National Coalition of Creative Arts Therapies Associations, its goals include: (1) developing an understanding of oneself and others through poetry and other forms of literature; (2) promoting creativity, self-expression, and greater self-esteem; (3) strengthening interpersonal and communication skills; (4) expressing overwhelming emotions and releasing tension; and (5) promoting change and increasing coping skills and adaptive functions (National Coalition of Creative Arts Therapies Associations, 2004a). It was established as a field by Jack Leedy, whose edited works in 1969 and 1973 gave rise to the Association for Poetry Therapy organization and the National Association for Poetry Therapy in 1981.

Poetry therapists assess the language development of the client and look for meaning in the rhythms and feelings of words, as well as in their signification (Lerner, 1994). Using words, poetry therapists help their clients discover their inner feelings and reframe their realities. They use metaphors to bring new perspectives and "maintain vitality in the face of our existential limitations of finiteness, aloneness, vulnerability, and mortality. Loss shadows every change. Nearly every poem—except some few that bespeak the philosophy of nihilism—affirms life in the face of death" (Gorelick, p. 123).

Approaches to poetry therapy include psychoanalytic, interpersonal, behavioral/cognitive, systems/metacommunication school, and humanistic/expressive (Gorelick, p. 124–125). All client populations are served, as well as a broad range of clinical issues. Poetry therapists work in major hospitals, in community settings, and in private practice. While there are formal university training programs in poetry therapy, qualified mental health professionals can study with an approved mentor in poetry therapy and work toward certification as a Registered Poetry Therapist or Certified Poetry Therapist. Stages of a poetry therapeutic process involve: recognition or absorption of the material; examination or exploration of responses; juxtaposition, or putting responses in context; and application to the self (Gorelick, 2005, p. 128). Ironically, while poetry therapy is one of the newest expressive therapies, archetypally it comes from the birth of human experience.

## Expressive Therapies

Expressive therapists believe that imagery can be expressed in any modality, and that it acquires its meaning by moving through art, movement, poetry, story, and whatever else moves the image toward understanding. The therapist is trained in a variety of modalities and how to creatively address presenting problems. Excellent training in degree programs or certificate programs can be found at Lesley University, California Institute for Integral Studies, and Tamalpa Institute. Recommended readings include *Principles and Practice of Expressive Arts Therapy* by Knill, Levine, & Levine (2005).

## CONCLUSION

The creative and expressive arts therapies are increasingly useful for mind/body health. They work effectively with groups in a wide variety of settings, and can be powerful in settings involving trauma and natural and man-made disasters. They can also be valuable to healing at the bedside, in medical clinics, and on interdisciplinary treatment teams. Arts therapists are trained to identify and build on people's innate strengths, creativity, and resourcefulness, traits skills desperately needed at this point in history.

## TOOL KIT FOR CHANGE

### Role and Perspective of the Healthcare Professional

1. The arts unite ancient healing practices and contemporary medical technology, using multiple modes of intelligence.
2. Arts can reduce stress and health complaints, improve immune function, provide both physical and psychological benefits, and even help people live longer. They can provide a diagnostic image of culture and the individual.
3. Arts therapies work effectively with groups in a wide variety of settings. They work with infants, children, adolescents, adults, and the elderly, and work with a wide range of emotional and physical challenges.

### Role and Perspective of the Participant

1. Art awakens the imagination and life force.
2. The arts therapies can address human anxieties, issues of grief and loss, and natural and man-made disasters.
3. The act of creation is a courageous affirmation of life in face of the void or death.

### Interconnection: The Global Perspective

1. The humanities connect people across different cultures and traditions to common aspects of the human condition.
2. The arts speak many languages and can communicate with many cultures.
3. The arts connect us to nature and to larger forces around us.

## REFERENCES

Abrams, Viven. (1997). [Review of the L. Silverstone book, *Art therapy the person-centered way: Art and the development of the person*]. *The Arts in Psychotherapy*, 389–390.

Adler, J. (1996). The collective body. *American Journal of Dance Therapy*, *18*(2), 81–94.

Adler, J. (2002). *Offering from the conscious body: The discipline of authentic movement.* Rochester, VT: Inner Traditions.

Aldridge, D. (1992). Two epistemologies: Music therapy and medicine in the treatment of dementia. *The Arts in Psychotherapy, 19,* 243–255.

Aldridge, D. (1998). Life as jazz: hope, meaning, and music therapy in the treatment of life-threatening illness. *Advances in Mind/Body Medicine, 14,* 271–282.

Alvin, J. (1975). *Music therapy.* New York: Basic Books.

Aristotle. (1961). *Poetics.* New York: Hill and Wang.

Arnheim, R. (1969). *Visual thinking.* Berkeley: University of California Press.

Berger, M. R. (1992). Isadora Duncan and the creative source of dance therapy. *American Journal of Dance Therapy, 14*(2), 95–105.

Betensky, M. (1995). *What do you see? Phenomenology of therapeutic art expression.* Bristol, PA: Jessica Kingsley Publishers.

Bruscia, K. (1998). *Defining music therapy.* Gilsum, NH: Barcelona.

Campbell, D. (1991). *Music physician for times to come.* Wheaton, IL: Quest Books.

Chace, M. (1993). Dance alone is not enough. In S. Sandel, S. Chaiklin, & A. Lohn (Eds.), *Foundations of dance/movement therapy: The life and work of Marian Chace* (pp. 75–97). Columbia, MD: Marian Chace Memorial Fund of the American Therapy Association.

Chaiklin, S. (1969). Dance therapy. In *American Dance Therapy Association Proceedings,* 25–31.

Chodorow, J. (1991). *Dance therapy and depth psychology: The moving imagination.* New York: Routledge.

Dyrud, J. (1970). *Marian Chace. American Dance Therapy Association Proceedings,* xiii.

Ederer-Schwartz, J. (1991). An interview with Elizabeth Polk. *American Journal of Dance Therapy, 13*(2), 81–99.

Elkins, D., & Stovall, K. (2000). American Art Therapy Association, Inc: 1998–1999 Membership Survey Report. Art Therapy. *Journal of the American Art Therapy Association, 17,* 41–46.

Emunah, R. (1994*). Acting for real: Drama therapy process technique, and performance.* New York: Brunner/Mazel.

Espenak, L. (1969). The use of dynamics as an approach to catharsis. *American Dance Therapy Association Proceedings,* 84–93.

Espenak, L. (1981). *Dance therapy.* St. Louis, MO: MMB Music, Inc.

Evans, B. (1991). The child's world: Its relation to dance pedagogy. Article 3: The link between. In R. Benov (Ed.), *The collected works by and about Blanche Evan* (pp. 57–60).

Available from the Blanche Evan Dance Foundation, 146 Fifth Avenue, San Francisco, CA 94118. (Original work published 1949)

Feder, B., & Feder, E. (1998). *The art and science of evaluation in the arts therapies: How do you know what's working?* Springfield, IL: Thomas.

Forinash, M. (2005). Music therapy. In C. Malchiodi (Ed.), *Expressive Therapies* (pp. 47–67). New York: Guilford Press.

Garai, J. (2001). A humanistic approach to art therapy. In J. Rubin (Ed.), *Approaches to art therapy* (pp. 243–253). New York: Brunner-Routledge.

Gardner, H. (1982). *Art, mind and brain: A cognitive approach to creativity.* New York: Basic Books.

Gersie, A. (1997). *Reflections on therapeutic storymaking.* Bristol, PA: Jessica Kingsley Publishers.

Goodenough, F. (1926). *Measurement of intelligence by drawings.* New York: Harcourt, Brace, & World.

Goodill, S. (2005). *An introduction to medical dance/movement therapy.* Bristol, PA: Jessica Kingsley Publishers.

Gorelick, K. (2005). Poetry therapy. In C. Malchiodi (Ed.), *Expressive Therapies* (pp. 117–140). New York: Guilford Press.

Graham-Pole, G. (2000). *Illness and the art of creative self-expression.* Oakland, CA: New Harbinger.

Grocke, D. (2002). *Opening remarks.* Tenth World Congress of Music Therapy. Oxford, United Kingdom.

Hawkins, A. (1991). Marion Chace Annual Lecture: The intuitive process as a force in change. *American Journal of Dance Therapy, 13*(2), 105–116.

Hervey, L. (2000). *Artistic inquiry in dance movement therapy: Creative alternatives for research.* Springfield, IL: Charles C. Thomas.

Hodges, D. (Ed.). (1996). *Handbook of music psychology.* St. Louis, MO: MMB Music.

Imber/Black, E., & Roberts, J. (1992). *Rituals for our times.* New York: Harper Collins.

Jennings, S. (1992). *Dramatherapy with families, groups and individuals.* Bristol, PA: Jessica Kingsley Publishers.

Johnson, D. (1998). On the therapeutic action of the creative arts therapies: The psychodynamic model. *The Arts in Psychotherapy, 25*(2), 85–90.

Jung, C. G. (1966). *On the relation of analytical psychology to poetry. The spirit in man, art and literature* (pp. 65–83). Princeton: Princeton University Press.

Kalish, B. (1973). Some thoughts on ADTA. *Proceedings of the Eighth Annual Conference of the American Dance Therapy Association: Dance therapist in dimension: Depth and diversity* (pp. 248–253) Columbia, MD: The American Dance Therapy Association.

Kiecolt-Glaser, J. K., McGuire, L., Robles, T., & Glaser, R. (2002). Psychoneuroimmunology and psychosomatic medicine: Back to the future. *Psychosomatic Medicine, 64,* 15–28.

Kestenberg, J. (1975). *Children and parents.* New York: Aronson.

Kramer, E. (2001). *Art as therapy: Collected papers.* London: Kingsley.

Knill, P., Levine, E., & Levine, S. (2005). *Principles and practice of expressive arts therapy: Toward a therapeutic aesthetics.* Philadelphia: Jessica Kingsley Publishers.

Knill, P., Barbra, H., & Fuchs, M. (1995). *Minstrels of the soul.* Toronto: Palmerston Press.

Landgarten, H. (1991). *Adult art psychotherapy.* St. Louis, MO: MMB Music.

Landy, R. (2005). Drama therapy and psychodrama. In C. Malchiodi (Ed.), *Expressive Therapies* (pp. 90–116). New York: Guilford Press..

Lerner, A. (1994). *Poetry in the therapeutic experience.* St. Louis, MO: MMB Music.

Levick, M. (1969). Art therapy. *American Dance Therapy Association Proceedings,*16–18. Fourth Annual Conference. October 31–November 2, 1969. Philadelphia, PA.

Levin, H. (1969). Music in therapy. *American Dance Therapy Association Proceedings,* 16–18.

Lewis, P. (Ed.) (1979). *Theoretical approaches in dance-movement therapy* (Vol. 1, pp. 61–85). Dubuque, IA: Kendall/Hunt.

Liebman, M. (1990). *Art therapy in practice.* Bristol, PA: Jessica Kingsley.

Loman, S. (1998). Employing a developmental model of movement patterns in dance/movement therapy with young children and their families. *American Journal of Dance Therapy, 20,*(2), 101–115.

Loman, S. (2005). Dance/movement therapy. In C. Malchiodi (Ed.), *Expressive therapies* (pp. 68–89). New York: The Guilford Press.

Lowenfield, M. (1969). *The world technique.* London: Allen & Unwin.

Malchiodo, C. (2005). *Expressive therapies.* New York: The Guildford Press.

May, R. (1975). *The courage to create.* New York: Bantam Books.

McNiff, S. (1998). *Art-Based Research.* Phil: Jessica Kingsley.

McNiff, S. (1981). *The arts and psychotherapy.* Springfield, IL: Charles C. Thomas.

McNiff, S. (1986). *Educating the creative arts therapist: A profile of the profession.* St. Louis, MO: MMB Music.

McNiff, S. (1988*). Art-based research.* Bristol, PA: Jessica Kingsley.

McNiff, S. (1992). *Art as medicine: Creating a therapy of the imagination.* Boston: Shambhala.

Moreno, J. L. (1946). *Psychodrama.* New York: Beacon House.

National Coalition of Creative Arts Therapies Associations. (2004a). *Poetry therapy.* Retrieved from www.nccata.org/poetry.html.

National Coalition of Creative Arts Therapies Associations. (2004b). *National Coalition of Creative Arts Therapies Associations* . Retrieved from www.nccata.org/.

Naumburg, M. (1966). *Dynamically-oriented art therapy: Its principles and practice.* New York: Grune & Stratton.

Pennebaker, J. W. (1990). *Opening up: The healing power of expressing emotions.* New York: The Guilford Press.

Pratt, R., & Tokuda, Y. (1997*). Arts medicine.* St. Louis, MO: MMB Music.

Robbins, A. (1989). *The psychoaesthetic experience: An approach to depth-oriented treatment.* New York: Human Sciences Press.

Robbins, A. (1994). *A multi-modal approach to creative art therapy.* Bristol, PA: Jessica Kingsley.

Rothstein, M. D. (1970). Movement characteristics of hospitalized psychiatric patients. In *American Dance Therapy Association Proceedings.*

Rhyne, J. (1995). *The Gestalt art experience.* Chicago: Magnolia Street.

Sandel, S., Chaiklin, S., & Lohn, A. (1993). *Foundations of dance/movement therapy: The life and work of Marian Chace.* Columbia, MD: Marian Chace Memorial Fund of the American Dance Therapy Association.

Schlitz, M., Amorok, T., & Micozzi, M. (2005). *Consciousness and healing: Integral approaches to mind/body medicine.* St. Louis, MO: Elsevier.

Schoop, T. (1974). *Won't you join the dance? A dancer's essay into the treatment of psychosis.* Palo Alto, CA: National Press Books.

Serlin, I. A., Classen, C., Frances, B., & Angell, K. (2000). Symposium: Support groups for women with breast cancer. *The Arts in Psychotherapy, 27*(2), 123–138.

Serlin, I. A. (1993). Root images of healing in dance therapy. *American Dance Therapy Journal, 15*(2), 65–75.

Serlin, I. A. (1996). Interview with Anna Halprin. *American Journal of Dance Therapy, 18*(2), 115–123.

Siegel, E. (1995). Psychoanalytic dance therapy: The bridge between psyche and soma. In *American Journal of Dance Therapy, 17*(2), 115–128.

Spintge, R., & Droh, R. (Eds.). (1996). *MusicMedicine.* St. Louis, MO: MMB Music.

Wadeson, H. (1980). *Art psychotherapy.* New York: John Wiley.

White, E. Q. (1973). An historical perspective of the registry. *Proceedings of the Eighth Annual Conference of the American Dance Therapy Association: Dance therapist in dimension: Depth and diversity* (pp. 253–261). *Proceedings of the Eighth Annual Conference.* Dance Therapy Association. October 18–21. Overland Park, Kansas.

Whitehouse, M. (1986). C. G. Jung and dance therapy: Two major principles. In P. Lewis (Ed.), *Theoretical approaches in dance-movement therapy* (pp. 61–85). Dubuque, IA: Kendall/Hunt.

Zinker, J. (1978). *Creative process in Gestalt therapy.* New York: Brunner/Mazel.

## RESOURCES

*American Art Therapy Association.* 1202 Allanson Road, Mundelein, IL 60060. (847) 949–6064.

*American Dance Therapy Association.* 2000 Century Plaza, Columbia, MD 21044. (410) 997–4040. http://www.adta.org, *American Journal of Dance Therapy.* New York: Human Sciences Press.

*Hospital Audiences, Inc.* 220 W. 42nd St., New York, NY 10036. http://www.hospitalaudiences.org

*International Journal of Arts Medicine.* MMB Music, Inc. (good resource for creative arts therapy materials). Contemporary Arts Building, 3526 Washington Ave., St. Louis, MO 63103–1019. Email:Mmbmusic@mmbmusic.com

*Society for the Arts in Healthcare.* 45 Lyme Rd., Suite 304, Hanover, NH 03755–1223. (603) 643–2325. HealthArts@aol.com. Publishes a newsletter listing events and resources, and sponsors a yearly interdisciplinary conference.

*Stern's Book Service.* 2004 W. Roscoe St., Chicago, IL 60618. (773) 883–5100. University of California Extension, Center for Media and Independent Learning. They carry many creative arts therapy books. Creative arts therapy videotapes for rent or purchase. 2000 Center Street, 4th Floor, Berkeley, CA 94704. (510) 642–0460.

Chapter Seven

# DANCE/MOVEMENT THERAPY FOR THE WHOLE PERSON

*Sherry Goodill, PhD, ADTR, NCC, LPC*
*and Dianne Dulicai, PhD, ADTR*

## INTRODUCTION

This chapter will acquaint the reader with dance/movement therapy (DMT) practice in clinical and wellness contexts. DMT is a therapy that considers the whole person, working towards self-integration, health, and well-being. We present elements of our profession to other clinicians who may wish to collaborate with dance/movement therapists for clinical work or research or integrate aspects of this approach into their own work with clients. Interested healthcare consumers will find information for making educated healthcare service choices for themselves. We will examine and describe dance/movement therapy within a framework informed by systems theory and focus on some of the major human systems that operate in this therapeutic approach. These systems—the movement system, the neurological and physiological systems, the family system and the social/community system—are part of the gestalt for any individual seeking wellness or clinical psychotherapy services. Clinical psychosocial assessment and interventions in dance/movement therapy address functioning in relation to all four of these systems, with varying emphases depending on the reasons for seeking therapy.

## HUMAN MOVEMENT IN A BIOPSYCHOSOCIAL AND DEVELOPMENTAL CONTEXT

We begin with an emphasis on seeing all humans in the contexts in which we are embedded. As we begin our life's journey, a sperm carrying millions of pieces of information joins a cell with its own DNA information to share. We have already begun as a system derived from both parents, influenced by genes and by the environment and culture of both contributors. Both parents have family systems reaching backwards through immediate ancestors to the origins of humankind. Each parent lives in this universe, on this planet, during this century, in a specific area of the earth, with people sharing an influencing culture. Accordingly, we begin, grow, and live within many systems—solar and social, cellular and cultural.

When we are ill, contract "dis-ease" or function poorly, it is important to remember that we all exist within systems that mutually act and react with each other—and multiple systems exist within each of us. Consider for example an ordinary stressor such as applying for a job, sitting for an exam, or speaking in public. All may produce varying degrees of anxiety to which your body may respond by increased pulse, sweating, or a dry mouth. Simply thinking about the event may have riveted your attention, initiating the brain stem functioning regulated by the limbic cortex (Vinogradova, 1969). Or perhaps on the way to the job interview you are reviewing an argument you had with a family member before leaving and your attention is interrupted continually, burdening your system with additional distraction. In these moments and phases of stress and distress, your central nervous system alerts the body through chemical signals in the form of hormones, and the system's homeostasis is changed, disrupted, by all the activity. Perhaps you have learned active ways to reduce or stabilize these changes and you begin deep breathing and thinking about details of what you want to say or remember, thereby initiating the frontal cortex again and quieting the fight-flight response. Complex interactions in the brain and body are activated in this common task. In a more disturbing example of how the micro and macro systems interact, actual brain structure and states are changed in children who live in continuous environments of trauma or extreme distress (Perry, Pollard, Blackley, Baker, & Vigilante, 1995). Thus, these children's brain-body interactions are not only a detriment to the children but are influenced by macrosystems such as state and local governments who have the responsibility for laws governing abuse and agencies assigned to help them.

Scientific theory and research have recently rendered the distinctions between brain, mind, and body increasingly diffuse (Klivington, 1997). Dance/movement therapy is perhaps a prototype for our modern understanding of the mind/body integration as it engages the mind/body connection as a reciprocal dynamic, respecting and harnessing the power of what we call the psyche to impact what we commonly consider the soma, and vice versa. Accordingly, to work with patients towards improved emotional, relational, psychological, and cognitive functioning is to facilitate good health in all spheres (Engel, 1977). In DMT, the psychosocial meets the psychomotor meets the psychophysiological.

# DANCE/MOVEMENT THERAPY: BACKGROUND, THEORY, AND PRACTICE

The use of dance as a healing art reaches back to community and ritual practices in primitive societies, when little differentiation was made between the social, religious, family, developmental, and health aspects of life (Hanna, 1995). Dance/movement therapy (DMT) emerged as a human service profession in the middle part of the twentieth century, when, following two world wars, Western societies found themselves in political turmoil and recovering from human tragedies on a global scale. The American Dance Therapy Association (ADTA) was established in 1966, and defines DMT as "the psychotherapeutic use of movement as a process which furthers the emotional, social, cognitive, and physical integration of the individual" (ADTA, 2005). This definition names integration as the primary goal of the therapy, signaling a holistic assumption about the nature of health; that is, a more integrated person is a healthier person. The founders of the ADTA cited integration of self in this definition of the work, bringing the emotional, the social, the cognitive, and the physical together in a unifying manner at a time when brain-behavior relationships were questioned and the sociocultural realm was often excluded from psychotherapy models. Their intuition about movement as related to the other aspects of human experience and functioning was innovative for its time.

## EDUCATION, CREDENTIALING, AND RESEARCH IN DANCE/MOVEMENT THERAPY

Dance/movement therapists are mental health specialists, educated at the master's level or above. DMT is one of the creative arts therapies, along with art therapy, music therapy, psychodrama, drama therapy, and poetry therapy. These experiential therapies tap the power of creative and artistic processes for facilitating the health and growth of individuals and groups. The creative arts therapy professions work together through the National Coalition of Arts Therapy Association (see www.nccata.org for more information). Currently, in the United States, there are two specialty credentials for dance/movement therapists: the entry-level DTR or Dance Therapist Registered, and the ADTR, signifying the individual is a member of the Academy of Dance Therapists Registered. In addition, many dance/movement therapists are also National Certified Counselors (a credential conferred by the National Board for Certified Counselors) and in many states, dance/movement therapists are licensed as counselors or as creative arts therapists. Over 200 working dance/movement therapists in the United States are also doctorally prepared, with degrees in related areas such as psychology, neuroscience, education, or interdisciplinary topics.

Since the 1960s DMT research has grown steadily in rigor, scale, and sophistication. DMT scholarship is published in two main journals, the *American Journal of Dance Therapy*, and *Arts in Psychotherapy: An International Journal*, as well as periodicals in complementary therapies, psychology, and counseling. The field has embraced a broad spectrum of research approaches (see Cruz & Berrol, 2004) with a research agenda that includes outcome studies on treatment efficacy, service program models and evaluation, clinical assessment strategies, and ongoing theory development.

## THE SCOPE OF PRACTICE AND RANGE OF APPLICATIONS

What distinguishes DMT among the abundant treatment options in the mental health, education, and mind/body therapy arenas is not *whom* the work serves, but *how* the therapy is conducted. The goals of psychotherapy, developmental enhancement, psychosocial support, and rehabilitation are accomplished through the integration of expressive, creative movement experiences and cognitive understanding of the self in the context of a therapeutic relationship. Movement is ubiquitous, and so the range of populations and life circumstances addressed through DMT is as broad as life itself. The modality appears to benefit nonpsychiatric or "normal" populations as well as those in treatment for behavioral and emotional problems (Cruz & Sabers, 1998; Ritter & Low, 1996). For example, dance/movement therapists work with infants and their parents (Murphy, 1998), young children (Tortora, 2005), normal school-aged children (Kornblum, 2003; Koshland & Wittaker, 2004) and those with serious learning disabilities such as autism (Erfer, 1995). Dance/movement therapists work with teens considered at risk (Duggan, 1995; Farr, 1997), adults with substance abuse disorders (Milliken, 1990), anxiety disorders (Erwin-Grabner, Goodill, Schelly, & VonNeida, 1999; Kierr, 1995), psychiatric diagnoses (Brooks and Stark, 1989; Erhardt, Hearne, & Novak, 1989), those who struggle with domestic violence (Leventhal & Chang, 1991), homelessness (Ginzberg, 1991), eating disorders (Krantz, 1999) and the debilitating sequelae of child abuse (Harvey, 1995; Mills & Daniluk, 2002; Weltman, 1986) and war torture (Gray, 2001). Dance/movement therapists work with children and adults who are coping with various medical conditions including cancer (Cohen & Walco, 1999; Dibbel-Hope, 2000; Ho, 2005; Mendelsohn, 1999; Sandel et al., 2005; Serlin, Classen, Frances, & Angell, 2000), pain conditions (Bullington, Nordemar, Nordemar, & Sjostrom-Flanagan, 2003), and other chronic health problems (Berrol, Ooi, & Katz, 1997; Goodill, 2005a, 2005b). Dance/movement therapists support those at the end of life as well, integrating DMT with palliative care (Cohen, 2004; Thompson-O'Maille & Kasayka, 2005).

## SOME THEORETICAL CONSTRUCTS THAT UNDERLIE DMT

The theory, research, and practice of DMT are an amalgam drawn from the arts and from science. One component of the amalgam is creativity—the freeing influence of creating options of behavior as well as art making.

Dance/movement therapy hypothesizes that *changes in movement can lead to changes in other behavior.* When, during the DMT process, a client tries moving differently in response to anxiety, conflict, difficult feelings, or impulses, he is learning new options for behavior. These changes may become new and healthier responses. With a very disorganized client who demonstrates fragmented movement, the therapist often introduces organization through rhythmic movement. To the extent that the better-organized movement enables the patient to function, attend to work and relationships, and move more efficiently, the movement intervention serves as an adjunct to psychoactive medication.

Important concepts underlying DMT also include insights regarding basic elements of dance as an art form, notably the phenomenon of *rhythm as an organizing factor* (Berrol, 1992; Condon, 1968) and the mobilization of body and mind (Bartenieff, 1980). Dance studies have taught us that synchronizing movement of people enhances their communication abilities and defines a group. This occurs even in everyday life. When you participate in a "wave" at your local football game, the players and you both know you are their group of supporters, part of something larger than yourself. The shared rhythmic activity brings about a sense of belonging, and the energy is infectious.

The relationship between therapist and client has long been understood to be the critical indicator of successful psychotherapy. In DMT, the relationship with the therapist provides a consistent interaction with one who is knowledgeable and is governed by ethical standards of practice. Initial rapport and the therapeutic alliance are formed through the nonverbal communication and the movement relationship (Schmais, 1974).

## INTEGRATION OF MOVEMENT AND WORDS
## IN DANCE/MOVEMENT THERAPY

To say that DMT is a nonverbal technique is inaccurate. DMT focuses primarily on the sensed, kinesthetic, and motoric, but goes beyond that. The integration of words and movement is essential to make full use of the power of movement to inform, communicate, and express. In the translation from the nondiscursive to the discursive and back again (often made through the use of metaphors, images, and sounds; Gorelick, 1989), the patient and the DMT together bring into awareness that which was buried in memories, or too difficult to discuss in verbal language alone. For the discoveries made in the creative movement state in a session to generalize into everyday life, the feelings, actions, interactions, and patterns seen and experienced in the nonverbal realm need to be discussed and actively connected to therapeutic goals and life's challenges.

## WHAT HAPPENS IN A DANCE/MOVEMENT THERAPY SESSION?

### The Structure of a DMT Session

The description to follow is commonly but not universally followed, and is drawn from works by Schmais (1981), Chaiklin and Schmais (1993), and the authors' clinical work. Individual therapists' work will vary according to therapeutic style and the needs of the clinical population or treatment setting. In addition, dance/movement therapists will almost always modify the session in response to the patients' observed needs and responses.

A DMT session begins with a warm-up: gentle stretching exercises and movement patterns that aim to mobilize body energy and help the patient or client tune in to bodily sensations in a safe way. The warm-up is holistic in focus: starting with attention to the body and building in awareness of emotional states, needs, and the interpersonal climate. During the warm-up, the therapist is observing and assessing the client's state, gathering data about movement phrases, dynamics, and the congruence of verbal and nonverbal expression. Using this information and the client or group's own intentions, the therapist progresses the session into theme development. In this middle part of the session, movement structures are offered by the therapist, or evolve more from the patients' ideas, or a combination of both. Generally, higher functioning patients are able to tolerate more ambiguity and follow the creative processes with lower levels of imposed structure and therapist input. Conversely, lower functioning patients usually need a higher degree of structure in order to be able to move authentically and purposefully in the session. Themes addressed are correlated to the treatment goals. As in the case examples below, these goals may be articulated at the movement level, or may be general behavioral objectives. The improvisational dance/movement tasks are designed to help patients creatively, even playfully, confront challenges, conflicts, losses, difficult emotions, and troubled relationships. In the movement patterns that develop, people will engage in problem solving, release tensions and try on new behaviors, and access untapped resources in themselves. Closure of a dance/movement therapy session includes a physical cool down, and guidance to reflect on the movement experiences. The therapist may direct exercises for centering and grounding, and for transitioning the mental state into a more secondary process thinking mode (Brenner, 1974).

## Clinical Methods in Dance/Movement Therapy

In clinical work, dance/movement therapists rely heavily on a few basic yet elegant techniques. The first, often known as "reflect and respond," is the deceptively simple process wherein the therapist uses his or her own moving body as a kinetic mirror of the patient's movement expression. Sandel (1993) described this process as "empathic reflection" and it is also referred to as kinesthetic empathy. In studies of nonverbal echoing and synchrony, Fraenkel (1983) found that instances of these shared behavior events between participants in counseling interactions are associated with the process of building empathy and with the successful communication of healthcare information between patients and providers (Fraenkel, 1986). In addition, Navarre (1981, 1982) reported that the sharing of similar postures by people in dyadic interviews, or postural mirroring, enables the development of rapport. Neuroscientists have recently found a scientific basis for this phenomenon. Gallese, Keysers, and Rizzolatti (2004) discovered the "mirror neuron." When we witness someone else's action, this neuron activates a network of areas that would have activated if we had actually performed the action ourselves. In building their theory towards a unifying neural hypothesis of the basis of social cognition, Gallese and colleagues state, "The human brain is endowed with structures that are active both during the first- and third- person experience of actions and emotions....By means of this activation, a bridge is created between ourselves and others" (p. 400). Specifically, the insula, anterior cingulated cortex, and basal ganglia were identified as "fundamentally motor structures involved in emotion expression and action control" (p. 401). Practical implications of findings like these are that when a dance/movement therapist reflects a movement in a group, and when patients are actively mirroring each other, we now understand that the movers and observers alike are experiencing the actions reflected. As more neurological research emerges about behavior, cognition, and emotional communication, we grow in respect for the validity of movement theory, constructed in earlier decades through experiential understanding.

When conducting a session, a dance/movement therapist leads and follows at the same time. Leading, he or she provides basic structures and guides the flow of movement from warm-up to theme development to closure phases. The therapist may actively move with the patients (Chaiklin & Schmais, 1993) or may assume the role of a "witness" to the client's movement process (Chodorow, 1991). Whether actively moving or actively witnessing, the therapist is also following: constantly observing for subtle shifts in energy, intensity, focus, facial and vocal expressions, emotion, posture, and gesture. These nuanced responses and initiations by the patient signal internal shifts and constitute opportunities for input from the therapist—opportunities to explore change.

Dance/movement therapy brings to life the concept of therapy as a process of change by using the artistic method of improvisation. Improvisation is not simply making it up as one goes along. Rather, in the hands of a therapist skilled in the art and craft of movement, it is about theme and variation (Nachmanovich, 1990), leading the patient through shifting activities, emphasis, quality, and structures in response to the patient's expressive initiations. When the client becomes familiar with the tool of seeing the relationship between the "free expression" of the movement and the internal state, he/she can successfully work toward insight and other therapeutic goals.

## Group and Interactional Processes in Movement

In group DMT, patients reap the inherent benefits of group therapy, enhanced by the unique properties and healing factors conferred through shared rhythmic activity and simultaneous experiencing with others. In addition to rhythm, discussed above, these include vitality, education about the mind/body relationship, and cohesion (Schmais, 1985). The group dynamic is manifest and explored in part through the use of different spatial formations in group DMT. The circle, an oft-used formation for the warm-up and closure parts of sessions (see below) facilitates a strong group boundary, encourages cohesion, and symbolically works as the container of feelings and experiences. For example, the ancient and well-known use of circles for rituals in primitive and modern-day cultural groups makes this formation a powerful nonverbal structure for therapy (Serlin, 1993). Other spatial patterns used in social and theatrical dances such as parallel or serpentine lines, scattered pathways, pairs, and subgroup clusters frame the group's exploration of power dynamics, affiliations, and interpersonal boundaries (Schmais, 1981).

Self-touch and interpersonal touch occur in DMT. This is not a "hands-on" therapy, but in the unfolding movement sequences and expressive experiences touch is initiated spontaneously between clients in group therapy contexts, or between client and therapist in individual therapy. This is always done within ethical limits, respecting privacy and volition. Dance/movement therapists will address issues of touch in the therapeutic contract, and in group settings outline the parameters for any interpersonal touch. Inasmuch as therapy is a context for learning how to live life more fully, the inclusion and permission to use touch is a part of the educational and "practicing" function of dance/movement therapy. Self-touch, through directed self-massage and in spontaneous nonverbal expression, heightens proprioception and the sense of self as perceived through the body's primary physical boundary, the skin.

Self-expression is a central focus of DMT and can be an important release for a client in therapy. However, there are times when a therapist would not encourage self-expression—when the client needs strengthening of defenses and coping resources before releasing deeply felt or threatening feelings. During that period of treatment, the therapist can bring in more elementary theoretical tenets such as increasing a sense of grounding (Bartenieff, 1980), rhythmic movement for organization, and increasing interaction synchronous movement for increased social affiliation.

Dance/movement therapy hypothesizes that changes in movement can lead to changes in behavior. In the DMT process, clients will explore moving differently in response to anxiety, conflict, or impulses. This is a way of learning new options for behavior; changes which may then become new and more adaptive responses.

The creative process in DMT is augmented by the use of props and musical accompaniment. Props such as flowing scarves, physioballs, or large stretch-bands can stimulate exploration of new movement qualities, support the use of imagery and development of therapeutic metaphors, and provide a physical bridge between group participants who may feel isolated but also not ready for direct physical contact. Carefully chosen music can set the emotional tone for the session and provide a supportive rhythmic base. Dance/movement therapists do not always work with music, but when they do, it is usually chosen on the spot based on the therapists' assessment of patients' energies and needs.

## LABAN MOVEMENT ANALYSIS AND HOLISTIC PSYCHOSOCIAL ASSESSMENT IN DMT

What methods do dance/movement therapists use to evaluate movement behavior and how has the research on DMT assessment developed? A major contributor was Rudolph Laban, who contributed a wealth of evidence about human movement and its significance to the understanding of the individual and community. His greatest contribution to the field of DMT was twofold: his hypothesis of the relationship of movement behavior to personality characteristics and his development of a system for notating the movement behavior. His motivation was to expand the use of movement components in the theater in both dance and drama (Laban, 1950). Application to other areas such as psychotherapy and education were to be fulfilled by his protégés Marion North, Lisa Ullmann, Valerie Preston Dunlop, Irmgard Bartenieff, and others. He directed his students to observe body level material such as parts of the body moved, the stance of the body when still and in motion, the transition between one phrase of movement to another, how the gesture accompanies full body action, and the shape the body forms in action. Other researchers used these elements in studying communication research, yet Laban's original contribution was to describe not only *what* happened in the body but *how* the movement happened. For this, he discovered and described a framework for the "Effort" elements of Space (between Direct and Flexible/Indirect), Weight (between firmness or Strength and gentle Lightness), time (between sudden/ Quickness and Sustainment), and Flow (between Bound and Free) (for more on the Efforts, see Dell, 1970; North, 1972).

Bartenieff fled from Germany to the United States in 1936 and combined her training as a physical therapist and dancer to develop application of her Laban training as therapeutic movement intervention. In 1943 she was invited to become a member of the Dance Notation Bureau in New York and with Martha Davis, a psychologist, and Forrestine Paulay, an anthropologist, started the Effort/Shape department there. To that end, she developed Bartenieff Fundamentals, a set of exercises that "reawaken awareness of muscles and joints…so that you can extend your movement possibilities in both energy and expressiveness" (Bartenieff, 1980, p. 230). She was hired at Bronx State Psychiatric Hospital to explore the use of this work with patients there, resulting in numerous collaborative publications and a new acceptance of DMT (Bartenieff & Davis, 1965/1973, 1968; Davis, 1970a, 1981). Bartenieff's theory of movement intervention is grounded solidly in the movement itself. She posited that in the process of extending the quality and range of one's body movement options, the experience will extend the quality of one's functional and emotional life and enhance the experience of living (Bartenieff, 1980).

Two major studies by Davis extended Bartenieff's work to adult psychiatric patients. The first describes the history of Laban's analysis and notation of movement and how the movement patterns can be interpreted psychologically. Movement case studies of hospitalized patients and a family therapy session are included (Bartenieff & Davis, 1965). A study of a group psychotherapy session follows, introducing the use of Effort dynamics and spatial characteristics and how they reveal kinds of relatedness and movement style (Bartenieff & Davis, 1968). Davis then developed a movement diagnostic scale, the Movement Psychodiagnostic Inventory, which revealed (1) a correlation between movement "fragmentation" and multiple hospitalizations, and (2) a relationship between high phenothiazine medication and reduced mobility (Davis, 1981). These findings inform DMT assessment and treatment. The therapist may, for example, observe fragmented movement in a highly disorganized patient, and facilitate organization through rhythmic movement. Should that individual appear more organized after these interventions, the DMT will have provided an adjunct to psychoactive medication. Davis continues to develop movement assessments most recently related to nondiagnosed persons as well as work developed to identify deception through movement (Davis &

Hadicks, 1990; Davis, Walters, Vorus, & Connors, 2000). One theoretical tenet of DMT is that movement reflects personality (Schmais, 1974). Freud himself described his patient's movements as a relevant source of information though he discouraged movement initiation in the patient (Freud, 1938). Today this concept is well accepted and in some cases exploited and simplified. Neuroscience advances allow us to understand more fully how the state of being, cognitive functioning, and emotional discharge are displayed in the movement behavior of us all.

North remained in England continuing and expanding Laban's research and testing his hypothesis about the association between movement and personality with two major studies: one with infants through five years (North, 1974) and the other with primary school children (North, 1972). Both of North's research projects used the indices developed by Laban and the 1972 study tested hypotheses correlating the movement behavior with Children's Apperception Tests (CAT), Stanford Benet IQ test, the educational psychologist report, Scale B of the test for maladjustment (Maudsley Hospital, London), and the classroom teacher's report (see Table 1). This study drew from 26 children whose parents gave permission for participation. An example of the correlations using information about one child is shown below.

Of a class of 26 children, 12 were randomly chosen to participate in the study, 6 boys and 6 girls. Participants were drawn from an underprivileged neighborhood. One child tested with a low IQ score. This study moved the hypothesis Laban presented closer to empirical evidence. Since North's study, hundreds of others have tested the validity of Laban's framework in numerous investigations (e.g., Dulicai, 1977, 1995). Results from North's 1974 study with infants, some of whom were followed to adulthood, will appear in a forthcoming publication, presently in progress.

Judith Kestenberg, another movement researcher and psychoanalyst, set out the theory that congenital motor rhythms observable in early infancy express normal developmental, psychosexual drives, and that they remain consistent

**Table 1.**
**Case 1: 8 Years, 3 Months; IQ: 114; Scale B Score: 15 (with High Neurotic Tendencies)**

| Movement report | Teacher's report | Scale B |
|---|---|---|
| Because of her lack of intuitive perception, her emotional insecurity, and her lack of rhythmical adaptablity, she has no confidence, sensitivity, or awareness to make easy relationships. | Generally cooperative with other children of same age and with those in authority. She avoids older children. Not popular, but not particularly shy. | Does not fight with other children. Is not much liked by other children. Does things alone. Does not bully other children. Does not destroy property of others. |

*Source:* Adapted from North (1972).

over time. Kestenberg (1975) postulated that the early motor rhythms reflect drive discharge to forms of regulation observable in what is termed the Flow of Tension. The kind of Flow patterns, and how they vary in intensity and duration, are correlated with various affects. The observed patterns and constructs of Tension Flow and Shape Flow have become the focus of numerous studies by Kestenberg and her colleagues. Kestenberg's daughter Janet Kestenberg Amighi, with colleagues Susan Loman, Penny Lewis, and K. Mark Sossin, published a comprehensive description of the Kestenberg Movement Profile (KMP; Amighi, Loman, Lewis, & Sossin, 1999). In their volume, major components of this developmentally sensitive assessment, which uses both Laban Movement Analysis (LMA) and tension flow rhythm writing, are presented clearly and with clinically relevant psychological, cognitive, and emotional correlates.

Parallel to this development, nonverbal communication research grew within the psychological and social sciences disciplines. Two major contributors, Ray Birdwhistell and Albert Scheflen, individually and jointly produced nonverbal research projects on movement and communication in individuals, families, and groups. The concept that nonverbal behavior was a major means of communication in humans as well as animals was new during the early 1970s. In addition they were able to define the units of behavior and correlate them with sociocultural norms as well as individual motivation (Birdwhistell, 1961, 1973; Scheflen, 1963, 1964; Scheflen & Scheflen, 1972). Another major contributor was William Condon, who presented his research findings on the relationship of language, rhythm, self-synchrony, and interpersonal synchrony to DMT practice (Condon, 1968).

From the initial work of Laban in the 1950s continuing through the groundwork developed by his students described here to young movement researchers today, we continue to refine and expand new insights drawn from movement studies.

## CLINICAL EXAMPLES

Three clinical examples from a range of populations and contexts are presented to illustrate how DMT assessment and/or treatment can address the "whole person" through integration of physical, social, cognitive, and emotional aspects. These brief narratives are derived from our clinical experience. Examples 1 and 2 are case histories from Dianne Dulicai's practice, and are narrated in the first person by this author (DD), while Example 3 is narrated by Sherry Goodill (SG). Movement descriptors drawn from the LMA system are capitalized. The identities of clients have been disguised, including place and time.

## Example 1: A Young Girl with Academic and Behavioral Problems

Earlier, the North research project with school children was presented. Using the same method for movement evaluation as used in this project, I (DD) assessed a young girl whose teacher had referred her due to her disruptive behavior and flagging grades. Her parents agreed and cooperated fully with the teacher's recommendations. The girl, who I will call Sally, had not received any therapeutic intervention previous to this time. Sally was an attractive and energetic 8-year-old. I observed her in a desk task at school, on the playground, and at home making cookies with her mother.

At her desk task, she directly focused on her work for a brief period in which she handled her paper with a Sustained, Light, sensitive touch, and gave a glimpse of good future development. After a few minutes, she lost her focus; she began to use Strong Weight, Free Flow, and overly large movements sufficient to tear the paper. Quickly she displayed anger and frustration and on the way to throw away her paper hit another child with the crumpled paper. Just as quickly, that movement dispersed. When not in distress, Sally used complex gestures that remained focused throughout, suggesting complex mental action. On the playground, Sally showed great pleasure in large motor activity and her disruptive behavior was less prominent. Though she enjoyed the large motor movement, they way she shaped the movement was more appropriate to a younger child and produced a lack of stability in her phrase completion. When she lost control, she used more infantile behavior such as falling to the ground and increasing muscle restraint to the point of shallow breathing, much like when a 3-year-old's temper tantrum is subsiding.

The assessment generated a twofold set of goals for the first session in order to support her strengths and offer other movement options when she was frustrated.

### Strengths

1. Use of Sustained, sensitive movement and Direct clear focus
2. Joy of large physical movement
3. Complex use of space

### Limitations

1. Poor Shaping of large spatial movements
2. Poor coping mechanisms for dealing with frustration and anger

And what does this look like in the DMT session? If you are an athlete or have taken an exercise class, it looks very much the same. The warm-up that mobilizes and warms the body for action gave me a way to check my assessment observations. Sally took to the movement activity with pleasure and wanted to show me some favorite movements from her movement classes.

The next part of the session is usually the part of the session in which the participant follows or leads movement of choice. This gave me the opportunity to begin the movement conversation with Sally. I could use, in my own body, some of the movement qualities identified as strengths, such as Sustained, very Light, Directly focused gestures, and watch her response. She could use a big strong movement that she liked and I could move with her and take over at the apex of the movement, introducing a new way to end it, all the time observing how she responds to my initiation. Always the session ends with closure: winding down, lowering the activity level and emotional quality so as to return to class.

At about the fourth week of seeing Sally one hour weekly, during the middle part of the session, Sally could not contain her Strong, Free Flow movement nor close it with stability. Rather, she fell to the floor. While we were on the floor, she explained that she lost control during school the previous day and had to have a "time out." This gave us the opportunity to talk about what she felt when she lost control at school—what she was feeling right before it started. Sally told me about how she disliked being the "youngest one of all." "I'm as smart as they are—smarter," she complained. I discovered that "they" represented not only her schoolmates, but more importantly, her half sister. Her self-awareness was improving and she was starting to put some of her feelings into words.

With only three months remaining in the school year, the rest of the work with Sally moved quickly and successfully. We found new more appropriate ways to express her feelings of frustration. She asked for and received a try in an advanced arithmetic class, rewarding and challenging her cognitive potential. More important, she gained the confidence to ask for things she thought she deserved. She auditioned for the beginning tennis team and was rewarded with acceptance. Changes in her behavior brought better relationships with her peers and teachers and her parents reported improvement in the relationship with her half sister.

Obviously, this therapeutic outcome is rewarding for the child and for a therapist, though it isn't often accomplished quite so readily with children who have difficulty changing behavior. All therapeutic challenges are not this easily resolved, but this case gives the reader a beginning look at how DMT can be used and how changes made initially in the DMT session generalize to other areas of functioning in the patient's life.

### Example 2: Case of Young Adult Man in Individual Movement Psychotherapy

Sam was a student in medical school, and it is important to understand the larger systems impacting his life. His father was the youngest of five siblings caught in Germany prior to World War II and the only one to survive. His mother, also from Germany, was an only child of parents who were both physicians. She came to the United States with an aunt after being hidden in a home in Brussels but left her ailing parents behind. Both parents had issues with abandonment, guilt, and loss, and had great expectations of their only son. As a young boy, Sam had met many of those expectations—good grades, good social skills, and respectful and loving ways with his parents. His first year at medical school was stressful and Sam didn't cope with stress well. In his early years he suffered from rashes and stomach problems during periods of stress and would withdraw into periods of isolation. As his first-year exams came close, Sam became more and more withdrawn, finally missing classes. His roommate later reported being concerned about Sam's halfhearted discussion of suicide. Sam went to the hospital clinic and was hospitalized with depression. The admitting physician had referred Sam to me (DD) for part of his treatment.

I saw Sam each day for the first three days, a schedule that allowed us to establish a relationship and permitted me to assess his movement characteristics and acquaint myself with his family history. This time also gave Sam the time to acquaint himself with what the body revealed and become aware of his nonverbal communication. During his fourth session, I asked about his first visit with his parents since coming to the clinic. His torso sank into the chair, his head dropped to his chest, and he said it was embarrassing, particularly the way his Dad felt. He started to explain but I quickly interrupted and asked him to show me, not talk about it.

Sam moved to the door and simulated the short statue of his father, one hand behind him and one hand curved to simulate holding a cigar and gesturing with each word. He walked firmly and directly to me without any other focus, jabbing at me strongly while -repeatedly saying, "Disappointing." When I asked him what he had done in response, he stood silently without an answer. Then his body sank and he retreated several steps. In a moment, his intelligence and insight came to bear and a smile crossed his face. He said, "I couldn't stand up for myself—I wasn't a disappointment!" We talked about what other response he could have used rather than backing down or being disrespectful. We spent some time exploring possibilities, but Sam said he needed to think it over until our session on following day. The next day when I arrived, he greeted me with a wide wry smile telling me that he had figured it out. When I role-played his dad entering as Sam had described, Sam brought out a cigar that he had asked a staff member to get for him, and stood very erect with a wide firm stance. He began to laugh, happy to tell me that his father had laughed as well. Just responding differently had allowed Sam to try a new behavior—standing up for himself—and allowed his father to accept a humorous response to assist him in listening to his son's words.

Sam continued his DMT sessions after being released from the hospital and he returned to his medical studies. He continued to find more constructive behavioral options that suited him in familial, social, and professional interactions. He also realized that actual physical movement was a useful, effective tool for him to mobilize when he felt he was withdrawing and he included a gym appointment throughout his time in school and into his professional years.

## Example 3: A DMT Support Group for Adults with Medical Conditions

A DMT-based support group for adults with chronic medical conditions shows how symbolizing one's experience in nonverbal bodily expression can enhance self-awareness and possibly self-care. A five-week program in an urban health center integrated DMT with knowledge from health psychology and nursing to focus on adherence, self-care, and group support for people with diabetes, asthma, arthritis, and/or hypertension. Attendees also cope with stressors stemming from poverty, racism, and a somewhat chaotic urban environment. In one session, I (SG) presented the group with a collection of everyday found objects and instructed people to select an object that symbolically represents a health challenge. They were then invited to develop a movement phrase or expressive sequence that uses the object and explores or shows the experience of living with or overcoming that challenge. A woman with chronic back pain took and held a gnarled and twisted gourd. She said, "This is how I feel when the pain is bad." Then with twisting, wringing motions translated the qualities of the object, and her pain, first into gestural movement and then in full body movement expression. As the other group members and I joined her and mirrored those movements, we found an empathic understanding of her pain, and she felt less alone in her bodily felt experience.

Another woman selected an eraser, and made large slow arm circles with the eraser in hand, saying she would erase all of her pain. Continuing, and in an expression of the group support, she said she would erase the pain of all present. Indeed, she would erase all the pain felt in the world. Here, the symbolic elements of an eraser became a way to physically convey not only her own bodily felt pain, but also her sense of the group, and her sense of benevolence towards all humanity. There was a transcendent quality to the way this sequence unfolded, and with music playing in the background, the group joined her in the repeating circular movement pattern, symbolically wiping away pain together.

In summary, dance/movement therapy theory and research come alive in moments and sequences like those described just above. With careful observation and assessment of qualitative changes in movement dynamics and employing the natural power of kinesthetic empathy, dance/movement therapists bring out their patients' nonverbal and verbal expression of feelings, needs, and ideas. In the context of therapeutic movement relationships, individuals can experience new ways of knowing themselves, explore their own mind/body dynamics, and practice change in the framework of creative improvisation. The clinical examples herein suggest the range of the work and how dance/movement therapy is essentially and inherently integrative of mind and body. As a complementary psychotherapy in the healthcare spectrum, DMT offers caregivers and patients a way to access the wisdom of the body while also addressing psychosocial needs and challenges.

## TOOL KIT FOR CHANGE

### Role and Perspective of the Healthcare Professional

1. Dance/Movement Therapy is defined by the American Dance Therapy Association as "the psychotherapeutic use of movement as a process which furthers the emotional, social, cognitive and physical integration of the individual" (see www. adta.org). The American Dance Therapy Association (ADTA) credentials dance/ movement therapists with the entry-level DTR (Dance Therapist Registered), or the advanced ADTR (Academy of Dance Therapists Registered). The ADTA maintains a code of ethics and has established standards of practice (www.adta. org). In many states in the United States, dance/movement therapists are also licensed as professional counselors, mental health counselors, or creative arts therapists.
2. Dance/movement therapists work on multidisciplinary treatment teams in a wide range of clinical, educational, rehabilitation, forensic, and wellness programs and facilities. They also work as consultants and in private practice.
3. Dance/movement therapy (DMT) is founded and practiced on the essential premise of the mind and body as inextricably linked, working with the bidirectionality of the psyche-soma relationship. Rhythm, imagery, and empathic reflection of nonverbal, creative expression support the natural mind/body dynamic in the direction of wholeness, self-awareness, and more integrated functioning.

### Role and Perspective of the Patient/Client

1. Primary goals of DMT concern behavioral, emotional, and psychosocial functioning, and total health from a holistic perspective. These goals are addressed through improvised and structured dance and movement tasks and activities in the context of a supportive psychotherapy relationship. Experiences in movement are integrated and applied to life challenges and issues through verbal exchange about themes, images, symbols, and interactions.
2. Dance/movement therapists are mental health professionals and creative arts therapy specialists. They are educated at the master's level or above. Educational standards for DMT professional preparation are established and upheld through the ADTA. Dance/movement therapists have background and skills in the

movement arts, with extensive coursework in psychology-related topics, and supervised clinical training.

3. A 1998 meta-analysis of dance/movement therapy effectiveness with a variety of populations (Cruz & Sabers, 1998) yielded ES (Effect Size) estimates for DMT outcomes that are comparable to those published for other medical and psycho-therapy treatments.

### Interconnection: The Global Perspective

1. Dance/movement therapy is a global discipline, with therapists working in 22 countries. Professional organizations for dance/movement therapists exist on every continent.

## REFERENCES

Amighi, J. K., Loman, S., Lewis, P., & Sossin, K. M. (1999). *The meaning of movement: Developmental and clinical perspectives of the Kestenberg Movement Profile.* The Netherlands: Gordon and Breach Publishers.

Bartenieff, I., & Davis, M. (1965/1973). *Research approaches to movement and personality.* New York: Arno Press.

Bartenieff, I., & Davis, M. (1968). An analysis of the movement behavior within a group psychotherapy session. Paper presented at the Conference of the American Group Psychotherapy Association, New Orleans, LA.

Bartenieff, I., with D. Lewis. (1980). *Body movement: Coping with the environment.* New York: Gordon & Breach Science Publishers.

Berrol, C. F. (1992). The neurophysiologic basis of the mind-body connection in dance/movement therapy. *American Journal of Dance Therapy, 14*(1), 19–29.

Berrol, C. F., Ooi, W. L., & Katz, S. S. (1997). Dance/Movement Therapy with older adults who have sustained neurological insult: A demonstration project. *American Journal of Dance Therapy, 19*(2), 135–160.

Birdwhistell, R. L. (1961) Paralanguage: 25 years after Sapir. In H. W. Brosin (Ed.), *Lectures on experimental psychiatry.* Pittsburgh: University of Pittsburgh Press.

Birdwhistell, R. L. (1973). *Kinesics and context: Essays on body-motion communication.* Harmondsworth: Penguin Books.

Brenner, C. (1974). *An elementary textbook of psychoanalysis.* New York: Anchor Books.

Brooks, D., & Stark, A. (1989). The effect of D/MT on affect: A pilot study. *American Journal of Dance Therapy, 11*(2), 101–111.

Bullington, J., Nordemar, R., Nordemar, K., & Sjostrom-Flanagan, C. (2003). Meaning out of chaos: A way to understand chronic pain. *Scandinavian Journal of Caring Sciences, 17*(4), 325–331.

Chaiklin, S., and Schmais, C. (1993) The Chace approach to dance therapy. In S. Sandel, S. Chaiklin, & A. Lohn (Eds.), *The foundations of dance/movement therapy: The life and work of Marian Chace.* Columbia, MD: American Dance Therapy Association.

Chodorow, J. (1991). *Dance therapy and depth psychology.* New York: Routledge.

Cohen, S. O. (2004). Holistic management of symptoms. In B. S. Carter & M. Levetown (Eds.), *Palliative care for infants, children and adolescents: A practical handbook.* Baltimore: The Johns Hopkins University Press.

Cohen, S. O., & Walco, G. A. (1999). Dance/Movement Therapy for children and adolescents with cancer. *Cancer Practice, 7*(1), 34–42.

Condon, W. S. (1968). *Linguistic-kinesic research and dance therapy.* Paper presented at the Third Annual Conference of the American Dance Therapy Association, Monograph No. 3, pp. 21–42.

Cruz, R. F., & Berrol, C. F. (Eds.). (2004). *Dance/movement therapists in action: A working guide to research options.* Springfield, IL: C.C. Thomas.

Cruz, R., & Sabers, D. (1998). Dance/movement therapy is more effective than previously reported. *The Arts in Psychotherapy, 25,* 101–104.

Davis, M. (1970a). Effort/Shape analysis: Evaluation of its logic and consistency and its systematic use in research. In I. Bartenieff, M. Davis, and F. Paulay (Eds.), *Four adaptations of effort theory in research and teaching.* New York: Dance Notation Bureau.

Davis, M. (11981)). Movement characteristics of hospitalized psychiatric patients. *American Journal of Dance Therapy, 4*(1), 52–71.

Davis, M., and Hadicks, D. (1990) Nonverbal behavior and client state change during psychotherapy. *Journal of Clinical Psychology, 46*(3), 340–350.

Davis, M., Walters, S. B., Vorus, N., & Connors, B. (2000). Defensive demeanor profiles. *American Journal of Dance Therapy 22*(2), 103–121.

Dell, C. (1970). *A primer for movement description: Using Effort/Shape and supplementary concepts.* New York: Dance Notation Bureau.

Dibbel-Hope, S. (2000). The use of dance/movement therapy in psychological adaptation to breast cancer. *The Arts in Psychotherapy: An International Journal, 27*(1), 51–68.

Duggan, D. (1995). The "4's": A dance therapy program for learning disabled adolescents. In Levy, F. J. (Ed.), *Dance and other expressive art therapies; When words are not enough.* New York: Routledge.

Dulicai, D. (1977). Nonverbal assessment of family systems: A preliminary study. *The Arts in Psychotherapy: An International Journal, 4,* 55–62.

Dulicai, B. D. (1995). *Movement indicators of attention and their role as identifiers of lead exposure.* Unpublished doctoral dissertation, The Union Institute, Cincinnati, OH.

Engel, G. L. (1977). The need for a new medical model: A challenge for biomedicine. *Science, 196*(4286), 129–136.

Erfer, T. (1995) Treating children with autism in a public school system. In F. J. Levy (Ed.), *Dance and other expressive art therapies: When words are not enough.* New York: Routledge.

Erhardt, B. T., Hearne, M. B., & Novak, C. (1989). Outpatient clients' attitudes towards healing processes in dance therapy. *American Journal of Dance Therapy, 11*(1), 39–60.

Erwin-Grabner, T., Goodill, S., Schelly Hill, E., & VonNeida, K. (1999). Effectiveness of Dance/Movement Therapy on reducing test anxiety. *American Journal of Dance Therapy, 21*(1).

Farr, M. (1997). The role of dance/movement therapy in treating at-risk African American adolescents. *Arts in Psychotherapy: An International Journal, 24*(2), 183–191.

Fraenkel, D. L. (1983). The relationship of empathy in movement to synchrony, echoing, and empathy in verbal interactions. *American Journal of Dance Therapy, 6,* 31–48.

Fraenkel, D. L. (1986). *The ins and outs of medical encounters: An interactional analysis of empathy, patient satisfaction, and information exchange.* Unpublished doctoral dissertation, University of Rochester, Rochester, NY.

Freud, S. (1938). Symptomatic and chance actions. In A. A. Brill (Ed.), *The Basic Writings of Sigmund Freud* (pp. 129–140). New York: Random House (Modern Library).

Gallese, V., Keysers, C., & Rizzolatti, G. (2004). A unifying view of the basis of social cognition. In *TRENDS in Cognitive Sciences, 8*(9), 396–403.

Ginzberg, J. (1991) In search of a voice: Working with homeless men. *American Journal of Dance Therapy, 13*(1), 33–48.

Goodill, S. (2005a). *An introduction to medical dance/movement therapy: Health care in motion.* London: Jessica Kingsley.

Goodill, S. (2005b). Research letter: Dance/movement therapy for adults with cystic fibrosis: Pilot data on mood and adherence. *Alternative Therapies in Health and Medicine, 11*(1), 76–77.

Gorelick, K. (1989). Perspective: Rapprochement between the arts and psychotherapies: Metaphor the mediator. *The Arts in Psychotherapy: An International Journal, 16*(3), 149–155.

Gray, A. (2001). The body remembers: Dance/movement therapy with an adult survivor of torture. *American Journal of Dance Therapy, 23*(1), 29–43.

Hanna, J. L. (1995). The power of dance: Health and healing. *Journal of Alternative and Complementary Medicine, 1,* 323–331.

Harvey, S. (1995). Sandra: The case of an adopted sexually abused child. In F. J. Levy (Ed.), *Dance and other expressive art therapies: When words are not enough.* New York: Routledge.

Ho, R. T. H. (2005) Effects of dance movement therapy on Chinese cancer patients: A pilot study in Hong Kong. *The Arts in Psychotherapy,* 337–345.

Kestenberg, J. (1975). *Children and parents: Psychoanalytic studies in development.* New York: Jason Aronson.

Kierr, S. (1995). Treating anxiety: Four case examples. In F. J. Levy (Ed.), *Dance and other expressive art therapies: When words are not enough.* New York: Routledge.

Klivington, K. (1997). Information, energy, and mind-body medicine. *ADVANCES: The Journal of Mind-Body Health, 13*(4), 3–42.

Kornblum, R. (2003). *Disarming the playground: Violence prevention through movement and pro-social skills.* Oklahoma City: Wood & Barnes.

Koshland, L., & Wittaker, J.W.B. (2004). PEACE through dance/movement: Evaluating a violence prevention program. *American Journal of Dance Therapy, 26*(2), 69–90.

Krantz, A. M. (1999) Growing into her body: Dance/movement therapy for women with eating disorders. *American Journal of Dance Therapy, 12*(2), 81–103.

Laban, R. (1950). *The mastery of movement.* Boston: Plays, Inc.

Leventhal, F., and Chang, M. (1991) Dance/movement therapy with battered women: A paradigm of action. *American Journal of Dance Therapy, 13*(2), 131–145.

Mendelsohn, J. (1999). Dance/movement therapy for hospitalized children. *American Journal of Dance Therapy, 21*(2), 65–80.

Milliken, R. (1990). Dance/movement therapy with the substance abuser. *Arts in psychotherapy, 17*(4), 309–317.

Mills, L. J., & Daniluk, J. C. (2002). Her body speaks: The experience of dance therapy for women survivors of child sexual abuse. *Journal of Counseling & Development, 80*(Winter), 77–85.

Murphy, J. M. (1998). Nonverbal interventions with infants and their parents. *American Journal of Dance Therapy, 20*(1), 37–54.

Nachmanovich, S. (1990). *Free play: Improvisation in life and arts.* New York: Penguin Putnam.

Navarre, D. (1981). *Posture sharing in the interview dyad.* Unpublished doctoral dissertation, State University of New York, Buffalo.

Navarre, D. (1982). Posture sharing in dyadic interaction. *American Journal of Dance Therapy, 5*(1), 28–42.

North, M. (1972). *Personality assessment through movement.* London: MacDonald and Evans.

North, M. (1974). *The emergence of purposive movement patterns in babies.* Unpublished doctoral dissertation, University of London.

Perry, B. D., Pollard, R. A., Blackley, T. L., Baker, W. L., & Vigilante, D. (1995). *Childhood trauma, the neurobiology of adaptation and use-dependent development of the brain: How states become traits.* Houston, TX: Childtrauma Academy Programs, Department of Psychiatry and Behavioral Sciences, Baylor College of Medicine.

Ritter, M., & Low, K. G. (1996). Effects of dance/movement therapy: A meta-analysis. *The Arts in Psychotherapy, 23*(3), 249–260.

Sandel, S. (1993). The process of empathic reflection in dance therapy. In S. L. Sandel, S. Chaiklin, & A. Lohn (Eds.), *The foundations of dance/movement therapy: The life and work of Marian Chace.* Columbia, MD: American Dance Therapy Association.

Sandel, S. L., Judge, J. O., Landry, N., Faria, L., Ouellette, R., and Majczak, M. (2005). Dance and movement program improves quality-of-life measures in breast cancer survivors. *Cancer Nursing, 28*(4): 301–309.

Scheflen, A. E. (1963). Communication and regulation in psychotherapy. In *Psychiatry, 26,* 126–136.

Scheflen, A. E. (1964). The significance of posture in communication systems. In *Psychiatry, 27,* 316–331.

Scheflen, A., & Scheflen, A. (1972). *Body language and the social order.* Englewood Cliffs, NJ: Prentice-Hall.

Schmais, C. (1974). Dance therapy in perspective. In K. C. Mason (Ed.), *Focus on dance: Vol. 4. Dance therapy* (p. 72). Washington, DC: AAHPERD/NEA.

Schmais, C. (1981). Group development and group formation in dance therapy. *The Arts in Psychotherapy: An International Journal, 8,* 103–107.

Schmais, C. (1985). Healing processes in group dance therapy. *American Journal of Dance Therapy, 8*(1), 17–36.

Serlin, I. A. (1993). Root images of healing in dance therapy. *American Journal of Dance Therapy, 15*(2), 65–76.

Serlin, I. A., Classen, C., Frances, B., & Angell, K. (2000). Symposium: Support groups for women with breast cancer: Traditional and alternative expressive approaches. *The Arts in Psychotherapy, 27*(2), 123–138.

Thompson-O'Maille, T., & Kasayka, R. E. (2005) Touching the spirit at the end of life. *Alzheimer's Care Quarterly, 6*(1): 62–70.

Tortora, S. (2005). *The dancing dialogue: Using the communicative power of movement with young children.* Baltimore, MD: Brookes Publishing Company.

Vinogradova, O. S. (1969). Functional properties of cortical neurons. In A. R. Luria (Ed.), *Higher cortical functions in man* (3rd ed., pp. 367–385). Moscow: Moscow University Press.

Chapter Eight

# DRAMA THERAPY: PAST, PRESENT, AND FUTURE

*Robert J. Landy, PhD, RDT-BCT, LCAT*

## WHAT IS DRAMA THERAPY?

Drama therapy is an aesthetic healing form that proceeds minimally as one takes on a role and tells a story in role. Oftentimes while engaged in drama therapy, one also enacts all or part of the story alone or with a group and then reflects upon the meaning of the story. In the reflection, clients make a connection between the fiction of the story and the reality of their everyday lives.

As in the other creative arts therapies—art, bibliotherapy, dance, music, poetry, photography, and psychodrama—drama therapy is holistic and integrative, involving the body as well as the intellect, the affective and spiritual qualities of a human being as well as the social. And as with the related creative arts therapies, its uniqueness among psychotherapies is that it stems from an expressive, aesthetic process—the art of drama and theater. The clients in drama therapy work through play and through all the imaginative capacities they can draw upon to create roles and to tell and enact stories in role.

It could be argued that all forms of dramatic activity, from the play of children to the theatrical performances of professional actors, are inherently therapeutic. For example, while engaging in drama, such effects as relaxation, spontaneity, insight, and catharsis can occur. Drama therapists, however, attempt to consciously apply the natural play and drama of individuals toward the realization of specific therapeutic goals. Unlike creative parents, drama teachers, and theater directors, drama therapists are trained in both the theory and practice of several psychotherapeutic and drama therapy approaches and are able to meet the academic, clinical, and ethical standards of their profession.

## THE GOALS OF DRAMA THERAPY

The goals of drama therapy can be understood according to a framework created by this author. In *Persona and Performance*, Landy (1993) identified 84 role types common to both dramatic literature and to the drama therapy experience. The role types are organized within six domains or categories reflecting human existence. These domains provide a clear framework for understanding drama therapy goals. The first domain is the somatic, pertaining to aspects concerning the body. In realizing somatic aims, drama therapists generally consider working toward relaxation, flexibility, ability to embody roles, and to tell and enact stories through movement.

The second domain is the cognitive. Cognitive aims would include the ability to attend and respond to a dramatic stimulus and to understand the difference between a fictional role and story and their everyday counterparts. Drama therapists aim toward helping clients view their dilemmas through the lens of their fictional creations. Once the connection is made, clients are able to gain awareness through an understanding that the character of Little Red Riding Hood, for example, is a representation of themselves. At a higher level, one can follow up on that insight with a plan of action to change the real life story.

In the affective domain, that pertaining to values and emotional experience, the drama therapist aims to provide a range of roles and stories that represent a full spectrum of emotions. In experiencing the primary emotions of joy and sadness, fear and love, surprise and disgust (see Ekman, 1992), clients have the ability to expand their emotional repertoire. In terms of values, the drama therapist also attempts to introduce a variety of role types so that clients can explore their own value systems through the frame of the roles.

The social domain is the fourth and it contains several goals. The most significant is for clients to experience their behavior in relation to others in their group. Drama therapists aim toward helping clients not only to assume a role, but to engage effectively and appropriately with others in their roles. Further, in drama therapy one can explore a social or political issue through role-play and storymaking, with the aim of helping a group examine the complex dimensions of that issue. For example, the group would not only play the role of Little Red Riding Hood in relation to the seductive wolf, but that of innocents in relation to seducers.

The fifth domain is that of the spiritual. It is interesting to note that in very early forms of ritual and theater, the roles most played were those of gods and supernatural powers (see Brockett & Hildy, 2003). In playing the roles, the celebrants and actors aimed to accomplish supernatural goals—to gain better control of the forces of nature and destiny that were most out of their control. In playing spiritual roles, clients in drama therapy attempt to take on a godlike power in order to experience a sense of transcendence.

The final domain is that of the aesthetic. The aesthetic pleasures can be similar to those of the spiritual—a sense of transcendence, calm, and peacefulness. Or the aesthetic experience can be more visceral and disturbing as one plays with roles and images of feared and despised figures. Within this domain, the drama therapist aims to provide a fully holistic experience, engaging the body and mind, the feelings and spirit in order to discover a means of expression that is spontaneous and integrative.

In spite of the fact that there are several forms of drama therapy, each with an overriding goal, most drama therapists would agree that their work helps clients discover a greater sense of playfulness, spontaneity, and balance among the roles they play, the stories they tell and enact.

## POPULATIONS

Drama therapy has been around as an organized profession in the United Kingdom and the United States, among other countries, since the 1970s. In that time, drama therapists have worked with an abundance of client populations, including the physically and developmentally disabled, the homeless and incarcerated, terminally ill adults, traumatized children, war veterans, dysfunctional families, and a full range of mentally ill people representing clinical Axis I and Axis II disorders. Drama therapists have also worked with a range of mood and adjustment problems affecting the general population such as reactions to lifestyle changes, poor school performance, natural disasters, divorce, and death. In the drama therapy literature, one can read that certain forms of drama therapy seem to be best suited for particular populations. One finds, for example, the use of expressive character masks with incarcerated felons (see Bergman & Hewish, 2003). With the same population, we find reference to highly effective work with Shakespearian plays (see Cox, 1992). For children experiencing chronic medical problems, the use of fairy tales is often highly therapeutic (see Bouzoukis, 2001).

## EDUCATION AND TRAINING IN DRAMA THERAPY

In drama therapy, most of the education and training occurs on the postgraduate level. In the United Kingdom and other countries, that training might lead to a certificate of completion. But increasingly, educational institutions are offering the master's degree (MA) as a terminal practitioner's degree. In North America, there are three MA university-based programs. The Drama Therapy Program at New York University is located within a performing arts department. The Drama Therapy Program at California Institute for Integral Studies is housed within a counseling psychology department. The program at Concordia University in Montreal, Canada, is part of a creative arts therapy department. Hunter College in New York City and Kansas State University in Manhattan, Kansas, also offer courses in drama therapy but do not grant a degree in the field.

We must remember that drama therapy is still a relatively new discipline and that its identity is often grounded in one of several disciplines—the arts, the social sciences, or the sister creative arts therapies. And yet, whatever the disciplinary base, the curriculum for these and other programs tends to be similar, with coursework in psychology and counseling, theater, and most essentially, drama therapy methods, practices, theory, and research. All programs require an extensive clinical internship. Most require a master's thesis that demonstrates a student's burgeoning knowledge of research skills in the discipline.

Aside from university training, a number of private training institutes have developed that are generally tied to one particular form of practice such as developmental transformations, narrative drama therapy, and transpersonal drama therapy. Institutes in the United States include the Drama Therapy Institute of Los Angeles, the Institute for Healing and Wellness and Omega Theatre in Boston, the Institutes for the Arts in Psychotherapy in New York City, and Stop-Gap Institute in California. A more recent and eclectic institute in New York City is called the Center for Creative Alternatives, a subsidiary of the long-standing Creative Alternatives, which has offered for more than 25 years drama therapy workshops in various medical, educational, and mental health facilities throughout metropolitan New York City. These institutes offer various degrees of training from beginning workshops and classes to more directed programs that potentially lead to a state or national credential.

There are also private organizations that practice drama therapy and offer training and supervision to drama therapists but refer generally to their work as educational or performance-based, such as Hospital Audiences, Inc. (HAI) and Enact, both located in New York City.

The professional organization that represents drama therapists in North America, and indeed internationally, is called the National Association for Drama Therapy. The organization is responsible for setting and monitoring standards of training, education, and professional ethics. On the international scene, there are a number of professional organizations also responsible for standards of training and education. The primary one in the United Kingdom is called the British Association of Drama Therapists. In Europe, several universities and private institutes educate students and professionals in the field. Most universities offer postgraduate diplomas.

In the United Kingdom, the University of Surrey at Roehampton is unique in that it offers an MA plus the only PhD in drama therapy in the world. Drama therapy is taught on the undergraduate level in the Netherlands. There are two private training programs in Athens, Greece: The Drama Therapy Center

Aeon and the Greek Institute of Playtherapy and Dramatherapy. There are two academic programs in Israel, the first at an affiliate of Lesley University, offering an MA, the other at Tel Hai College, offering a certification in drama therapy. There are also a number of training opportunities offered by private institutes in Northern Ireland, Cyprus, Italy, Germany, the Czech Republic, and Finland. Although there is great interest in drama therapy in the Far East, and a handful of professionals trained in the Western drama therapy programs, there are no formal training or educational programs in drama therapy with the exception of institutes sponsoring psychodrama in Japan, Taiwan, and Hong Kong.

## THE ANCIENT ROOTS OF DRAMA THERAPY

In ancient times, healers believed that people became ill because they offended certain spirits or strictures. Throughout human history, healers of all kinds have known that treatment of a sick person proceeds through the body. And because many believed that the body was inhabited by spirits and a mind, these healers developed ways to purge the offending spirits, to cajole and placate the unquiet mind.

In preindustrial times healers intuited that to treat the sick body, one had to engage directly with the patient, not only in prescriptive words and therapeutic touch, but also in expressive forms of movement and sound, of word and image making, in order to make contact with the spirit world that exists both within and beyond the body. Ancient Indian and Chinese healers, believing illness to be an imbalance in one's vital life energy or chi, worked on the body through herbal medicine and acupuncture, and on the spirit through such expressive activities as body movement, meditation, chant, and visual depiction of symbolic images. Traditional shamanic healers throughout the world moved spirits in and out of the body through a mix of hypnotic trance, symbolic dance, song, storytelling, and dramatic enactment.

Drama and related arts as therapy have been traced back to the early days of shamanism and healing rituals (Lewis, 1993; Pendzik, 1988; Serlin, 1993; Snow, 2000). Drama as healing has roots in early ritual practices in ancient Egypt and the Near East, in India and China, then later in Greece and Rome (see Brockett & Hildy, 2003). The first Western forms of theater evolved from the dithyramb, an improvised dramatic rite enacted through song, story, and movement, to honor the god, Dionysus. In Aristotle's (1954) *Poetics*, we find a reference to tragedy as evolving from the dithyramb and comedy evolving from equally mysterious rites, which Aristotle referred to as phallic performances. Translated from ancient Greek, the word *tragedy* means *goat song*, another reference to an ancient rite of sacrifice probably connected to the Dionysian rituals. In observing contemporary shamanic healing rituals, we can clearly see how those roots have supported strong and persistent traditions.

Drama therapy is indeed ancient, a descendant of traditional healing, shamanism, and ritual practices whose purpose was to heal individuals and to provide a sense of community within a group of villagers. As an ancient healing form, dramatic practice was fully holistic, integrating the body and mind and spirit, incorporating many of the expressive arts of movement, song, story, and meditation.

## THE MODERN ROOTS OF DRAMA THERAPY

As a form of action psychotherapy, drama therapy originated in the practice and theory of J. L. Moreno, an Austrian psychiatrist who began to experiment with action methods in Vienna in the 1920s. Moreno's early experimentation concerned the development of a theater of spontaneity, the first modern example of improvisation performed before an audience. In Moreno's Stegreiftheater, actors were encouraged to experiment with various themes suggested by the audience and by their director, Moreno. Further, actors would improvise scenes based upon current events. Moreno called this work the Living Newspaper and used it as a forum not only to debate the important issues of the day, but to bring them to life through dramatization. Moreno's theater became therapeutic as he realized its potential to bring personal, interpersonal, and social issues to awareness and to move toward change.

The early psychodramas in Moreno's theater of spontaneity evolved into the full-blown work that he and his later wife and colleague, Zerka Moreno, developed in the United States. Psychodrama is a form of group psychotherapy where clients dramatize rather than speak about their problems. Psychodrama is practiced within a modified theatrical setting. The main client, called the protagonist, works on an open stage with an embedded problem and chooses others in the group, called auxiliaries, to represent figures within the problematic drama. The director helps the protagonist deepen his understanding of the problem and find ways to confront the appropriate auxiliary figures and to then move toward a resolution of the problem. The psychodrama director uses many techniques in exploring problems, some of which will be discussed below.

Moreno was also responsible for creating social forms of therapeutic drama, which he called sociodrama and sociometry. The former proceeded through methods similar to psychodrama, although the subject was generally a social theme rather than a personal one. Sociometry (see Moreno, 1960) is the study of group relationships and dynamics. Moreno became rather adept at charting the intricate social webs within families, organizations, and other social structures.

Another key figure in the development of drama therapy was Fritz Perls (1969), the founder of Gestalt therapy with his wife, Laura. Laura Perls understood

Gestalt as "an aesthetic philosophy" (Serlin and Shane, 1999). Perls borrowed many of his technical approaches to therapy from Moreno, including role reversal and work with the empty chair. Perls worked in groups, like Moreno, but did not involve the group as much in sharing personal reflections. His work tended to be less reality-based than Moreno's in that he would facilitate dialogues between a client and fantasy figures or objects. Perls became known for his dream work in which each figure and object in the dream represented a split-off part of the personality. As a Gestalt therapist, Perls aimed toward an integration of the split-off parts and would thus encourage his clients to play out all of the figures in the dream.

Both Moreno and Perls were influential to drama therapy in their insistence upon drama as the primary therapeutic modality, upon action as the precursor of cognition, upon role taking, role playing, and role reversal as the essential forms of the dramatization, and upon the importance of empathy and spontaneity as the goals of all action-based therapies.

The line between Moreno and Perls and the contemporary drama therapists can be seen more fully when drawn backward into the work of the early psychoanalysts who broke from the orthodoxy of Freud. Although there is only enough space to discuss their work briefly, Carl Jung, Otto Rank, Sandor Ferenczi, and Wilhelm Reich all fought tirelessly to identify the essential benefits of working therapeutically through visual images, through stories and dramatizations, through movement and manipulation of the body, and through active engagement with patients. They all did this at a great risk of being banished from the inner circle of classical psychoanalysis as they dared to defy Freud. They all agreed that despite Freud's brilliant explorations of the psyche and the unconscious mind, he failed to take a more holistic position and ultimately reduced his treatment method to logical analysis, a rational means toward uncovering an irrational psychological structure.

The most important developments of these early pioneers that led to the discoveries of Moreno and Perls and later drama therapists included Jung's active imagination, Rank and Ferenczi's active therapy, Rank's work with myth and story, Ferenczi's mutual therapy, and Reich's movement and body work. All would be later incorporated into the practice of drama therapy, although few would be referenced.

The development of the profession of drama therapy is fairly brief, with two major trends in the United Kingdom and the United States. In the United Kingdom, Peter Slade (1954, 1995) is generally viewed as the first to coin the phrase *dramatherapy* as one word in the early 1950s, extending from his pioneering work in child drama. Sue Jennings (1974), who began to develop remedial drama for use with handicapped and disabled populations, was influenced by Slade and other British pioneers of drama education. But she also created her own form of dramatherapy (Jennings, 1987, 1990, 1997) over some

35 years of practice, defining the concepts of the nascent field and providing clear technical descriptions of the process with a wide variety of populations from normal neurotics to incarcerated felons.

Marion Lindkvist also pioneered the early profession of dramatherapy in England, opening up a center of drama and movement called Sesame and training generations of practitioners. Jennings and Lindquist were followed by such important practitioners and thinkers as Alida Gersie and Ann Catternach and then by Phil Jones and Roger Grainger, as well as a host of other second- and third-generation pioneers.

In the United States, the field was pioneered by a number of practitioners including the child psychoanalyst, Eleanor Irwin, the clinical psychologist, David Read Johnson, the Sesame-trained René Emunah, and the theater-trained Robert Landy. In the anthology *Current Approaches in Drama Therapy* (Lewis & Johnson, 2000), some 17 drama therapists are featured, whose work ranges from analytically based to spiritually based.

David Read Johnson (2000) has created a diagram, "The Historical Roots of Drama Therapy Approaches," placing the major figures in American drama therapy within the context of three original domains—psychotherapy, psychiatric care, and theater. Taken together, all these modern roots and branches grow from the two major components of drama therapy. The drama part derives from the art form of theater. The most significant theater models are those of Stanislavski, in the primacy of affective experience and physical action; Brecht, in the primacy of theatrical distancing and social-political action; and Grotowski, in the primacy of somatic experience and psychophysical action. The therapy part derives from the early psychoanalysts, especially those who broke from Freud's purely rational approach and began to look at the primacy of imagination, affect, and action. And it also derives from the radical experimentation of J. L. Moreno, who imagined and then implemented a full-blown therapy of action.

## THREE APPROACHES TO DRAMA THERAPY

Drama therapy as a discipline is practiced in many forms. In the book *Current Approaches in Drama Therapy* (Lewis & Johnson, 2000), 16 different approaches are featured. The most prominent forms, those based in clear theory and practice and represented by a growing research literature, are associated with major figures in the field who are either university professors or founders of private institutes.

In a recent film (Landy, 2005), three major approaches to drama therapy are highlighted: role method, psychodrama, and developmental transformations. Psychodrama, developed by J. L. Moreno, is a discipline unto itself, but can also be seen as an action or dramatic therapy as it is fully based in role enactment.

In this section, we will explore these three approaches, looking at theory, clinical practice, and research.

## Role Method

Role method is tied to the role theory of drama therapy. Role theory begins with a complex understanding of role as based in both theater and in social science. For one, role is a unit of personality, representing certain discrete qualities of an individual, rather than the individual as a whole. Role can also be understood as a theatrical metaphor viewing the person as an actor who has the ability to take on and play out a wide range of parts.

As a human being develops, roles are given, taken, played out, and generated. Human beings are given certain biologically based roles at birth through their DNA. Roles concerning gender and ethnicity, abilities and disabilities, become part of one's early role repertoire. Roles are taken from significant social models. The developing child internalizes qualities of mother and father, for example, learning not only what it means to be a mother and father, but also what it means to be a child in relationship to parents. Having internalized a range of roles from the social world, people play out their own versions of those roles and their counterparts. People, however, are not only role players, but also creators or generators of unique roles. Although a person might come from a family of working-class extroverts who have little connection to intellectual or aesthetic pursuits, for example, he might discover a way to create a prominent role of introverted artist, based only in part upon his identification with role models outside the family.

The concept of role derives from the theater. In creating a model for understanding the dimensions of roles available, Landy (1993) created a systematic taxonomy of roles, categorizing 158 roles and subroles according to their qualities, functions, and styles of enactment. In his role theory, Landy speculates that the taxonomy represents, in part, roles available to be taken on by all individuals, similar to Jung's system of archetypes. At the heart of role theory is the postmodern notion that in the absence of a core self the personality is comprised of a system of interrelated, dynamic roles.

In his early work, Landy (1993) postulated an interaction between polarities represented by role and counterrole. The former is the part of the person that, like a protagonist in a play, is in search for greater understanding. The counterrole, like the antagonist, is the part of the person that either blocks the journey or simply stands on the other side, a foil to the initial role. Between role and counterrole is a transitional figure called the guide. The guide functions to integrate the role polarities. Initially represented by one's parents or caregivers who lead the developing child along the path toward independence, the guide works to contain the client's ambivalences as represented in polar roles.

Like Virgil leading Dante to the Inferno, the guide helps to lead clients to the source of their problems and to encourage them to take the risky voyage to discovery.

The goal of role theory is balance, for people to discover a way to live among their polarities, represented by role and counterrole, mediated by the guide. In moving toward that goal, Landy developed the role method (2000) of drama therapy, which proceeds according to the following eight steps:

1. Invoking the role
2. Naming the role
3. Playing out/working through the role
4. Exploring relationships of role to counterrole and guide
5. Reflecting upon the role play: discovering role qualities, functions, and styles inherent in the role
6. Relating the fictional role to everyday life
7. Integrating roles to create a functional role system
8. Social modeling: discovering ways that clients' behavior in role affects others in their social environments

Although clients do not necessarily follow the steps chronologically, there is an internal logic to each step. One can either work individually or as part of a drama therapy group through the role method. The work usually begins as clients warm up their bodies and prepare their imaginations for the experience. The therapist helps the clients to discover a role to be taken on and played out in the session. This step is called invoking the role as clients bring to life a figure from their imaginations. As an example, Sue, a 65-year-old woman, recently widowed, is part of a drama therapy group. Sue is a pseudonym based upon several real clients.

The therapist invites the group as an initial warm-up to stretch out their bodies and to reach out toward some figure. While doing so, Sue imagines that she is reaching for the hand of her grandmother.

In the next step, the therapist asks the client to name the role, in order to provide more specificity and clarity. In that the role method most often proceeds through fictional characters, the therapist asks the client to imagine the role as a fictional character. She names the figure Grandmother from Little Red Riding Hood.

The third step involves the beginning of the dramatization. In our example, Sue is asked to embody the role of Grandmother and to speak a monologue introducing herself. As she works, it becomes clear that there are other characters within the drama. Sue identifies them as the granddaughter, whom she names Little Red, and Peter Wolf. Throughout her dramatization, she explores the relationship of the role of Grandmother to those of Little Red and Peter Wolf. In working, the therapist views Grandmother and Little Red as role and counterrole. Peter Wolf, the sexually charged young man, becomes a guide figure standing between the aging woman, fearful of losing her youth and sexuality, and the innocence of the young girl, who is about to take a dangerous journey into the woods of experience. This part of the work reflects step four as the interrelationships of the three primary roles are explored.

Following the enactment, the client is encouraged to reflect upon the fictional drama. In step five, Sue, for example, is asked to consider her feelings and thoughts about the three characters of Grandmother, Little Red, and Peter Wolf. Who are they? What do they want? How do they present themselves in terms of degrees of emotion and distance?

And then, bringing the fiction back to reality, Sue is asked to speak about the parts of herself that are similar to and different from those of the three fictional roles. How does she see herself as an aging grandmother, an innocent young girl, a sexually aggressive wolf?

During the next, related stage, Sue is asked to imagine the three roles working together. Is she able, for example, to tolerate the contradictory pulls of age and innocence, mediated by sexuality? If not, what does she do to resolve her ambivalence? What if the wolf is not the guide, but a counterrole? Who then would be the guide? Is a guide available? These kinds of questions inform the process of reflection which, at best, can lead to integration and balance, the primary goals of the role method. In Sue's case, she comes to the realization that Peter Wolf, being too predatory, is not the true guide. The true guide, according to Sue, had been left out of her story. When questioned by the group, she says that neither female figure was able to internalize the malevolent power of the wolf. The one male figure that was needed was that of the woodsman, the one in the fictional story who has the power to kill the wolf. Once she identified the woodsman, she was able to see him as a dormant part of herself that is positive and potent, capable of holding together the two parts of herself that had been split by the death of her husband. And then she realized that the grandmother figure was actually the widow, a new and difficult role that had been suddenly thrust upon her. It was a powerful realization that provided a sense of relief in accepting her new life situation.

The final stage, that of social modeling, concerns what Sue does with her new awareness outside of the group. The more Sue can live with her role polarities, the better she can model that balance for others in her social world. Soon after the death of her husband, Sue moved to a retirement community. Among her peers, many of whom were widows, Sue was eventually able to demonstrate the positive benefits of living fully without denying her youthful energy, her power, and her wisdom, all qualities of Little Red, the woodsman, and the grandmother.

Role theory and role method have been developed primarily by Robert Landy and his students and colleagues at New York University. Landy (1993,

1994, 2000) and his colleagues have published a number of books and articles further developing the conceptual and theoretical base of the field. They have worked with the taxonomy of roles, creating assessment instruments and testing them out with a number of different subjects (Landy, 2001a, 2001b; Landy, Luck, Conner, & McMullian, 2003). And finally, through case studies (Landy, 1996, 2000), Landy and others have demonstrated how and why role method is an effective means of treatment through drama.

## Psychodrama

In his major work in psychodrama, Moreno (1946) defined the concept of role as "the actual and tangible forms which the self takes" (p. 153). Moreno would go on to write numerous books, monographs, and articles explaining both the theory and practice of psychodrama and its related fields of sociodrama and sociometry. The theory remained incomplete, but throughout all his work there remained a clear sense that a role-playing approach facilitates a cathartic release of repressed emotion and moves the protagonist closer to Moreno's primary goal—that of spontaneity, the ability to respond to an old stimulus with some novelty and a new stimulus fully in the moment. Moreno focused upon four specific goals within his version of the ABCS, that is, Affect, Behavior, Cognition, and Spirituality, similar to four of the six domains given by Landy (1993).

Within the realm of affect, Moreno's goal was catharsis. Moreno referred to two kinds of catharsis. The first, catharsis of abreaction, concerned the release of feelings associated with a difficult time in one's life. The second, catharsis of integration, concerned one's ability to link feeling with thought, moving the client closer to a new course of action.

Behavioral goals in psychodrama concerned one's ability to practice alternative ways of behaving in difficult life circumstances. Although cognitive goals are about insight, Moreno conceived of insight as expressed through the body as well as the mind. The final area, spirituality, concerns an integration not only of self and other, but also of the group in relationship to a higher power. Moreno's writings are imbued with spiritual metaphors linking the ability to play God with the ability to be spontaneous and creative. In seeking levels of spiritual integration and in acting as if one were taking on the procreative power of supernatural beings, one achieves the highest psychodramatic goals.

Although Moreno's (1946) role theory was incomplete, he did identify four types of roles:

1. Psychosomatic or physiological roles, which relate to the body. These roles include eater, sleeper, eliminator, and mover.

2. Psychodramatic or fantasy roles, which relate to the imagination. These roles include gods, devils, and animals. They can also include roles that one wishes for, such as those concerning success and power.
3. Social roles, which relate to relationships with others. They include family, gender, and work-based roles.
4. Cultural roles, which arise in response to the demands of a given environment and relate to means of enacting particular family, gender, and work roles.

In the practice of psychodrama and sociodrama, Moreno developed a three-part structure of warm-up, action, and closure. The warm-up is intended to identify one protagonist within the psychodrama group who is ready to work on a particular issue. It also prepares the full group to engage with the protagonist in an auxiliary capacity. As auxiliaries, group members will take on the roles of significant figures within the protagonist's drama. The therapist, known as the director, works with the protagonist, the auxiliaries, and the full group to deepen the role-playing during the action phase and to help the protagonist fully express and resolve the dilemma. Following the action, the full group enters into the closure phase, sharing feelings and impressions stimulated by the psychodrama for the purpose of helping the protagonist cool down and integrate the experience, as well as helping others who have identified with the dilemma of the protagonist do the same.

Within psychodrama, there are many production techniques developed by Moreno that are now commonplace to many methods of psychotherapy. Zerka T. Moreno (1965), Moreno's wife and longtime collaborator, identified five of the most significant. They are the soliloquy, the double, the aside, role reversal, and the mirror. In soliloquy, the protagonist is asked to speak out his internal thoughts. This is usually done within the action phase of the session and includes gesture and movement, as well as words. The function of the soliloquy is to help the protagonist deepen his role and reach down further into feelings associated with the role.

The aside, as in theater, is a remark made by the protagonist to the audience, sharing some additional information not directly communicated in the drama. The purpose of the aside is to help the protagonist better integrate his thoughts and feelings.

The double is the best known of psychodramatic techniques. It is an alter ego expressed tangibly in action representing several unexpressed parts of the protagonist. The double can be played by the director, by a person chosen from the audience by the protagonist, or by a person who emerges spontaneously from the group. The double can amplify or tone down the protagonist's voice or action. Or the double might express the feeling, thought, or action underlying that given by the protagonist in the moment. The purpose of the double is to help the protagonist more fully express himself.

Role reversal, another very common psychodramatic technique, occurs when the protagonist changes parts with an auxiliary. If, for example, Sue was engaged in a scene expressing some anger toward her dead husband for leaving her alone in the world, the director might ask her to reverse roles with the auxiliary actor who was playing the husband. In the role of husband, Sue might be better able to view her new role as widow from a distance, better accepting the reality of death.

And finally, the mirror is a figure chosen from the group who stands in for the protagonist and enacts an alternative way to play out a role or a scene. The function of the mirror is to help the protagonist view new options of action. When the protagonist is blocked, over-flooded with feeling or dissociated from feeling, the mirror can provide a solid model that can often get the protagonist back on track.

In working psychodramatically, rather than delineating characters in a fictional story, Sue would focus upon an actual problem in her everyday life. On the other hand, she might choose to confront her dead husband, as exemplified above, expressing the anger she is not able to contain in the present.

As an example, Sue is warmed up in a group when asked to reach out for someone with whom there is unfinished business. She chooses her dead husband and verbalizes that she is angry at him for leaving her unprepared to take care of herself. The director asks Sue to imagine a scene between her and her husband. With some prompting, Sue settles on a coffee shop they frequented when they needed to talk things out. After setting up the bare bones of the coffee shop, the director asks Sue to choose a person from the group to play the husband. Sue chooses Charlie, a young man who has always energized the group.

As the scene begins, the director asks Sue to take on the role of the husband, instructing Charlie how to embody his physical, vocal, and emotional presence. In a role reversal, Sue is back to herself and confronts Charlie as the husband. Part of the dialogue is given below:

**Sue:** You left me with all your bills and debts and paperwork and bank accounts and I don't know what. What the hell am I supposed to do?

**Charlie:** Pay the bills. Take control. What's the problem?

**Sue:** I don't know how, that's the problem.

**Charlie:** So learn.

**Sue:** You never taught me.

**Charlie:** What are you, a 12-year-old?

Sue becomes very quiet. As this point, the director asks Sue to choose someone in the group as a double. Sue chooses Randi, whom she perceives as a strong young woman. Randi begins by imitating Sue's hunched-over posture and whiney voice. Sue becomes uncomfortable with what she hears and asks the director for help. The director instructs Randi to mirror an alternative response to the husband. This is Randi's response:

**Randi, as Sue**: I'm a grown woman, an adult who has wiped myself out too many times and given up too much power in this relationship. I behaved like a little girl, because you have treated me like that in the past and I resent you for it. But right now, I'm not holding onto the anger. I feel strong enough to do the paperwork. It doesn't take a brain surgeon to pay the bills. The harder part is living without you. I miss you so much. I wasn't ready to let you go. You had to know that. I just miss you so much.

The director asks Sue if she feels ready to do the scene herself. She is reluctant. The director has her reverse roles with Charlie and Charlie, as Sue, says: "I am afraid to say this in front of the group. I'm afraid to let out my feelings. What if I cry? My pain is so big, I don't know if anyone can help me."

With the urging of the director and the support of Randi, who has become Sue's supportive double, Sue plays out the scene as Charlie had modeled. When she does, she is full of feeling and allows her tears to flow. As she ends her scene, she expresses an awareness that her feeling of loss and deep sadness are much more important than her fear of not being able to balance the books.

During the closure, the group gathers around Sue and compliments her for being brave enough to express her pain and to get beneath the surface of her feelings of incompetence. Some share their own stories of loss and of finding the strength to express their pain and to move forward in building new relationships and a new life. Sue feels comforted and contained by the group.

J. L. Moreno (1946, 1960, 1963, 1969) has performed the lion's share of research and written the major books and articles in the field of psychodrama, sociodrama, and sociometry. However, a vast literature in the field has grown up around him. The *Journal of Group Psychotherapy, Psychodrama and Sociometry* has offered hundreds of research studies. As psychodrama has become very much an international phenomenon, researchers and practitioners have reported their findings in many cultures. However, like role method and most other forms of action drama therapy, psychodrama does not easily lend itself to quantifiable methodologies and thus the research tends to be more descriptive and clinical than empirical.

## Developmental Transformations

Developmental transformations is a form of drama therapy defined by its founder, David Read Johnson (2000) as "an embodied encounter in the playspace" (p. 87). In the film, *Three Approaches to Drama Therapy*, Johnson speaks about the theory and practice of developmental transformations:

> The basis of developmental transformations is the creation and maintenance of the playspace between the client and the therapist. This is an imaginative space that is created and maintained in a dramatic realm....One of the more important and unique elements to developmental transformations is the role of the therapist where the therapist puts himself in the therapeutic playspace with the client, allowing his body to be available for play with the client....As this process unfolds the therapist is going to be applying various kinds of techniques to try to loosen the grip of the clients on various forms that they have attached themselves to. We believe that...ill health or sickness is often associated with trying to hold on to previous forms that are no longer working. So the therapist basically is going to try...to encourage the client to move from a state of seriousness about themselves to a state of play and allow them to transform...

The goal of developmental transformations is to facilitate a process of flow, a term somewhat synonymous to that of Moreno's spontaneity. The spontaneous flow occurs within the client, between the client and others in the group, and in relationship to a Source. Although Johnson (2000) does not clearly define Source, he views it as connected to emanation theory wherein "the world is understood to be emanating from (i.e., flowing out) a fundamental Source of existence that remains beyond comprehension" (p. 88). This more spiritual notion of an essential Source is different from the conceptual base of role theory and psychodrama. In developmental transformations, all roles emanate from a Source and are, by nature, impermanent. The role-players are not necessarily the creators of the roles they play, but rather are vessels through which the roles are expressed and then let go. In role theory and psychodrama, role forms are more permanent, defined by essential human attributes pertaining to body, mind, emotion, social relationship, spirit, and creative expression. There is no Source or central core self, but rather the capacity of all human beings to be both creative and spontaneous.

Developmental transformations proceed in several phases, beginning with surface play, where both client and therapist play with roles and issues in somewhat of a stereotypical, light way, warming themselves up to engage on a deeper level. The next phase, persona play, involves engagement on the client's part with more personal issues from the past. In describing this phase, Johnson (2000) writes: "Every possible action toward significant people in their lives and themselves are portrayed, including those secretly held for years as well as new ones, never before conceived" (p. 92).

The third phase is that of intimate play, focused on the client's feelings toward the therapist. Many fantasies and wishes are enacted in this phase, and the therapist helps the client to express, as fully as possible, aspects of the relationship that feel risky and even forbidden. In the final phase, that of deep play, "client and therapist are intensely aware of each other and their bodies, and are freed up enough to work on their feelings of being bound or restrained by each other in play" (Johnson, 2000, p. 92). This final phase is one of intimacy and acceptance of one another apart from their roles. Johnson mentions that for developmental transformations to be successful, clients do not need to proceed to deep play. On any of the levels, one can work toward discovering a better way to release inhibitions, to become more playful and in the flow of relationship to self, to other, and to Source.

In developmental transformations, the therapist at times removes herself from the action and sits in a witnessing circle, a round piece of carpet placed at the fringe of the playspace. While there, she witnesses the play of the client and might engage with her verbally but not physically. When she returns, the reciprocal play resumes. The therapist and client contract to engage with one another for a specified time during each session. At the end of the time, the therapist says to the client: "Take a minute." There is no verbal processing. All reflective moments are intended to occur within the action of the session. She then leaves the room and the session ends.

Sue was very reluctant to engage in developmental transformations, fearing a loss of control and fearing that she would be infantilized by the therapist. However, she agreed to work for one session with a very engaging and playful young woman named Lee, who reminded her of herself before she had children.

They begin by stretching and shaking out their bodies, then walking around the space. Lee suggests that Sue lets out spontaneous sounds and movements. Then Lee asks Sue to sculpt her body in any position she chooses and to place her own body in relationship. Sue sculpts Lee as a scary figure, shaping her hands as claws, arms open wide, her face expressionless, with eyes closed. She turns her back on the figure and places herself within the arms of the figure. Sue expresses fear and Lee begins to make guttural noises, suggesting a fearful object. Sue withers and falls to the ground. Lee pats her head with her claws and says, ironically: "It's alright, my dear, I won't hurt you."

**Sue:**   But you did. You destroyed my life.
**Lee:**   Everyone feels that way about me. I'm really pretty cozy once you get to know me.
**Sue:**   You came too early. You're from the wrong story, you witch.
**Lee:**   Witch? Which?

As Lee plays with the word, transforming "witch" to "which," she lightens the tone of the scene. Sue picks up on it and engages in a playful exchange of questions:

**Sue:**   Which?
**Lee:**   Which?
**Sue:**   I know. That one over there.

Sue crosses the room and picks up her sweater, which she had discarded at the beginning of the session. She holds it in front of her and contemplates it.

**Lee:**    Looks good.
**Sue:**    Bright.
**Lee:**    Very bright.
**Sue:**    Red.
**Lee:**    Very red.
**Sue:**    It's hers. She lost it.
**Lee:**    She always does that, poor girl. She should know better.
**Sue:**    No, she shouldn't. She's just a little girl. How could she possibly know?
**Lee:**    All girls know that they shouldn't go into the woods alone, that they could be attacked by predators. Raped. Killed.
**Sue:**    We have to find her before it's too late.

Both women search throughout the room, Sue holding on tight to her sweater. At some point, Sue reaches out for Lee's hand.

**Lee:**    You want my hand?
**Sue:**    I don't know if I can trust you.
**Lee:**    Come on, sweetie, let's take a walk.

Sue takes Lee's hand, reluctantly at first, but then willingly, and they walk around the room, in silence. Sue is full of feeling. As they walk, she begins to cry.

**Sue:**    Who are you?
**Lee:**    I am your friend.
**Sue:**    I feel so alone these days.
**Lee:**    I'm here.
**Sue:**    Walk with me a little longer.

They walk. Sue comes to a point where she stops. She lets go of Lee's hand. Lee moves away and comes to rest in a small carpet-lined circle. She says to Sue: "Take a minute." Sue is alone with her thoughts. Lee leaves the room and the session is over.

The major research and published work in the area of developmental transformations has been done by David Read Johnson and his colleagues at the Institute for Developmental Transformations in New York City. Johnson continues to be a prolific writer who has published in many academic journals and books since the 1980s. The most comprehensive collection of papers is the *Developmental Transformations Papers, 1982–2006.*

## THE FUTURE OF DRAMA THERAPY

The field of drama therapy is heterogeneous, with training programs in private institutes and universities, set academically within departments of performing arts, creative arts therapy, and counseling psychology. There are several theories and many different approaches. Unlike psychodrama, a field onto itself, drama therapy is the product of a number of different pioneers, each coming from a different background. And yet, in spite of the differences, the field holds together in its commitment to work through the creative process of improvisation, storymaking, and role playing.

As the field looks toward the future, it needs to address a number of issues both from the inside and the outside. In a recent paper (Landy, 2006) the following issues were identified: developing a self-critical attitude; collaborating with colleagues in the related professions of psychology, creative arts therapy, and applied theater; addressing splits in the field and ruptures within society; facilitating effective research and mentoring; and reviving a playful, creative spirit, essential to the impulse that led to the creation of the profession. To address all these issues demands an attention to the most basic of dramatic processes, that of dialogue, literally a reasoning through, a commitment to engaging with others from different drama therapy cultures and from related fields of arts therapy, expressive therapy, performing arts, counseling, social work, and psychology. In imagining a bright future, many of these dialogues will continue and will lead to the building of further interdisciplinary bridges.

The idea of drama therapy began tens of thousands of years ago in a traditional and holistic understanding of the inseparable connection of psyche and soma. Wellness was a matter of balance between the natural and supernatural worlds, sustained by the grace of the spirits who favored the human beings who created them. Illness was a rent in the great curtain of being, requiring a performative cure to please the restless spirits. Although drama therapists are no longer shamans, they can return to the future with their ancient understanding intact—to achieve the goals of spontaneity, balance, flow within the unquiet mind, one needs to work through a form of action creative enough to summon together the full complements of the human being—mind and body and spirit.

## TOOL KIT FOR CHANGE

### Role and Perspective of the Drama Therapist

1. The drama therapist is a guide who helps clients engage in a process of role playing and storymaking. in order to discover a more balanced life.
2. The drama therapist works as director of the client's drama and sometimes coactor, encouraging embodied expression through improvisation and play.
3. The drama therapist works through action and reflection, engaging the client's mind, body, and spirit.

### Role and Perspective of the Client

1. The client engages in a playful process of healing.
2. The client experiences his/her process through assuming fictional roles and telling and enacting stories in roles. Following the fictional role enactment, the client reflects upon the fiction and relates it back to everyday life.

### Global Perspective

1. Drama therapy is based in traditional healing forms of shamanism practiced throughout the world. In its practice, it incorporates aspects of traditional healing through body work, puppetry, sound, and movement to invoke roles from the imaginal realm.
2. The aim of drama therapy, like that of many traditional forms of healing, is harmony and balance among the polarities of mind and body, emotion and cognition.
3. The language of performance is recognizable throughout the world as a means of expressing cultural, social, and personal issues to a receptive audience.
4. In dramatizing and witnessing the dramatization of social, cultural, and political issues, people with different perspectives have the opportunity to engage in effective dialogue in the service of exploring and resolving conflicts.

## REFERENCES

Aristotle. (1954). *Poetics* (I. Bywater, trans.) New York: Modern Library.

Bergman, J., & Hewish, S. (2003). *Challenging experience: An experiential approach to the treatment of serious offenders.* Oklahoma City: Wood 'N' Barnes Publishers.

Brockett, O., & Hildy, F. (2003). *History of the theatre* (9th ed.). Boston: Allyn & Bacon.

Bouzoukis, C. (2001). *Pediatric dramatherapy: They couldn't run, so they learned to fly.* London: Jessica Kingsley.

Cox, M. (1992). *Shakespeare comes to Broadmoor.* London: Jessica Kingsley.

Ekman, P. (1992). Are there basic emotions? *Psychological Review, 99,* 550–553.

Institute for Developmental Transformations. (2006). *Developmental transformations: Papers, 1982–2006.* New York: Institute for Developmental Transformations.

Jennings, S. (1974). *Remedial drama.* London: Pitman.

Jennings, S. (1987). Ed. *Dramatherapy, theory and practice for teachers and clinicians, 1.* London: Routledge.

Jennings, S. (1990). *Dramatherapy with families, groups and individuals: Waiting in the wings.* London: Jessica Kingsley.

Jennings, S. (1997). *Introduction to dramatherapy: Ariadne's ball of thread.* London: Jessica Kingsley.

Johnson, D. R. (2000). *Developmental transformations: Toward the body as presence.* In P. Lewis & D. R. Johnson (Eds.), *Current approaches in drama therapy.* Springfield, IL: Charles C. Thomas.

Landy, R. (1993). *Persona and performance: The meaning of role in drama, therapy and everyday life.* New York: Guilford Press.

Landy, R. (1994). *Drama therapy: Concepts, theories and practices* (2nd ed.). Springfield, IL: Charles C. Thomas.

Landy, R. (1996). *Essays in drama therapy: The double life.* London: Jessica Kingsley.

Landy, R. (2000). Role theory and the role method of drama therapy. In P. Lewis & D. R. Johnson (Eds.), *Current approaches in drama therapy.* Springfield, IL: Charles C. Thomas.

Landy, R. (2001a). Tell-A-Story—A new assessment in drama therapy. In R. Landy, *New essays in drama therapy—Unfinished business.* Springfield, IL: Charles C. Thomas.

Landy, R. (2001b). Role profiles—An assessment instrument. In R. Landy, *New essays in drama therapy—Unfinished business.* Springfield, IL: Charles C. Thomas.

Landy, R., Luck, B., Conner, E., & McMullian, S. (2003). Role profiles: A drama therapy assessment instrument. *The Arts in Psychotherapy, 30*(3), 151–161.

Landy, R. (Producer). (2005). *Three approaches to drama therapy.* DVD and VHS videotape. NY: New York University.

Landy, R. (2006). The future of drama therapy. *The Arts in Psychotherapy, 32*(2), 135–142.

Lewis, P. (1993). *Creative transformation: The healing power of the arts.* Wilmette, IL: Chiron Publications.

Lewis, P., and Johnson, D. R. (Eds.). *Current approaches in drama therapy.* Springfield, IL: Charles C. Thomas.

Moreno, J. L. (1946). *Psychodrama* (Vol. 1). Beacon, NY: Beacon House.

Moreno, J. L. (1960). *The Sociometry Reader.* Glencoe, IL: The Free Press.

Moreno, J. L. (1963). *Who Shall Survive?* Beacon, NY: Beacon House.

Moreno, J. L. (1969). *Psychodrama.* (Vol. 3). Beacon, NY: Beacon House.

Moreno, Z. T. (1965). Psychodramatic rules, techniques, and adjunctive methods. *Group Psychotherapy, 18,* 73–86.

Pendzik, S. (1988). Drama therapy as a form of modern shamanism. *Journal of Transpersonal Psychology, 20,* 81–92.

Perls, F. (1969). *Gestalt therapy verbatim.* Moab, Utah: Real People Press.

Serlin, I. A. (1993). Root images of healing in dance therapy. *American Dance Therapy Journal, 15*(2), 65–75.

Serlin, I. A., & Shane, P. (1999). Laura Perls and Gestalt therapy: her life and values. In D. Moss (Ed.), *The pursuit of human potential: A sourcebook of Humanistic and Transpersonal psychology* (pp. 375–384). Westport, CT: Greenwood Press.

Slade, P. (1954). *Child drama.* London: University Press.

Slade, P. ( 1995). *Child play.* London: Jessica Kingsley.

Snow, S. (2000). Ritual/theater/therapy. In P. Lewis & D.R. Johnson, (Eds.), *Current approaches in drama therapy.* Springfield, IL: Charles C. Thomas.

Chapter Nine

# POETRY THERAPY: RECLAMATION OF DEEP LANGUAGE

*John Fox, CPT*

> The ritual chants and incantations of shamanism, the healing songs and magic of primitive people with their rich core of poetry, illustrate the vital role of art in ancient medicine. Poetry is indeed a force, an act of human magic, that alters the way we see our lives and so changes us. (Morrison, 1978, p. 94)

Plato said that beautiful language induces *sophrosyne,* a condition of stability and integration in psychic life. Beautiful language was given names by the Greeks of *epode* and *theklerian*—charms and spells to evoke in the listener the experience of calm and well-being (Morrison, 1978, p. 94).

This idea that the right words can heal is not a fantastic assertion without any basis. It is not merely a wistful hope that these reports from an ancient time, a time no longer relevant to our own situation, *might* still prove true. It is a wisdom that little children know and use to delight themselves and self-soothe. This perennial wisdom about the creative arts is part of cultures found across the planet, and is a wisdom that remains available to us today.

Poetry is a natural medicine; it is like a homeopathic tincture derived from the stuff of life itself—*your experience.* Poems distill experience into the essentials. Our personal experiences touch the common ground we share with others. The exciting part of this process is that poetry used in this healing way helps individuals integrate the disparate, even fragmented, parts of their lives. Poetic essences of sound, metaphor, image, feeling, and rhythm act as remedies that can elegantly strengthen our whole system—physical, mental, and spiritual (Fox, 1997, p. 3).

A person does not need to self-identify as a poet. Creative arts therapists believe individuals have the natural capacity to express themselves. Given useful tools, skillful support, and a safe, nonjudgmental environment that nurtures playfulness and depth, much is possible.

Poems speak to us when nothing else will. Poetry helps us to *feel* our lives rather than be numb. The page, touched with one's poem, becomes a place for painful feelings to be held, explored, and transformed. Writing and reading poems is a way of seeing and naming where we have been, where we are, and where we are going with our lives. Poetry provides guidance, revealing what you did not know you knew before you wrote or read the poem. This moment of surprising yourself with your own words of wisdom or of being surprised by the poems of others is at the heart of poetry as healer. "Poetic form provides the necessary veils and disguises that circumvent resistance to expression. By facilitating the expression of repressed emotion, the poem helps to secure therapeutic release and assists in the resolution of the poet's conflict" (Morrison, 1985, p. 35).

In many cultures older than our own quite young American one, there remains a close connection to, or at least a vivid memory of, this healing potential of words, indeed of a language that induces *sophrosyne*. Contemporary Greek poet Odysseas Elytis, winner of the Nobel Prize for Literature in 1979, in his book of essays, *Open Papers,* speaks of the medicinal and protective power of language and words of which he was aware even in childhood:

> ...until a few years ago our island nurses, with utter seriousness, chased evil spirits from above our cradles by uttering words without meaning, holding a tiny leaf of a modest herb which received God knows what strange powers exclusively from the innocence of its own nature. Poetry is precisely this tiny leaf with the unknown powers of innocence and the strange words which accompany it. (Elytis, 1995)

## LIFE AS THEATER-IN-THE-ROUND

To consider the value of poetry as a way to respond to pain and trauma, it is important to remember there was a time when poetry was a natural part of daily life for people. The fact that the arts were a central part of community experience is extremely significant in the context of the value of the creative arts and in the larger consideration of whole-person psychology.

Psychiatrist Ken Gorelick, a founding member (in the middle 1970s) of the original biblio/poetry therapy round table that occurred at St. Elisabeth's Hospital in Washington, DC, wrote a brief and brilliant essay that appeared in *The Journal of Poetry Therapy* in 1987, entitled "Greek Tragedy and Ancient Healing: Poems as Theater and Asclepian Temple in Miniature." Gorelick compares modern-day use of "poetry as healer (Leedy, 1985,

p. xxii)" to the presentation of tragedies in ancient Greek theater-in-the-round:

> ...the arts collaborated with the actors in bringing the story to life, the poetic feeling of a profoundly moving story was the mainspring of the power to touch and move the audience. If the theater experience was personally and deeply felt, it would carry over to personal life beyond the theatrical space. (Gorelick, 1987, p. 40)

He writes further:

> The group psychotherapy setting is a miniature theater-in-the-round. The participants take dual roles of protagonist and audience as they reflect and create a here-and-now reality for one another. Group members shuttle between the role of sufferer-participant and empathizer-observer, as in the audience Aristotle described. As group members examine the poem and are drawn into its depths, they are like the sufferers seeking their healing dream in the depths of Asclepian temples. The poem creates a frame in which each person's dream for himself/herself can arise. Drawn into the depths of the poem, the group members are simultaneously drawn into the depths of their lives to find an open space in which they can transform themselves, shape new lives and create new destinies. (Gorelick, 1987, p. 42)

The activity of poem-making and hearing poems (or prayers), as a way to tend to deep wounds, express a full range of emotional and life circumstance, and reclaim wholeness has been with us for a very long time. This intuitive and somatic sense of wholeness is often deeply rooted in a spiritual and transpersonal dimension. Aldous Huxley called this intrinsic wisdom the perennial philosophy: "The world is poetical intrinsically and what it means is simply itself. Its significance is the enormous mystery of its existence and of our awareness of its existence."

## RECLAIMING WHOLENESS: CRYING OUT

The root of the word reclaim is Latin, *reclamare*, and means *to cry out*. The emotionally and spiritually rich Psalms of David give voice to this crying out:

**Psalm 86**

*Bow down Your ear, O Lord,*
*hear me;*
*For I am poor and needy.*
*Preserve my life, for I am holy;*
*You are my God;*
*Save Your servant who trusts in You!*
*Be merciful to me, O Lord,*
*For I cry to You all day long.*
*Rejoice the soul of Your servant,*
*For You, O Lord, are good,*

*and ready to forgive,*
*And abundant in mercy to all those*
*who call upon You.*

(King David, Old Testament)

In *Poetic Medicine: The Healing Art of Poem-making,* I follow the poem-making path of the late Roberta de Kay, a woman at midlife, coping with a diagnosis of advanced cancer. Like David, the psalmist, Roberta felt that at some especially painful stages of her journey the form of spiritual poetry modeled by the Psalms was the only way she could express her needs to God.

In a chapter I call "When God Sighs: Making Poems About Loss, Illness and Death," I have described how Roberta felt that David's *Psalms* gave her permission to wail. She started to write her own series of psalms that dealt with emotional and spiritual issues of her illness.

### Psalm 13

*Oh Lord, I am sinking in despair*
*fearing you have forgotten me.*
*How long will my mind be confused*
*and my heart in grief?*
*Turn towards me, mothering Healer, bring*
*light to move from despair before my*
*heart closes.*
*Gently comes your healing hand*
*across my mind bringing what was needed*
*before I knew myself.*
*Trust in your mercy opens my heart*
*and I realize again your grace.*
*I am richly renewed.*
*Your mercy is deeper than my despair.*

(Fox, 1997, p. 177)

After writing these psalms, Roberta began to write about subjects and experiences other than cancer. Poem-making was an important way for her to remember that she is much more than illness and, even more important, that her love of beauty and intense perceptions of life transcend that illness and are a more accurate description of who she really is and what she offers to the world.

Ray McGinnis, in his excellent book *Writing the Sacred: A Psalm Inspired Path to Appreciating and Writing Sacred Poetry,* discusses the therapeutic value of the psalm form:

The challenge of finding ways of expressing what we think and feel, and of revealing to the Holy One our joys, sorrows, dark nights of the soul, and our restoration, remains with us no matter what our age. Psalm-writing offers us one way to listen afresh to our experience in the present moment. While the spiritual moods and themes found in the Psalms can awaken us to our own story, writing new psalms can help us shed light on our contemporary situation, much like writing prayers can. (McGinnis, 2005, p. 15)

The sudden writing of a poem as an act of crying out by someone in grief—someone who has not written a poem since high school—suggests to me that writing poems is, at essence and beyond linguistic skill, a spontaneous, natural action, comparable to the function of our immune system and connected with healing. On any given morning in the dark at 2 a.m., someone is up and trying to find words for the unspeakable. The poet Phillip Levine describes this crying out with words that express the somatic and existential imperative of self-awareness:

> ... my
> jaws ache for release, for
> words that will say
>
> anything. I force myself
> to remember
> who I am, what I am, and
> why I am here...

(Levine, P., 1984, p. 22)

What Phillip Levine is writing about—that urge to express—has existed since humans could cry out. The Greek wisdom culture with its tragedies, the enlightened society of India with its deep immersion in Vedic scripture written in the vibratory language of Sanskrit, the insight of the poetic *Tao Te Ching* in China, Native American peoples with their spirit of interconnection—all use healing words and the creative imagination (metaphor, image, and symbol) as a way to prepare and sustain a healing container and cultivate an environment for the purpose of rebalancing the mental, physical, and spiritual aspects of being human.

Here is a story to illustrate how writing can create such a container, how it can be used as a catalyst for crying out within the frame of therapeutic work.

Cathy wrote the following poem at the age of 34. For several years, Cathy suffered from severe lower back pain that persisted despite various medical treatments. Cathy's need to "cry out" almost as David does in some of the Psalms was because of intense physical pain and her longing for relief from that pain.

When Cathy attended the workshop I gave with the guidance of my mentor and poetry therapy pioneer, Joy Shieman, she had not written a poem since high school. But that evening, in a 12-minute freewrite, she composed this poem:

> *Pain's terrorwide eye*
> *stares at me unblinking*
> *lidless*
> *as summer noontime sun.*
>
> *I barely dare to dream*
> *of escape.*
> *The eye might see my pluck*
> *and sear its stare*
> *into my back forever.*
>
> *Twinkling love-lit star eyes,*
> *motherlove my longing for your gaze*
> *shapes the faceless space*
> *I call my heart, breaks*
> *like fever, aches*
>
> *into my consciousness     mama, mama    pain*
> *is for heroes not little girls or grown women*
> *to bear      nowhere*
>
> *my shadeless heart to hide.*

(Fox, 1986, p. 15)

She begins—and it is important to say she *begins* with this poem—to give a name to what hurts. Cathy describes her pain in her own words. Her images are powerful and unmistakable: The pain is relentless as a sun at high noon.

She uses the creative language and image of a "terrorwide eye" to describe feeling trapped by the pain, yet there is a longing to heal, a longing for the solace "twinkling love lit star eyes, motherlove" could provide. These words, *terrorwide* and *motherlove,* do not pass unnoticed through my spell checker because they are not dictionary words, they are made words, they are put together by the writer in a creative act, and through this creative act they become tremendously evocative, personal, and creative in their construction.

The Greek word for poetry is *poeisis,* which means *to make.* In creating this poem, Cathy begins to get a sense for herself as someone who makes, who creates. She is, by this definition, a poet and an artist. These images, when held in the container of the poem, have potency and meaning. The creative force of them, unhindered by attempts to explain this pain in a discursive way, allows for a breakthrough of speaking her truth to begin.

Through poetry, the discursive, intellectualizing mind drops into the intuitive, feeling heart (Levine, S., 1979). Here, a listener can connect more deeply, more empathically, with another's truth. Insight can begin to evolve from the level of honest feeling. The poem, when written on the page, can be returned to and reflected upon. The insights given voice by writing can be recognized and integrated over time. The poem becomes a vessel for discovery, a safe object that acts as a catalyst for self-disclosure, a place where empathy and insight can be shared.

At other times, once it is slammed down on the page, it may be appropriate simply to let the poem go, to discard the poem and go on. The poem may also be released more formally, in a kind of ritual, such as a fire ceremony, that honors the courage it took to write anything at all.

Cathy takes steps in her poem to call for help. She recognizes a need for solace. It is a way to begin to mother herself, to tend to her pain and offer herself greater care. Especially when it is spoken aloud, this poem expresses a force of longing that can break her fever.

Cathy uses vivid—even archetypal—images, makes line breaks and rhythms, joins words in powerful juxtaposition, calls upon a healing force that reminds us, as Morris R. Morrison says in his essay, "The Use of Poetry in the Treatment of Emotional Dysfunction," published in *Arts & Psychotherapy*, "Poetry is indeed a force, an act of human magic" (Morrison, 1978, p. 97).

## EMPATHY AND THE WHOLE BODY OF A POEM

Words like *container* and *vessel* are appropriate ways to describe a poem, but, really, the poem is like a body. In fact, as a tangible, made thing that is like a body, it has a shape that reveals insights and holds feelings, that has rhythm and movement. It has a permeable quality that allows the whole system to breathe. Poetic language, language that comes from the heart, has the potential, the natural ability, in fact, to circulate everywhere. The nuance of metaphor becomes a revived capillary that relieves numbness and returns feeling to one's life. Sometimes a poem acts as a system of both digestion and elimination.

Galway Kinnell says, "Writing a poem is like making an artifact. It is making something physical out of words." Stanley Kunitz says, "Poetry has a great digestive system and can consume and recycle almost anything" (Moyers, 1996, p. 244).

This body, full of movement, sound, breath, rhythm, sensory experience, meaning, and feeling, can allow this expression, this discovery, to make and take up a place in space. When spoken aloud, the poem is infused with breath—or sometimes the breath feels withheld—and words are spoken into the air. The poems reveal a somatically felt understanding—healing begins as fever breaks.

The key therapeutic factor is that the poem written by a person using it for healing and/or therapeutic purposes is rarely a finished product. What a poem offers to both client and poetry therapist when they attend to it is *a process* to discover renewing and unfolding layers of insight.

The poem on the page and spoken into the air is a laboratory to explore whole-body psychology. This is critical for understanding poetry therapy and for any poetry therapist or client to understand, so that critique and literary analysis are, in the context of the healing encounter, set aside.

What is not set aside is recognition that poetic elements, what I call "poetic medicine," help bring a poem alive, particularly through image and metaphor. As a poetry therapist, I am interested in introducing, by skillful means, these elements into the writing process. How do I do this? First, I have great faith that in a nonjudgmental environment much will come naturally to a person and to a group. Second, I believe it can also come through the example provided by preexisting poems.

## PREEXISTING POEMS AS CATALYST

Exploration of a preexisting poem (Mazza, 1999, p. 25) brings at least two benefits. The poem facilitates therapeutic discussion, and, secondarily, but with great benefit, without making it an intellectual exercise that will pull participants away from their feeling responses, a poem can help individuals get a handle on what kind of materials they can draw upon to create their own poetic palette of "colors."

Nicholas Mazza, professor of social work at University of Florida Tallahassee and author of *Poetry Therapy: Interface of the Arts in Psychology*, writes:

> The use of pre-existing poems for the purpose of prompting verbalization is often nonthreatening. Clients are invited to share their reactions to the poem as a whole or to a particular line or image. While ostensibly talking about a poem, inevitably the client reveals aspects of self. The external object provides a degree of security to the client. Poetry therapy, therefore, can promote engagement of the client in offering an element of control to the client by means of his or her interpretation of the poem. (Mazza, 1999, p. 25)

The client's or participant's engagement is not only with the poetry therapist and the group in the exploration of self and one's relationship to the world through the medium of the poem, but can also be an engagement with the self and the blank page upon which he or she may write through the recognition of metaphor, image, sound, and other poetic elements found in the poem. The poem can act as a catalyst to help individuals to find their own images. Preexisting poems are used to facilitate the finding of one's own creative voice.

Cathy's poem about the pain in her back employs compelling literary devices such as juxtaposition of words, metaphor, line break, spacing and symbol. In the therapeutic and healing environment, those are treated not as literary devices to analyze in an evaluative—good or bad—way, but as sacred material for healing work. This deep shift in relationship to artistic expression, this non-judgmental acceptance and, indeed, genuine curiosity and empathy required of the poetry therapist for both the poem and the poem maker, is essential to moving toward a healing outcome.

The poetry therapist will find that empathy is essential to facilitating that movement. What role does empathy play in responding to creative expression? How can empathy benefit the therapeutic process of creative expression?

## EMPATHY

The late Arleen Hynes, OSB and poetry therapist, created in 1976 the first study group for poetry therapy at St. Elisabeth's Hospital in Washington, DC. Hynes, perhaps the leading theorist in poetry therapy, writes in her classic *Biblio/Poetry Therapy: The Interactive Process. A Handbook,*

> Empathy is defined as the capacity to understand intellectually or imaginatively another's feelings or thoughts without actually experiencing them oneself. For the biblio/poetry therapist, this quality involves both the ability to *perceive* accurately what the participant feels and means and the capacity to communicate back to the participant an understanding and an acceptance of the other's private inner feelings and thoughts. Although not all theories of therapeutic communication stress empathy, we agree, for example, with that of Carkhuff (1969), who sees empathy as the variable "from which all other dimensions flow in the helping process." (Hynes & Hynes-Berry, 1986, p. 118)

I encouraged Cathy to work more with her poem. I specifically asked her if she would read her poem to the counselor she had just begun to see. She agreed to do this. Cathy reported the following about her poem, the writing of it, and her experience of sharing it with this therapist:

> Until I wrote this poem I did not know how much the constant pain had frightened me. I didn't know there could be words for the pain, because it felt like a disaster of unspeakable proportions. I remember taking the poem to a therapist whom I had sought out for help with the feelings that surrounded the knife-like pain which had persisted in my lower back.
>
> I felt self-conscious as I read this poem out loud to her, keeping my eyes on the paper. I hardly knew this person nor she me. We had met only once or twice before. When I looked up I saw tears filling her eyes, and in an instant, I fell headlong into a world I had felt separated from by intense physical pain; the world of being known, seen, understood and cared for.
>
> After writing this poem and reading it to this therapist, something changed. I didn't feel helplessly speechless about hurting even though I still had pain.
>
> Sometimes today, even years later, it is hard for me to tolerate seeing the nakedness of longing for comfort that I expressed in this poem, but when I push through my

embarrassment and share it anyway, people usually respond with deep understanding. So the not being alone is a world I keep getting to visit like a great gift that keeps on happening and surprising me. (Fox, 1997, p. 16)

The raw energy of her poem serves as a point of empathic connection with her therapist and provides an increased self-awareness resonant with the ideas of whole-person psychology. The privilege of caring for those who are ill and in need of support includes the great responsibility of speaking and listening in a healing way. Poetry is a great tool for learning more about and improving these skills of both speaking and listening.

## THE WORDS THE HEALER SPEAKS

This 1993 poem by Joseph Bruchac reminds us that the words a healer speaks matter. Bruchac's Abenaki heritage informs his worldview:

### The Remedies

*Half on the Earth, half in the heart,*
*the remedies for all the things*
*which grieve us wait for those who know the words to use to find them.*
*Penobscott people used to make*
*a medicine for cancer from Mayapple*
*and South American people knew*
*the quinine cure for malaria*
*a thousand years ago.*
*But it is not just in the roots,*

*the stems, the leaves,*
*the thousand flowers*
*that healing lies.*
*Half of it lives within the words*
*the healer speaks.*
*And when the final time has come*
*for one to leave this Earth*
*there are no cures,*
*for Death is only*
*part of Life, not a disease.*

*Half on the Earth, half in the heart,*
*the remedies for all our pains*
*wait for the songs of healing.*

Joseph Bruchac (Fox, 1997, p. 58)

It seems to many interested in the value of whole person psychology that—because of our reliance on technology, drugs, and a professional distance made more acute within the confines of a managed care system that does not take the nature of the human heart into much account—we have lost the connection to the earth wisdom that guides us to a deeper understanding and appreciation of what it means to *stay with* another person in a healing way and in a way where the poetry therapist, or any counselor, for that matter, can speak words that heal.

Psychologist Lauren Slater writes in her remarkable memoir *Welcome to My Country: A Therapist's Memoir of Madness,* says,

> Especially in this time of managed care, more emphasis seems to be placed upon medication and the quick amelioration of symptoms, short-term work and privatized, profit-making clinics, than upon the lovely and mysterious alchemy that comprises the cords between people, the cords that soothe some terrors and help us heal. (Slater, 1996, p. xiii)

Dr. Michael Okun, neurologist, Medical Director of the National Parkinson Foundation, and codirector of the Center for Movement Disorders at the University of Florida's Shands Hospital in Gainesville, says this about the value of art in a medical setting, in an exquisite documentary produced by Dr. David Watts, *Healing Words: Poetry & the Art of Medicine:*

> The interface between art and medicine is natural. It's always been there. The reason it has been there is because we don't have all the answers. So the doctor or the bedside physician is left to interpret to the best of his or her ability and help the patient to make very important and life-changing decisions. At the same time you are trying to deliver to that patient the best possible medical advice and the best possible medical care. But when you do that, you realize it is not a cookie-cutter approach—not everyone can have the same thing or needs the same thing to get better or to heal whether that means getting better or not getting better. Because of that you realize that the practice of medicine is an interface between art and medicine. Sometimes there is more art and other times more medicine—but if you leave one or the other out then you ultimately fail with your patient. (Watts, 2006)

The reason poetry and the other creative arts are currently peripheral as treatment modalities, when it comes to both mental and physical health, may have more to do with a serious misreading of the history and intention of healing than with any actual truth that their peripheral role is a result of better and more modern advancements. Australian poet Judith Wright makes her fierce point about this:

> Since poetry has so small an audience, the notion has begun to grow up that it is a kind of survival from more primitive times, a form of communication no longer needed by modern man. The fact is rather that modern man is something like a survival of poetry, which once shaped and interpreted his world through language and the creative imagination. When poetry withers in us, the greater part of experience and reality wither too; and when this happens, we live in a desolate world of facts, not of truth—a world scarcely worth the trouble of living in. (Wright, 1983, p. 10)

## WHAT CHILDREN BRING: A FRAGILE GIFT

Children, generally speaking, through their willingness to play, mess around, experiment, through their lack of cynicism and/or sense of irony, through their sheer enjoyment and pleasure in the sound of words, through flashes of wisdom that remind us of Wordsworth's line that children come "trailing clouds of glory," through a spirit of spontaneity, have a natural connection to creative language and the creative imagination.

Do you sense a magic charm inside this poem written by a first grader? I included this poem in my book *Poetic Medicine: The Healing Art of Poem-making:*

> *Inside a bubble*
> *There is a sea of petals*
> *And a wind of water*

Greta Weiss (Fox, 1997, p. 96)

And yet many children (and by this I also mean all the adults that I meet!) either withstand indifference to their voices, are denied the faith to support their words and the encouragement that their words matter, experience criticism, or have to survive the intense intellectual scrutiny whose supposedly "educational" glare is too bright and inappropriate to appreciate the more intuitive, heartfelt, imaginative, somatic, rhythmic, and even symbolic relationship with language that may well begin in the womb and when a baby is breast-feeding or rests his or her head next to the steady sound of the mother's heart.

Joost A. M. Meerloo, MD, anthologized in *Poetry As Healer: Mending the Troubled Mind,* edited by Jack Leedy, MD, wrote in his seminal poetry therapy essay "The Universal Language of Rhythm":

> Observation of fetal movements as reaction to sounds, combined with the knowledge that amniotic fluid is a better sound conductor than air, makes the existence of a prenatal syncopated rhythmic sound world more than likely. We can imitate the whole physical uterine plant and reproduce the various sounds in this experiential setting by holding the head under water and hearing the pre-birth world. This experiment makes it easier to understand why there is in later life such a strong universal spontaneous reaction to syncopated music. The fact is that an old mnemonic pattern has been invoked with all its unconscious associations with previous nirvanic joys. (Meerloo, in Leedy, 1985, p. 6)

And, further, he wrote

> Rhythm can completely revolutionize our body system. Rhythm is the integration of chaotic inner and outer events into one's own "musical" experience. (Meerloo, in Leedy, 1985, p. 15)

So much depends on how we listen and the kind of questions we ask children at this time when their creative voice is in bud. Criticism can wound a child's connection with his creative spark for the rest of his life. Any creative arts therapist is especially aware of and sensitive to these stories. We know that welcoming gestures of curiosity and believing in a child, as expressed in open-ended questions or mirroring lines of a child's poem and in appreciation for what is shared, can create for the child an entirely different experience whose effects can last a lifetime.

Barbara McEnerney's poem, "As They Are," is very helpful when I want to reach that creative place in people's hearts and get them to talk about their experience about wounds to their creative spirit and how they feel about expressing themselves creatively. The poem offers this exploration: What happened to you as a child when you expressed yourself creatively?

Barbara's poem addresses the issue of self-criticism. It opens the door for the wounds experienced through the disregard of others, whether that came from teachers or parents, to be shared. It also reflects, through an image like "rambling along" a "weedy path" on the joys and blessings of "foolin' with words" (Moyers, 1999). I ask people: When you read and hear *As They Are*, what lines attract you the most? Which images in this poem speak to your feelings and attitudes about your own creativity?

## As They Are

*And what if my words,*
*my fledgling poems,*
*were children, were toddlers*
*trying first steps,*
*tumbling, skinning knees,*
*squealing with glee,*
*splashing mud,*
*making a mess,*
*discovering themselves?*

*Would I hold them*
*at arm's distance,*
*disown them, hide them,*
*say what I imagine*
*others will think—*
*that, after all, they*
*really aren't very good?*

*And could that be*
*a way of protecting them—*
*shielding, holding back?*

*I know the mockery*
*odd children can face.*

*Instead, could I let*
*them ramble along weedy*
*paths only they know?*
*Lean close to hear*
*them whisper secrets,*
*learn what they*
*need from me?*
*Could I love them*
*as they are,*
*give them room*
*to grow, a chance*
*to shine?*

Barbara McEnerney (1997)

What can children show us adults about exploring our creativity? One day, working in a classroom of fifth graders, I asked the children to choose from among a table full of common everyday items and make a poem. I was inviting them to approach these "everyday" objects with some freshness and curiosity. The objects included a pair of running shoes, a bouquet of flowers, a skillet, and a bar of soap. Elizabeth chose the soap bar, and, after some encouragement through hearing a poem by Pablo Neruda called "Ode to My Socks," she applied to a blank page her own imagination, senses, intuition, and experience. Within a few minutes, her poem emerged in exactly the shape it is presented here:

### Bar of Soap

*The bar of soap*
*is so much more*
*than it appears*
*to be. The little*
*package washes*
*you clean, like*
*a dream, the*
*slightest sound*
*can wash it away.*
*Its shape and*
*size make all*
*the difference.*
*It has no*
*outer shell.*
*Just smooth*
*white slippery*
*solid. Dreams*
*do not require*
*a shell. Nothing*

*protects them.*
*There is nothing*
*to break through.*
*You fall asleep*
*the dream is there,*
*you pour the*
*water over*
*it, the soap*
*substance*
*is there.*
*It appears*
*so little yet*
*does so*
*much.*

Elizabeth, fifth grade (Fox, 1997, pp. 62–63)

Recognition and respect for this child's creative voice can make a lifetime of difference. Such respect will help the child maintain access to his or her creativity as a source for lifelong learning, healing, and empowerment through creativity. While visiting a classroom of fourth graders in Fredericksburg, Texas, I was determined not to teach the children anything about poetry. I wanted instead to learn from them about poetry.

It was a strategy to help me develop trust between us, but my intention was based on the conviction I have that each person comes to this life with a creative spark and, further, an innate creative and unique sensibility about the world that comes from that creative spark. I believe the more that spark is met, encouraged, nurtured, and celebrated at a young age, the greater is the possibility for a person to maintain a connection with it throughout his or her lifespan.

I asked the children this question: "What would human beings lose in our world if we did not have poetry?" Within 10 seconds I received these exact answers and in this order from both boys and girls:

**Feeling**          **Imagination**          **Music**          **Memory**

What a deep range of responses! What a high bar that had set for me! They were, at the age of nine, already tuned in to the essentials of both poetry and the values of a rich inner life. They deserve so much and have so much to give! I want those children to have continuing access to this awareness when they reach midlife.

## WHEN SOMEONE DEEPLY LISTENS

What is the standard of excellence for which all poetry therapists should strive? There is first the difficult to describe, but absolutely clear, commitment to deeply listen to a client or group of people. Listening happens best—and, really, only—when we are able to still the mind chatter and be present.

Deep listening, Taoistic in nature, which Abraham Maslow describes so well, is a foundation upon which trust can be built. Maslow writes:

> In order to be able to hear the fact-voices, it is necessary to be very quiet, to listen very receptively—in a Taoistic fashion. That is, if we wish to permit the facts to tell us their oughtiness, we must learn to listen to them in a very specific way which can be called Taoistic—silently, hushed, quietly, fully listening, noninterfering, receptive, patient, respectful of the matter-in-hand, courteous to the matter-in-hand. (Maslow, 1971, p. 120)

What the arts provide, and poetry as healer and poem-making certainly offers, is a container that makes this deep listening clear. It begins to feel like the spiritual practice of giving witness. This listening is not static. I believe it is more than even positive regard, as powerful as that is. Listening is a verb that is alive.

I believe trust is nurtured, deepens, and grows in this gradual, unfolding quality of listening. Listening permeates the healing container with a silence that honors and sacralizes the space in which the relationship takes place. This woven quality of silence and listening is important for both client and therapist because it is generative (Ueland, 1938) of the creative process, and that generativity contributes to self-discovery, especially in the context of the creative arts.

Poetry therapists also learn the value of empathic silence. Both the facilitator and other group members may find quiet sympathy to be the best acknowledgement of a deeply felt statement or a painfully won insight. Of course, empathic silence may be accompanied by other nonverbals such as a nod, a murmur, or, if appropriate, a light touch (Hynes & Hynes-Berry, 1986, p. 162).

Twenty-two years ago, when I was first working at El Camino Hospital in Mountain View, California, with the great pioneer in poetry therapy, Joy Shieman, I asked myself, "How can I listen better?" And this poem came to me.

### When Someone Deeply Listens To You

*When someone deeply listens to you*
*it is like holding out a dented cup*
*you've had since childhood*
*and watching it fill up with*
*cold, fresh water.*
*When it balances on top of the brim,*
*you are understood.*
*When it overflows and touches your skin,*
*you are loved.*

*When someone deeply listens to you,*
*the room where you stay*
*starts a new life*
*and the place where you wrote*
*your first poem*
*begins to glow in your mind's eye.*
*It is as if gold has been discovered!*

*When someone deeply listens to you,*
*your bare feet are on the earth*
*and a beloved land that seemed distant*
*is now at home within you.*

John Fox

## BEAUTY AND THE NEWS

*It is difficult to get the news from poems,*
*yet men die miserably every day*
*for lack of what is found there.*
William Carlos Williams (1969, from "Asphodel, That Greeny Flower")

What responsibility do we, as people committed to helping others, have if not to help provide an environment where the creative expression of feeling, imagination, music, and memory can be used to heal, inform, and help renew our human experience? The creative arts are one of the best ways I know to create such an environment.

If I read the newspaper, I find that horrendous loss is written in our headlines of war, poverty, environmental degradation, business corruption, and religious discord. What will feed us as human beings is not found in the empty calories of the political or market-manipulated sound bite. And I believe this profound loss of, and subsequent longing for, meaning, a treasure so difficult to find in our consumer culture, shows up in clients in our offices and participants in workshops, is presented by those in drug and alcohol rehab centers, and is felt acutely by patients in our hospitals dealing with illnesses and by so many others in need.

What pediatrician William Carlos Williams is saying is that the "news" of poetry is a language uniquely suited to helping a person to recognize two imperatives: to value what's true and to appreciate our capacity as human beings to savor beauty (Williams, 1969). The poetry therapist recognizes this, too:

The poetry therapist looks for literature that is universal enough, beautiful enough, profound but true enough to touch each individual in a group; he or she also facilitates the discussion to make the most of the material's potential. Ultimately, however, recognition cannot be programmed. The human heart is too singular. (Hynes & Hynes-Berry, 1986, p. 30)

John Wright, retired endocrinologist, wrote a poem that looks at the healing sources that helped him deal with and overcome depression. It comprises his recognizing:

> *his truth and appreciation*
> *the value of human warmth and touch in healing*
> *that beauty is integral to his wellbeing.*

He dedicates this poem to his psychiatrist:

### Therapy

*to Phillip*

*You attribute my recovery*
*to nor trip tyline—*
*its effects on neurotransmitters,*
*on the a myg dala.*

*You barely nod towards your worth—*
*insisting on blood levels,*
*on a therapeutic dose.*

*While I credit half our success*
*to pear trees blossoming white*
*beyond your left shoulder,*

*to the wisteria—*
*its pink flowers hanging*
*lush and fragrant*
*over the portico,*

*to the warmth of your hand.*

John Wright, MD (2005, p. 43)

John uses scientific words he is familiar with, *amygdala* and *nortriptyline,* and he brings to them a creative voice, rather than merely a clinical designation. He approaches these words playfully by writing them out in syllables. He calls attention to them in this way, helping a reader to enter these words, showing them as a kind of music.

> *nor trip tyline    a myg dala*

More importantly, John recognizes that beauty—through the powerful image of lush pear trees, blossoming wisteria, and the empathy felt in the warmth of Phillip's hand—make a great difference in his therapy. "I credit half our success," he says. He wants his psychiatrist to know this. He would like him to notice, too.

The malleable nature of words being placed on the page (because you can change words, rearrange them) gives a poem its unique form, a creative shape. A poem is where one does not have to write all the way across the page (Stafford, 1978). That allows John to put that very last line on its own, in its own space, giving the warmth of that hand greater depth and recognition.

It is difficult not to be touched by the compelling loveliness of this language, which is what Plato is speaking of when he uses that word *sophrosyne*, "beautiful language," as something "that can return stability and integration to psychic life" (Morrison, 1978).

James Hillman, in his fine book *The Soul's Code: In Search of Character and Calling*, says beauty is given short shrift in psychological practice and ought instead to be an integral and valuable part of psychology and of the therapeutic encounter:

> The longing in the human heart for beauty must be recognized by the field that claims the human heart to be its province. Psychology must find its way back to beauty, if only to keep itself alive. (Hillman, 1996, p. 38)

Hillman speaks fiercely about what the loss of beauty in therapy or disregard of it by psychology has meant:

> ...psychology, without beauty becomes victim of its own cognitive strictures, all passion spent in pushing for publication and position. Without beauty, there's little fun and less humor. (Hillman, 1996, p. 36)

Again, Arleen Hynes says:

> Where beauty is perceived an integration of self takes place. The integrated personality by definition, has achieved the ability to be—free from the need to possess, to want, to demand for self alone. The same kind of freedom characterizes the recognition of beauty and makes it an integrating experience. (Hynes & Hynes-Berry, 1986, p. 27)

Western medicine and psychology increasingly recognize the arts as a valuable tool for tending to our wounds and expressing ourselves as whole persons. Bringing together the healing arts, and, in the case of this chapter, poetry, is a way to treat a full range of mental health problems, and it offers each person an opportunity to express truth, beauty, and meaning.

While beauty and meaning do not represent everything necessary for healing or to support the needs of a whole person, they do speak to what psychotherapy and the medical field in general could use more of. What ancient cultures once knew about treating the whole person is coming alive again through the creative healing arts.

## WHERE DID POETRY THERAPY OF TODAY BEGIN?

> We human beings are at our best when we enjoy poetry. Sometimes all you need is
> to reflect in your mind one poem that says, "I can make it through."
>
> —Maya Angelou

In the mid-seventeenth century an American physician named Benjamin Rush introduced poetry as a form of therapy at Pennsylvania Hospital. We don't know exactly what form "poetry therapy" took at that time, but the very use of poetry to treat mental illness is an indication that, from a very early time in psychology, practitioners have recognized the power of words to heal. Over 250 years later, poetry therapy is still employed at Pennsylvania Hospital.

In the late 1920s, a Brooklyn pharmacist named Eli Greifer included poems or "poetic prescriptions" with the medicinal prescriptions people had him fill. Greifer recognized that truth, beauty, and meaning could make a difference in the life of his customers.

In 1928 he opened the "Remedy Rhyme Gallery" in Greenwich Village in New York City. Greifer believed that memorization of poems was particularly useful for a process of healing he called "psychosurgery." He believed it was possible to "psychograft" or, through memorization, integrate the thoughts and feelings of great people into one's own psyche. Methods of poetry therapy have developed and expanded since Greifer's time, but in discussing his "psychografting" memorization technique, in speaking of the elements of poetry, Greifer sounds more like shaman than pharmacist:

> We have here no less than a psychograft by memorization in the inmost reaches of
> the brain, where the soul can allow the soul-stuff of stalwart poet-prophets to "take"
> and to become one with the spirit of the patient.
>
> Here is insight. Here is introjection. Here is ennoblement of the spirit of man...by
> blood transfusing the personality with the greatest insights of all the greatest souled
> poets of all ages...beautiful figures of speech, the melody of rhythm and meter and
> assonance...painted scenes...dramatic episodes, love's pervasiveness—all are conse-
> crated by the master poets to gently enter and transfuse the ailing subconscious, the
> abraded and suffering personality. (Greifer, 1963, p. 2)

In 1958, Eli Greifer met Dr. Jack Leedy, who was the directing psychiatrist at Cumberland Hospital in Brooklyn, New York, where Dr. Leedy worked most frequently with people suffering from drug addiction. It was an auspicious meeting for the future of poetry therapy. Leedy, inspired by Greifer's ideas and ignoring the disdain of many colleagues, became an ardent advocate for the use of poetry in therapy.

Jack Leedy was, through his compassion, charm, and drive, a major force in bringing the use of poetry to the attention of the mental health profession. Dr. Leedy founded the Association for Poetry Therapy in 1969.

Sherry Reiter, director of the Creative Righting Center in Brooklyn, a clinical social worker and registered poetry therapist, was a colleague of Dr. Leedy's in the mid-1970s. She recalls with some amusement her first meeting with him:

> Jack encouraged me to go to the United Nations and invite each embassy to the next National Poetry Therapy Conference, feeling that in fact the conference was meant to be a World Poetry Therapy Conference. He was so convincing that I *almost* did it! I have, however, become deeply involved in this work since that time. (Reiter, in Fox, 1997, p. 215)

Many others besides Leedy and Greifer have done important pioneering work in this healing art since the mid-1950s. These practitioners include Arthur Lerner, MD, Morrison R. Morrison, PhD, and Doris Gendelman, CPT. My mentor, Joy Shieman, RPT, is also one of those pioneers. She began her groundbreaking work on the mental health wing at El Camino Hospital in Mountain View, California in 1962, long before poetry therapy was a recognized field of practice.

Sherry Reiter, RPT, recalls an historic milestone of the poetry therapy movement:

> By 1980 poetry therapy as a healing tool was flourishing in different parts of the country. In order to unite everybody and share our collective wisdom, I called a gathering at the New School for Social Research, the place I had earlier taught courses with Dr. Leedy. It was incredible to call together such a diverse group of people. (Reiter, 1997, in Fox, p. 215)

In 1981, the association further developed professional standards for ethics, training, and certifications. Training is done by the Federation for Biblio/Poetry Therapy. The membership organization is called The National Association for Poetry Therapy. Funding for poetry therapy projects is provided by the National Association for Poetry Therapy Foundation. Association members comprise a wide range of professional experience, schools of therapy, educational affiliations, medical fields, pastoral care, artistic disciplines, and other areas of practice in both mental and physical health.

But in recognizing the significance of poetry as healer, the psychological community is not discovering something new. It is actually returning to its true home. James Hillman writes in Re-Visioning Psychology:

> Here I am working toward a psychology of soul that is based in a psychology of image. Here I am suggesting both a *poetic basis of mind* and a psychology that starts neither in the physiology of the brain, the structure of language, the organization of society, nor the analysis of behavior, but in the processes of imagination. (Hillman, 1992, p. xvii).

## TOOL KIT FOR CHANGE

### Role and Perspective of the Healthcare Professional

1. Poetry therapy is an interactive process with three essential components: literature, a trained facilitator, and the client.
2. A poetry therapist is a professional who is well grounded in psychology and literature, as well as group dynamics.
3. A poetry therapist creates a gentle, nonthreatening atmosphere where people feel safe and are invited to share feelings openly and honestly.

### Role and Perspective of the Patient/Participant

1. People have a natural capacity for expression; no previous experience with poetry is required, only a desire to discover and explore a creative space.
2. The hearing and writing of poems can act as a healing catalyst. Poem-making is a way to reclaim one's truth, feelings, and voice.
3. While writing expressively, the patient is encouraged to treat words as if they were paint, clay, or wood; to allow words to be a physical material to shape, mold, chisel, and blend. The goal is to liberate simple, seemingly ordinary words from the prison of habit and free those words to breathe fresh air together.

### Interconnection: The Global Perspective

1. Poetry therapists around the world effect positive change in the practice of religion and spirituality, medicine, healthcare, psychology, education, the reclaiming of indigenous traditions, community life, politics, social action, justice, environmental protection, and peacemaking.
2. Poem-making and the encouragement of the creative spirit help people to discover, consider, and integrate new and more useful ways of expression.

## REFERENCES

Elytis, O. (1995). *Open papers: Selected essays* (Olga Broumas & T. Begley, Trans.). Port Townsend: Copper Canyon.

Fox, J. (1997). *Poetic medicine: The healing art of poem-making.* New York: Putnam.

Gorelick, K. (1987). Greek tragedy and ancient healing: Poems as theater and Asclepian temple in miniature. *Journal of Poetry Therapy, 1*(1), 38–43.

Greifer, Eli. (1963). *Principles of poetry therapy.* New York: Poetry Therapy Center.

Hillman, J. (1992). *Re-visioning psychology.* New York: HarperCollins.

Hillman, J. (1996). *The soul's code: In search of character and calling.* New York: Random House.

Hynes, A. M., & Hynes-Berry, M. (1986). *Bibliotherapy: The interactive process. A handbook.* St. Cloud, MN: North Star Press.

Leedy, J. J. (Ed.). (1985). *Poetry as healer: Mending the troubled mind.* New York: Vanguard Press.

Levine, P. (1984). Selected poems. *Silent in America.* New York: Atheneum.

Levine, S. (1979). *A gradual awakening.* London: Rider & Co.

Levine, S. (1982). *Who dies? An investigation of conscious living and conscious dying.* Garden City, NY: Anchor Books.

Maslow, A. (1971). *The farthest reaches of human nature.* New York: Penguin Books.

Mazza, N. (1999). *Poetry therapy: Interface of the arts and psychology.* Boca Raton: CRC Press.

McEnerney, Barbara. (1997). "As They Are." Unpublished.

McGinnis, R. (2005). *Writing the sacred: A psalm-inspired path.* Kelowna, British Columbia, Canada: Woodlake.

Morrison, M. R. (1985) The use of poetry in the treatment of emotional dysfunction. *Arts in Psychotherapy, 5*(2), 60.

Moyers, B. (1996). *The language of life: A festival of poets.* New York: Doubleday.

Moyers, B. (1999). *Fooling with words: A celebration of poets and their craft.* New York: William Morrow.

Slater, L. (1996). *Welcome to my country.* New York: Random House.

Stafford, W. (1978). *Writing the Australian crawl: Views on the writer's vocation.* Ann Arbor: University of Michigan.

Ueland, B. (1938). *If you want to write: A book about art, independence and spirit.* New York: G. P. Putnam's Sons.

Watts, D., Baranow, J., Cavenaugh, J., Chaban, Vi., producers. Edited and Directed by Baranow, J., Cavenaugh, J. and Drewry, D. (2006). Film, DVD: *Healing words: Poetry & the art of medicine.* Mill Valley, CA: Ma Goose.

Williams, W. C. (1969). *Selected poems.* New York: New Directions.

Wright, J. (1982). *Epiphany journal: Nature and the poetic intuition.* San Francisco, CA: Epiphany Press.

Wright, J. L. (2005). *Beginning of love: Poems.* Edmonds, WA: Bluestone.

Chapter Ten

# SPIRITUALITY, HOPE, AND MUSIC THERAPY IN PALLIATIVE CARE

*David Aldridge, PhD*

Our spirit is the real part of us, our body its garment. A man would not find peace at the tailor's because his coat comes from there: neither can the spirit obtain true happiness from the earth just because his body belongs to earth.

—Khan (1979, p. 76)

Behind us all is one spirit and one life. How then can we be happy if our neighbour is not also happy?

—Khan (1979, p. 123)

I am taking the risk in this paper of using terms like *spirituality, hope,* and *creativity,* not commonly voiced in the world of medicine. However, palliative care has a tradition of breadth in its understanding of healthcare needs and we find throughout the medical and nursing literature that the spiritual needs of patients are mentioned. My argument is that a time has come when such considerations can be voiced within the culture of the creative arts therapies. It is a careful, sober consideration of spirituality that I want to elaborate upon here, linking the promotion of hope to working creatively with music. While accepting that society is built upon the foundation of science and art, it would be a folly to ignore those streams of thought that refer to the spirit of humankind. Within these pages I hope to demonstrate that talking about spirituality can be brought into the discourse of patient care. By ignoring a concern of the very patients with whom we work, we are failing to meet their needs.

What I am proposing is that, in working with the dying and the chronically ill, we need to consider that which helps us to transcend our daily lives. Note that I am not separating practitioners and patients here, for we all surely face the great questions of life: "What is the meaning of life, what is the nature of suffering, why me, what can I do?" Even though it is a fact that is often forgotten, we are all facing death and in doing so we are all asked the question of how to live.

When we look at our lives from the perspective of how to live, we are faced with a crisis. I am using *crisis* here in a broad sense, to mean a judgment or discernment. Indeed, the difficulty faced in caring for dying patients is that although the problem appears to be that of chronic illness, in reality the challenges are acute and appear as a series of crises (Alter, 1994). Each crisis with a dying patient is a matter of identity—"Who am I? What will become of me?" (Simon & Haney, 1993).

We now have two questions, one concerned with existence and one with identity, and these questions have been the fundamental questions of all spiritual traditions. The practical ramifications of these questions are related to how we care for each other and how we recognize each other's quality as a person. To answer these questions we need to be alive to a new consciousness (Atnally, 1993).

The main emphasis of spirituality has always been that it will help us to achieve this new consciousness by transcending the moment. So, too, with the concept of hope, there is the expectation of a leap forward. In music therapy this transcending, expectant leap is made through the creative act. Through creative play, we can distinguish the inner world of ourselves. In this sense, consciousness is realized by doing.

Creativity occurs in the realization of an idea as created form. In the same way that the thoughts and ideas presented here have their own architecture realized in words and, as the architecture of the cathedral is realized in stone, the architecture of music is realized in sounds. We can also be the architects of hope. By transcending the moment of suffering, a new consciousness is created. This new consciousness is realized concretely in the performance of music. We sing and play what we are. There is no precocious need to identify this as an emotional experience, rather to savor the experience in the moment itself.

Perhaps it is important to state here the main idea underlying my thinking regarding music. Our human identity is that of a piece of symphonic music continually being composed in the moment. In contrast to a mechanistic metaphor of humanity that sees the body as an entity to be repaired, this view sees each being as vital and open to creation. We are improvised as a fresh identity according to every one of life's contingencies. Our very identities are created anew although the theme may be repeated, and it is this repetition that gives us coherence as a personality. Put another way, we are each a song that is continually being sung. What sings that song is a matter of personal belief.

Music therapy is an activity that promotes the expression of this song. Each person is given the opportunity to creatively define themselves as they wish to be.

What the person will become and how a personal future is defined, a future that is admittedly restricted and often tragically curtailed, are matters for joint therapeutic endeavor between therapist and patient (Aldridge, 1991b). The interaction between patient and therapist is creative in the sense that it is in interaction where momentary choices are made (Abra, 1994). It is possible to realize ourselves in the moment not solely as a body restricted by infirmity, but transcended as a soul realizable in the music. Even so, the end stage of our therapeutic endeavor is that the patient will die.

We know from clinical practice that the will to live is an important factor. Purpose and meaning in life are vital and all too often are not questioned when we are in good health. But should we fall ill, then purpose and meaning become crucial to survival. Illness may be seen as a step on life's way that brings us in contact with who we really are. The positive aspect of suffering has been neglected in our modern scientific culture so that we, as practitioners and patients, often search for immediate relief. Although the management of cancer pain has been a major contribution of the hospice movement, the understanding of suffering is still elusive in the literature. I am not suggesting that we actively seek out suffering or deny that pain is debilitating, rather to remind us that part of the human condition is indeed to suffer. In seeking to relieve suffering we can value the opportunity it brings to learn. It may well be that the difficulties reported in effectively relieving pain are the result of the failure to identify suffering.

We are all asked the ultimate question of what meaning and purpose our lives would have had if we were to die now. Most of our activities cut us off from this brutal confrontation except in the field in which we are working. Though the management of pain is often a scientific and technical task, the relief of suffering is an existential task. In the major spiritual traditions suffering has always had the potential to transform the individual. As Tournier (1981) reminded us, it is love that has the power to change the sign of suffering from negative to positive.

## WHAT IS SPIRITUALITY?

The natural science base of modern medicine often ignores the spiritual factors associated with health. Health invariably becomes defined in the anatomical or physiological, psychological, or social terms. Rarely do we find diagnoses that include the relationship between patients and their God. The descriptions we invoke have implications for the treatment strategies we suggest and the way in which we understand how people can be encouraged to become healthy. Patience, grace, prayer, meditation, hope, forgiveness, and fellowship are as important in many of our health initiatives as medication, hospitalization, incarceration, or surgery. It is these spiritual elements of experience that help us to rise above the matters at hand so that in the face of suffering we can find purpose, meaning and hope.

Working as a psychiatrist, Hiatt (1986) offered an understanding of the spiritual in medicine that can also be worked with in psychological terms. "Spirit refers to that non corporeal and non mental dimension of the person that is the source of unity and meaning, and 'spirituality' refers to the concepts, attitudes, and behaviours that derive from one's experience of that dimension." He suggested that by taking such a framework, we can discuss and use spiritual healing "within a modified western framework (of medicine)" (p. 742).

In recent years the word *spiritual* has appeared increasingly in the nursing literature (see table 1) where spiritual needs have been differentiated from religious needs (Boutell & Bozett, 1990; Burkhardt, 1989; Clark, Cross, Deane, & Lowry, 1991; Emblen, 1992; Grasser & Craft, 1984; Labun, 1988; May, 1992; Reed, 1987; Stuart, Deckro, & Mandle, 1989). Within these approaches there is a core of opinion that accepts suffering and pain as part of a larger life experience and that these, too, can have meaning for the patient and for the carer(s) (Nagai Jacobson & Burkhardt, 1989). The emphasis is placed upon persons' concept of God, sources of strength and hope, the significance of religious practices and rituals for the patients, and their belief system (Soeken & Carson, 1987). Spiritual well-being is also proposed as a hedge against suicide, providing some people with a reason for living (Ellis & Smith, 1991) and as a mediator of depression (Fehring, Brennan, & Kellar, 1987).

**Table 1.**
**Meanings of Spirituality**

| Author | Description |
| --- | --- |
| Emblen, J. (1992) | "…helping people to identify meaning and purpose in their lives, maintain personal relationships and transcend a given moment." |
| Hiatt, J. (1986) | "…that aspect of the person concerned with meaning and the search for absolute reality that underlies the world of the senses and the mind and, as such, is distinct from adherence to a religious system." |
| Kuhn, C. (1988) | "…those capacities that enable a human being to rise above or transcend any experience at hand. They are characterized by the capacity to seek meaning and purpose, to have faith, to love, to forgive, to pray, to meditate, to worship, and to see beyond present circumstances." |
| Smyth, P. (1988) | "…that life has a purpose, of the search for meaning, of the attempt to interpret their personal illness in a way that makes sense of their world view." |

Spirituality, characterized by the idea of transcendence, has a broader perspective than religion. Religious care means helping people maintain their belief systems and worship practices. Spiritual care helps people to maintain personal relationships and relationship to a higher authority, God, or life force (as defined by that individual), identify meaning and purpose in life, and transcend a given moment. This idea of transcendence, the ability to extend the self beyond the immediate context to achieve new perspectives, is seen as important in the last phases of life where dying patients are encouraged to maintain a sense of well-being in the face of imminent biological and social loss. Ross (1994) noted three necessary components to spirituality—the need to find meaning and purpose; the need for hope; and the need for faith in self, others, and God.

Reed's study (1987) of spirituality and well-being in terminally ill hospitalized patients hypothesized that terminally ill patients would indicate a significantly greater spiritual perspective than nonterminally ill hospitalized adults with problems that were not typically life-threatening and healthy nonhospitalized adults. For the terminally ill patients there was a shift toward greater spirituality, as indicated by a stronger faith and increased prayer.

Doctors, nurses, and clergy have worked together to care for the dying (Conrad, 1985; Reed, 1987; Roche, 1989), and a community approach that includes the families of the patients and their friends appears to be beneficial (Aldridge, 1987a). These benefits are a lessening of anxiety, general improvement in feelings of well-being, and an increasing spiritual awareness for the dying persons (Kaczorowski, 1989). In addition, comprehensive treatment programs for people with AIDS recommend that the spiritual welfare of the patients, and its influence on their well-being, be included (Belcher, Dettmore, & Holzemer, 1989; Flaskerud & Rush, 1989; Gutterman, 1990; Ribble, 1989).

It is not only for the dying that spirituality plays a role. For the widow who must adapt to the loss of a partner, the ability to express her spirituality can, along with other criteria, play an important role in enhancing well-being. For young and old groups of widows, attention to spiritual needs, physical exercise, and a willingness to be self-indulgent all contributed to satisfy emotional and sexual needs.

Spirituality and religion, then, appear to be meditating factors for coping with an impending loss of life and to be positive factors for maintaining well-being, particularly in older patients. When we consider patients in palliative care, it is appropriate to consider what we can also do for their families and friends. Our patients rarely die alone, and surely the caregivers (familial, filial, and professional) must be included for they, too, suffer and it is they, too, who must transcend the moment.

## MAINTAINING INTEGRITY AND HOPE

The true joy of every soul is in the realisation of the divine spirit; the absence of realisation keeps the soul in despair.

—Khan (1979, p. 105)

Positive emotions, which include the qualitative aspects of life—hope, joy, beauty and unconditional love—are known to be beneficial for the process of coping with the diagnosis of cancer during the course of treatment and for postoperative recovery. This realm of positive emotion is precisely the ground in which the creative arts generally can have their own being. Patients can express themselves in a way that is creative and not limited by their disease. From such a perspective we may expect that, although physical parameters may fluctuate or deteriorate, life-quality measures or existential indicators will show improvement.

A significant beneficial factor in enhancing the quality of life is hope. Hope has been identified as a multifaceted phenomenon that is a valuable human response even in the face of a severe reduction in life expectation. Yates (1993) offered six dimensions of hope: the sensations and emotions of expectancy and confidence, a cognitive dimension that comprises positive perceptions, a belief that a desired outcome is realistically possible, a behavioral dimension where patients act on their desires, a contextual dimension that links expectations with those of the family and friends, and a temporal dimension looking forward or even backward.

Hope was defined by the nurse-researcher Herth (1990) as an "inner power directed toward enrichment of 'being.'" With the exception of those diagnosed with AIDS, overall hope levels among subjects were high and were found to remain stable over time. Seven hope-fostering categories (interpersonal connectedness, attainable aims, spiritual base, personal attributes, light-heartedness, uplifting memories, and affirmation of worth) and three hope-hindering categories (abandonment and isolation, uncontrollable pain and discomfort, devaluation of personhood) were identified. Of the hope-fostering categories, we can translate six of them into activities pertinent to the creative music therapy situation (see table 2).

Hope, like prayer (Saudia, Kinney, Brown, & Young, 1991), is a coping strategy used by those confronted with a chronic illness that involves an expectation going beyond visible facts and is seen as a motivating force to achieve inner goals. These goals change. Although a distant future of life expectancy no longer exists for AIDS patients, life aims can be redefined and refocused. With the progression of physical deterioration, the future becomes less defined in terms of the body and time, but more defined in the meaning attached to life events in relationship with family and friends. In later stages there is a shift toward less concrete goals and a refocusing on

Table 2.
Dimensions for Fostering Hope

| Dimension of Hope* | Music Therapy Context |
| --- | --- |
| Interpersonal context, relationship with others | Therapeutic relationship |
| Beliefs and cognition, identifying attainable aims | |
| Spiritual base | Uplifting music, the traditional role of sacred music, transcending the moment |
| Personal attributes | Being creative, being musical |
| Light-heartedness | Play in therapy |
| Uplifting memories | Listening to music, playing and singing remembered songs |
| Affirmation of worth | Activity of mutual music making |

*After Herth (1990).

the self to include the inner peace and serenity necessary for dying (Herth, 1990).

The true meaning of hope is that of an inclination toward something that we do not know. There is a longing for the unknown. We are all waiting for a change, even if it is a material change of circumstance, and this expectation is hope. Such hope cannot be touched and often not understood. It is an attainment that may be described as beyond happiness and above death.

## MUSIC THERAPY AND THE CREATIVE ACT

Each individual composes the music of his own life. If he injures another he breaks the harmony, and there is discord in the melody of life.

—Khan (1979, p. 65)

Music therapy, with its ability to offer an experience of time that is qualitatively rich and not chronologically determined, is a valuable intervention. We are aware that music has soothing properties and is employed successfully as an anxiolytic (Aldridge, 1993a, 1993b). Yet music can also be inspiring and uplifting (see table 3). In its sacred practice, music has been used to transport the listener to other realms of consciousness and is used thusly in the final stages of dying (Schroeder-Sheker, 1993). Indeed, the power of music is that it has the ability to calm us or to stir us in so many dimensions (Khan, 1983).

Music therapy, with the potential for bringing form out of chaos, should offer hope in situations of seeming hopelessness and, therefore, a means of transcendence. This idea of transcendence, the ability to extend the self beyond the immediate context to achieve new perspectives, is seen as important in the

**Table 3.**
**Different Dimensions of Music**

| | |
|---|---|
| Popular | Inducing motions of the body |
| Technical | Satisfying the intellect |
| Artistic | Tending toward beauty and grace |
| Appealing | Piercing the heart |
| Uplifting | Enabling the soul to hear the harmony of the spheres |

last phases of life where dying patients are encouraged to maintain a sense of well-being in the face of imminent biological and social loss. Even in the midst of suffering it is possible to create something that is beautiful. This aesthetic expectation of self-in-relationship is positive; it is hope made manifest.

Significantly for many AIDS patients, personal relationships are deteriorating. Either friends die of the same illness or social pressures urge an increasing isolation. Spontaneous contacts are frowned upon and the intimacy of contact is likely to be that of the clinician rather than the friend. Music therapy offers an opportunity for intimacy within a creative relationship.

This relationship is both nonjudgmental and equal. The patient is encouraged to creatively form a new identity that is aesthetic even in the face of disfigurement.

Working together in a creative way to enhance the quality of living can help patients make sense of dying (Aldridge, 1987b, 1987c). It is important for the dying, or those with terminal illness, that approaches that integrate the physical, psychological, social, and spiritual dimensions of their being are used (Feifel, 1990; Gary, 1992; Herth, 1990). In addition, how we care for the sick and dying, no matter how they contracted their disease, is a matter of our own personal responsibility and a collective measure of our humanity (Aldridge, 1987a, 1987b, 1991a, 1991b).

In music therapy, patients are required to be active self-defining agents. The requirement is that they are moral (i.e., actively partaking and self-defining) when they are sick and suffering, not that they be subjected to our morality and definition.

Music therapy, with its emphases on personal contact and the value of the patients as creative productive human beings, has a significant role to play in the fostering of hope. Hope involves feelings and thoughts and requires action (i.e., like music, it is dynamic and susceptible to human influence). Stimulating the awareness of living, in the face of dying, is a feature of the hospice movement where being becomes more important than having. The opportunity, offered by music therapy, for patients to be remade anew in the moment, to assert an identity that is aesthetic, in the context of another person, separate yet not abandoned, is an activity invested with that vital quality of hope. Hope, when submitted to the scrutiny of the psychologist and not conforming to an established reality, can easily be interpreted as denial. For the therapist, hope is a replacement for therapeutic nihilism, enabling us to offer constructive effort and sound expectations (Menninger, 1959).

Any therapeutic tasks must concentrate on the restoration of hope, accommodating feelings of loss, isolation, and abandonment, understanding suffering, forgiving others, accepting dependency while remaining independent, and making sense of dying. Music therapy can be a powerful tool in this process of change. Change can be accommodated within the overall rubric "quality of life." Although the elusive life qualities inherent in creative activities—joy, release, satisfaction, simply being—are not readily susceptible to rating scales; we can hear them when they are played and feel them when they are expressed.

Music therapy appears to open up a unique possibility to take an initiative in coping with disease or to find a level to cope with near death. It is this opening up of the possibilities that is at the core of existential therapies (Dreyfus, 1987). Rather than patients living in the realm of pathology alone, they are encouraged to find the realm of their own creative being—and that is in the music.

## CONCLUSION

If the progress of disease is an increasing personal isolation, then the music-therapeutic relationship is an important one for maintaining interpersonal contact, a contact that is morally nonjudgmental, where the ground of that contact is aesthetic. For the sick, maimed, disfigured, and stigmatized, the opportunity to partake in a greater beauty is important. Furthermore, the therapeutic question is not, "What am I?" (a question that lies in the realm of categorization and cognition), but "How am I?" (which is one of being).

It is necessary to emphasize how important it is to keep our idea of creativity broad. A patient, when asked about the values of the various arts therapies he had recently had, commented, "I did not want to be so intensely creative (as in the art therapy), but I did enjoy the music therapy where I could sing." If being creative is used as a metaphor for new growth and understood solely in its material implications, no wonder that it will be rejected by some patients for whom new growth is a sign of a deterioration in health. Creativity can be used in the nonmaterial sense, as in making music, as transcending the moment. In this transcendence, the essence of spirituality, we take a leap, which is hope, into a new consciousness. That this new consciousness is not bound up with our bodies, our instincts, our motor impulses, nor our emotions, awakens our awareness to another purpose within us.

Finally, in our treatment initiatives and research projects, it appears prudent to include the caregivers of the patients. Although this may be alien to some individual therapeutic directions, the overwhelming burden of care and suffering of daily living lies outside the clinic. If we consider the course of life, which includes dying, as a developmental process, that process will have a personal ecology. This ecology is relationship.

To return from where I began, when hospice care becomes necessary, we must include ourselves and colleagues, too, in that ecology as we accompany our patients, in faith and hope, on that long journey that awaits us all.

## REFERENCES

Abra, J. (1994). Collaboration in creative work: An initiative for investigation. *Creativity Research Journal, 7*(1), 1–20.

Aldridge, D. (1987a). Families, cancer and dying. *Family Practice, 4,* 212–218.

Aldridge, D. (1987b). A team approach to terminal cam: Personal implications for patients and practitioners. *Journal of the Royal College of General Practitioners, 37,* 364.

Aldridge, D. (1987c). *One body: A guide to healing in the Church.* London: Society for the Propagation of Christian Knowledge.

Aldridge, D. (1991a). Meaning and expression: The pursuit of the aesthetics in research. *Holistic Medicine, 5,* 177–186.

Aldridge, D. (1991b). Spirituality, healing and medicine. *Journal of British General Practice, 41,* 425–427.

Aldridge, D. (1993a). Music therapy research I. A review of music therapy research as presented in the medical literature. *The Arts in Psychotherapy, 20*(1), 11–35.

Aldridge, D. (1993b). The music of the body. Music therapy in medical settings. *Advances, 9*(1), 17–35.

Alter, C. (1994, February). Redefining hope in the second decade of AIDS. A psychiatrist's experience. *Aids Patient Care,* 2–5.

Atnally, R. (1993). The human trinity: The three consciousnesses of man. *The Mankind Quarterly, 34*(1&2), 3–26.

Belcher, A., Dettmore, D., & Holzemer, S. (1989). Spirituality and sense of well-being in persons with AIDS. *Holistic Nurse Practitioner, 3*(4), 16–25.

Boutell, K., & Bozett, F. (1990). Nurses' assessment of patients' spirituality: Continuing education implications. *J-Confin-Educ-Nurs., 21*(4), 172–176.

Burkhardt, M. (1989). Spirituality: An analysis of the concept. *Holistic Nurse Practitioner, 3*(3), 69–77.

Clark, C. C., Cross, I. R., Deane, D. M., & Lowry, L. W. (1991). Spirituality: Integral to quality care. *Holistic Nurse Practitioner, 5*(3), 67–76.

Conrad, N. (1985). Spiritual support for the dying. *Nursing Clinics of North America, 20*(2), 415–426.

Dreyfus, H. (1987). Foucault's critique of psychiatric medicine. *The Journal of Medicine and Philosophy, 12,* 311–333.

Ellis, J. B., & Smith, P. C. (1991). Spiritual well-being, social desirability and reasons for living: Is there a connection? *International Journal of Social Psychiatry, 37*(1), 57–63.

Emblen, J. D. (1992). Religion and spirituality defined according to current use in nursing literature. *Journal of Professional Nursing, 8*(1), 41–47.

Fehring, R., Brennan, P., & Keller, M. (1987). Psychological and spiritual well-being in college students. *Researching Nurse Health, 10*(6), 391–398.

Feifel, H. (1990). Psychology and death. Meaningful rediscovery. *American Psychologist, 45*(4), 537–543.

Flaskerud, J., & Rush, C. (1989). AIDS and traditional health beliefs and practices of black women. *Nursing Research, 38*(4), 210–215.

Gary, G. A. (1992). Facing terminal illness in children with AIDS. Developing a philosophy of care for patients, families, and caregivers. *Home Health Nurse, 10*(2), 40–43.

Grasser, C., & Craft, B. (1984). The patient's approach to wellness. *Nursing Clinics of North America, 19*(2), 207–218.

Gutterman, L. (1990, March). A day treatment program for persons with AIDS. *American Journal of Occupational Therapy, 44*(3), 234–237.

Herth, K. (1990). Fostering hope in terminally-ill people. *Journal of Advanced Nursing, 15*(11), 1250–1259.

Hiatt, J. (1986). Spirituality, medicine, and healing. *Southern Medical Journal, 79*(6), 736–743.

Kaczorowski, J. (1989). Spiritual well-being and anxiety in adults diagnosed with cancer. *Hospital Journal, 5*(3–4), 105–116.

Khan, I. (1979). *The bowl of Saki.* Geneva: Sufi.

Khan, I. (1983). *The music of life.* Santa Fe, NM: Omega Press.

Kuhn, C. (1988). A spiritual inventory of the medically ill patient. *Psychiatric Med., 6*(2), 87–100.

Labun, E. (1988). Spiritual care: An element in nursing care planning. *Journal of Advanced Nursing, 13*(3), 314–320.

May, C. (1992). *Individual* care? Power and subjectivity in therapeutic relationships. *Sociology, the Journal of the British Sociological Association, 26*(4), 589–602.

Menninger, K. (1959). Hope. *The American Journal of Psychiatry, 116*(12), 481–491.

Nagai Jacobson, M., & Burkhardt, M. (1989). Spirituality: Cornerstone of holistic nursing practice. *Holistic Nurse Practitioner 3*(3), 18–26.

Reed, P. (1987). Spirituality and well-being in terminally ill hospitalized adults. *Researching Nurse Health, 10*(5), 335–344.

Ribble, D. (1989). Psychosocial support groups for people with HIV infection and AIDS. *Holistic Nurse Practitioner, 3*(4), 52–62.

Roche, J. (1989). Spirituality and the ALS patient. *Rehabilitation Nursing, 14*(3), 139–141.

Ross, L. (1994). Spiritual aspects of nursing. *Journal of Advanced Nursing, 19,* 439–447.

Saudia, T. L., Kinney, M. R., Brown, K. C., & Young, W. L. (1991). Health locus of control and helpfulness of prayer. *Heart Lung, 20*(1), 60–65.

Schroeder-Sheker, T. (1993). Music for the dying: The new field of music thanatology. *Advances, 9*(1), 36–48.

Simon, W., & Haney, C. A. (1993). The postmodernization of death and dying. *Symbolic Interaction, 16*(4), 411–426.

Smyth, P., & Bellemare, D. (1988). Spirituality, pastoral care and religion: The need for clear distinctions. *Journal of Palliative Care, 4,* 86–88.

Soeken, K., & Carson, V. (1987). Responding to the spiritual needs of the chronically ill. *Nursing Clinics of North America, 22*(3), 603–611.

Stuart, E., Deckro, J., & Mandle, C. (1989). Spirituality in health and healing: A clinical program. *Holistic Nurse Practitioner, 3*(3), 35–46.

Tournier, P. (1981). *Creative suffering.* London: SCM Press.

Yates, P. (1993). Towards a reconceptualization of hope for patients with a diagnosis of cancer. *Journal of Advanced Nursing, 18,* 701–706.

## Chapter Eleven

# EXPRESSIVE DANCE, WRITING, TRAUMA, AND HEALTH: WHEN WORDS HAVE A BODY

*Anne M. Krantz, PhD, ADTR and James W. Pennebaker, PhD*

The impact of trauma and stressful life events on psychological and physical health has been a focus of clinicians and researchers since the time of Freud. Complex relationships between extreme states of emotional stress and common mental and physical health problems suggest a need for models that integrate mind and body. The art of dance originates in human experience that is not primarily verbal, where movements tell a story for which language has no words. The approach of dance therapy (Evan & Rifkin-Gainer, 1982) uses nonverbal and verbal expression to contain, express, and regulate strong emotional states. The capacity to tolerate, reflect on, and express previously repressed or inhibited emotion and thought appears central to coping with stressful life events. There is reason to believe that when people integrate multiple levels of stressful experience and express themselves in emotionally meaningful ways, they not only feel better but also improve on a number of psychological and physical indices.

Traumatic life experiences and emotional upsets can profoundly impact the individual's physical, emotional, and mental health at all stages of life. In infancy, the experience of disruptive, intrusive, and upsetting interactions with caregivers leads to intense dysregulation of physiological and emotional states that correspond with neurological and structural changes affecting development of the self and subsequent emotional and cognitive resilience (Schore, 2003). Young children who witness domestic violence are at risk for developing post-traumatic stress disorder (PTSD) with long-term negative effects on emotional, cognitive, social, behavioral, and self-development (Lieberman & Van Horn,

1998). Trauma researchers have noted that overwhelming experiences associated with extremely stressful and intense emotions are stored at a somatosensory level, such as visual images or physical sensations, and are expressed as changes in the biological stress response that are often impervious to conscious memory, cognitive organization, and integration by verbal means alone (Sykes Wylie, 2004; van der Kolk, 1994). If coping with traumatic experience relies on individual emotional resilience, the regulation of strong emotion, and a capacity for self-reflection of the experience, then approaches are needed that help people to process potentially overwhelming affects which impact their psychosomatic, emotional, cognitive, and behavioral functioning (Fonagy, Gergely, Jurist, & Target, 2002; van der Kolk, Roth, Pelcovitz, Sunday, & Spinazzola, 2005). The question of how to use both verbal and nonverbal methodologies to access extreme emotional states has been a concern to clinicians and researchers from diverse theoretical backgrounds.

Pennebaker (1997) has spent years investigating the influence of verbal disclosure of emotional upheavals on physical and mental health. He and others have repeatedly found that expressing thoughts and feelings through writing or talking about traumatic events and emotions has a beneficial effect on health. Many studies indicate that when people transform their experiences of emotional upheavals into language, they show significant improvements in a range of social, psychological, behavioral, and biological measures (Pennebaker & Chung, 2006). Efforts to understand the underlying mechanisms of why verbal expression affects health have led to many inquiries into linguistic, cognitive, situational, and personality factors. While no single reason has been found to explain the effectiveness of writing about trauma, the power of expression through words has been demonstrated repeatedly and convincingly (Pennebaker, 1993). The question remained whether nonverbal expression of emotion and active confrontation of life traumas, as occurs in dance/movement therapy, would have positive effects on health. In this context, dance is understood as a personal psychophysical expression, simultaneously psychological and physical, uniting feeling and thought through action (Krantz, 1993). In dance/movement therapy, nonverbal expression of experiences such as sensation, imagery, thought, and memory, leads toward outlet and awareness of feeling states, and their subsequent integration into verbal modes of cognition and expression.

The premise of this chapter is that dance therapy, as a model of clinical practice that integrates body and mind, has much to contribute to effective processing of emotionally stressful experience. Support for this premise will come from three sources: (1) an exploratory study (Krantz, 1993) that looked at the effects of expressive dance and writing on health within the theoretical paradigm developed by Pennebaker (1997); (2) three clinical vignettes illustrating how treatment integrating body and words is conducted; and (3) treatment implications of using both nonverbal and verbal interventions to promote health. Such an integration may be particularly indicated where effects of traumatic or stressful life events are affecting areas of the brain and body which are not accessible to or modulated by cognition or verbal expression (Schore, 2003; van der Kolk, 1994). Most models of psychotherapy have traditionally been oriented toward verbal expression and interaction, with little or no emphasis on direct bodily intervention. The body-oriented psychotherapies have primarily been oriented toward psychophysical intervention, with less attention to the use of words. The approach of Blanche Evan's dance/movement/word therapy (Evan & Rifkin-Gainer, 1982) emphasizes the importance of integrating both.

## TREATING TRAUMA

The act of confiding deeply personal feelings and thoughts in the context of a therapeutic relationship is basic to most psychotherapy approaches. Different models of psychotherapy, however, emphasize competing strategies based on their conceptual frameworks for how change occurs. Analytic and cognitive psychotherapies focus on changing emotional and cognitive states with talking and thinking about problems as a way of confronting and resolving them. These linguistically based processes emphasize the role of gaining insight into the traumatic experience in order to understand and correctly assimilate it. In the early psychoanalytic treatment of hysterical patients, Freud and Breuer (1895/1966) emphasized the role of emotional expression of repressed affect. They assumed that abreaction, the mental reliving of a situation, and catharsis would release traumatic memories, leading to conscious integration of the trauma and thus, symptom resolution.

Modern psychoanalytic technique has adopted a more limited view of the curative role of catharsis (Greenson, 1967), with a greater emphasis on the role of therapy in helping persons to reconstruct their traumatic histories (Smith, 2004; Spezzano, 1993). Contemporary psychoanalysis views the role of the therapeutic relationship as central in regulating the traumatized patient's overwhelming affective states, so that painful thoughts and feelings can be tolerated safely in order to be worked through (Davies & Frawley, 1994). Building self-reflective capacity, that is, the ability to think about and make sense of one's own and other's mental states, in the context of one's life situations and relationships is seen as an important outcome of successful therapeutic work (Fonagy et al., 2002). The idea is that self-reflection is a basic component for emotional resilience needed to cope with trauma, and may even prevent the transmission of traumatic states from parent to child (Main & Hesse, 2000).

The interface of nonverbal and verbal aspects of the therapeutic relationship is being examined in the light of developmental research on infant-parent interactions. It has been demonstrated that moment-to-moment nonverbal interactions between mother and infant influence brain, behavior, and self-development (Beebe, Lachmann, & Jaffe, 1997; Stern, 1985), long-term attachment and relationship patterns (Main, 2000), and even the nature of verbal discourse and self-reflection during adulthood (Main & Hesse, 2000). Complex mind/body interactions that are established in our earliest relationships are the basis of affective self-regulation, required during routine stressful experiences early in life, such as separations and reunions, and subsequent regulation of emotion, physiology, and behavior during extremely upsetting or disruptive interactions and events. Neuroscientists have mapped brain/body pathways embedded in processing and linking of behavior, feeling, thought, and self-experience, so that verbal and nonverbal expression, as well as conscious and unconscious experience, are now being examined as interrelated systems rather than as separate domains of human experience (Damasio, 1999; Schore, 2001). These areas of mind/body research have much to contribute to how we understand human experience, particularly trauma, and how we conduct psychotherapy.

In another approach, cognitive therapists have focused attention on coping strategies related to changing beliefs and attitudes about events and how they are understood. Coping may depend on interventions that help to reorganize cognitive structures to assimilate, understand, or find meaning in the traumatic experience (Lazarus & Folkman, 1984). For example, understanding individuals' rational explanations of events by constructing adaptive narratives may influence their reactions to stressful events (Meichanbaum & Fong, 1993). It has further been suggested (Epstein, 1990) that since traumatic experiences produce such disorientation to one's sense of reality and basic view of oneself and the world, psychotherapeutic approaches that can address both language-based cognitive/rational and action-oriented emotional/experiential processes would facilitate resolving a trauma. Also, the active reexperiencing of traumatic memories and triggers through exposure therapy (Foa, Keane, & Freidman, 2000) facilitates mastery as well as cognitive appraisal of the events as they are experienced in the context of safe therapeutic support.

Irrespective of therapists' theoretical orientations, both verbal and nonverbal expression is used in psychotherapies in which emotional experience is viewed as a central aspect of the healing process (Scheff, 1979; Stern, 2004). While the effectiveness of active and physical emotional expression has been demonstrated in the context of brief psychotherapy (Nichols, 1974), evidence suggests that emotional expression alone is not sufficient for therapeutic change (Murray, Lamnin, & Carver, 1989; Pennebaker & Beall, 1986). Rather, expression seems to facilitate cognitive reappraisal and insight, leading to affective, attitudinal, and behavioral change. Leading trauma researchers and clinicians (Levine & Frederick, 1997; van der Kolk, 2004) suggest that a multimodal approach including the body, emotion, cognition, and behavior in intervention is essential in targeting unconscious triggers and defenses such as dissociation, which are impervious to memory or verbal discourse and resistant to change. Movement and body-oriented therapies, such as dance movement therapy (Levy, 1988) and somatic therapy (Ogden, Minton, & Pain, 2006), have evolved based on the assumption of the totality of the human being from birth (Evan & Rifkin-Gainer, 1982). These holistic approaches have developed interventions targeting multiple dimensions of body, mind, and spirit as substrates of human experience and expression.

Traumatic events can directly and suddenly affect physical well-being as well as emotional and cognitive states. Certain traumatic experiences (e.g., rape, physical abuse, or assault) involve serious harm or injury, and may provoke fear, loss, or social stigmas of punishment as an outcome of self-disclosure. The process of hiding one's true emotions requires active suppression of facial and bodily expression, language, and thoughts, as well as changes in overall bodily comportment and behavior. Defense mechanisms such as repression, denial, or dissociation may push disturbing thoughts or feelings from consciousness, resulting in pathological symptoms and behaviors. The act of keeping important emotion-laden experiences from consciousness prevents their understanding as well as their cognitive integration. The physiological work of suppressing bodily expression and concealing upsetting thoughts and feelings may be a cumulative stressor with adverse effects on physical and psychological health. Conversely, expressing and confronting such feelings may lead to working them through, and may be beneficial to long-term health (Pennebaker, 1997; Pennebaker & Hoover, 1985; Pennebaker and Susman, 1988).

## DISCLOSURE OF TRAUMA, WRITING, AND HEALTH

One strategy that has been found to produce positive effects in coping with trauma is writing. Since people are often resistant to disclosing highly emotional or traumatic experiences to others, the use of writing as an individual, self-contained mode of expression has been explored by several researchers using an expressive writing paradigm, developed by James Pennebaker (1989). In the basic paradigm, participants are randomly assigned to one of two or more groups and are asked to write about assigned topics for one to five consecutive days, from 15 to 30 minutes per day. The control condition is asked to write about superficial topics, such as what they did that day. Participants in the experimental group are asked to write about their deepest thoughts and feelings regarding the most traumatic or upsetting experience of their life. They are explicitly instructed to freely explore and express their emotions and thoughts in their own way and without regard to writing structure or form. The power of this method has been repeatedly demonstrated by consistent significant health benefits on a variety of subjective and objective psychological, physiological, and behavioral measures. Also, the personal nature of the writing has impressed researchers for its emotional range and depth, as well as its self-reported value and meaning to the participants.

Over two hundred studies using variations of this method have been published since 1986. Numerous experiments have demonstrated that when people write or talk about previously suppressed traumatic events and emotions, improvements are obtained in measures of overall health (Greenberg, Wortman, & Stone, 1996; Pennebaker & Beall, 1986), including reductions in physician visits and improved immune system functioning (Esterling, Antoni, Fletcher, Margulies, & Schneiderman, 1994; Lepore & Smyth, 2002; Pennebaker & Graybeal, 2001; Pennebaker, Kiecolt-Glaser, & Glaser, 1988; Sloan & Marx, 2004); cognition and coping (Murray, Lamnin, & Carver, 1989; Pennebaker, Colder, & Sharp, 1990), and behavioral markers, such as school performance and employment status (Lumley & Provenzano, 2003; Spera, Buhrfeind, & Pennebaker, 1994). Whereas the majority of writing studies have used non-clinical populations, the few studies on clinical samples show stronger effects for physical than psychological health outcomes. It is also notable that writing was less successful for psychiatric than physical illness populations (Frisina, Borod, & Lepore, 2004). Nonetheless, there is an abundance of evidence that in the laboratory setting, writing or talking about extremely upsetting personal experiences can lead to consistent significant health improvements for an impressive range of subject populations and outcome measures (Pennebaker & Chung, 2006).

Pennebaker (1989; 1993) initially explained these results by positing a psychosomatic theory of inhibition. According to this approach, actively confronting traumatic life experiences through writing or talking can help people to cope with the negative impact of these events. The idea is that the work of actively holding back or restricting thoughts, feelings, and behaviors can serve as a cumulative psychological and physical stressor that ultimately increases the probability of illness and other stress-related problems (Selye, 1956). Conversely, by confronting personal upheavals through actively dealing with the traumatic experiences and emotions through writing or talking, physiological and cognitive stress is lowered, leading to a lower probability of illness. Further, a coherent expression of the trauma assists in assimilating and integrating the experience into a narrative with a broader perspective of the impact of life events.

To better understand the underlying physiologic processes of writing about trauma which may be affecting health, Pennebaker, Mayne, and Francis (1997) investigated relationships between the linguistic content (e.g., the actual words and story structures) of trauma essays and long-term measures of health, including changes in physician visits and immune function activity. Analyses indicated that people whose health improved used a moderate amount of negative emotion words and more insight, causal, and reflective words. Both expressive emotion and insightful cognition appear to be necessary in order to predict improvements in health and changes in autonomic activity. This strategy, then, suggests that therapeutic changes in health may be determined by how words are used and on the impact of language on emotional processing, cognition, and the individual's perspective of the significant life events about which they wrote.

In an extensive review of the expressive writing paradigm, Pennebaker and Chung (2006) suggest that its effectiveness cannot be explained by a single cause, such as originally hypothesized by inhibition theory. Based on specific linguistic analyses of writing samples and health outcomes, they suggest that translating emotional experiences into language is an important feature of understanding the meaning of events and assigning coherence and structure to emotions. They posit that what is helpful about language is the translation of an analog (nonverbal emotional experiential) to a digital (represented through words) format, at which point cognition takes over. Concise, descriptive, and emotionally accurate language allows for assimilation and cognitive processing of strong or overwhelming affects, providing another explanation for why the writing process is useful to people. Being able to understand their emotional responses to stressful life events helps people plan for the future and develop adaptive coping strategies. There is growing evidence that those who have the ability to write a coherent, well-organized narrative that constructs meaning over the intervention period are most likely to benefit from the writing method. In order to build a coherent narrative, people must be able to cognitively process emotional events and gain some perspective on their lives in a self-reflective way.

These findings have important relationships to ongoing investigations by developmental and psychoanalytic clinicians and researchers who are working to understand the somatic, nonverbal, and implicit domains of experience so germane to working with traumatized patients. For example, Main and Hesse (2000) have found that adults who have been traumatized early in life have difficulty communicating coherently organized narratives about their relationships, personal history, and emotional life. Interpersonal trauma is disorganizing to their relationships and cognition, leading to dissociation, confusion, lack of meaningful behavior and expression, and emotional, behavioral, and cognitive incoherence. As adults, they lack self-reflective capacity and are unable to verbally communicate with emotional depth and clarity about past events and memories. It is unlikely that such an individual would be capable of writing a coherent narrative about his or her traumatic life events.

Also relevant is the use of dissociation as a common defense to overwhelming and unregulated emotional states evoked in trauma. By effectively disconnecting or blocking off neural pathways in brain areas that process cognitive, physical, and emotional information, dissociation prevents processing and integration of these experiences through the usual routes of memory retrieval, cognition, or verbalization. The phrase "there are no words" is in our lexicon for such emotionally overwhelming responses and experiences. The work of van der Kolk (2003) and others emphasizes physiological responses well known in high anxiety and posttraumatic stress states, where people cannot say what it is that they feel or think. The interface between verbal and nonverbal aspects of experience and their functioning is central to understanding the substrates of the human mind, that is, how it is that we know what we feel and who we are. The premise is that knowing oneself, even what one feels and experiences, does not take place verbally, but on an implicit nonverbal level, both in and out of our direct appraisal or conscious awareness (Damasio, 1999). Extending our consciousness as we think about things, we translate such experiences into verbal analogs of thought and words, which then changes our way of experiencing events. We can then hold in mind many images and thoughts as they become more explicit. The interface between verbal and nonverbal, implicit and explicit, realms of experience is basic to catching nuances in relationships, therapy, and communication about our deepest sense of self and the most meaningful and challenging experiences of our lives. A more precise recognition of the role of the body and nonverbal communication would enhance the limitations of language to describe such human experience. In other words, drawing attention to the relationship between narratives and the experiences they are constructed to represent has clinical relevance (Stern, 2004; Knoblauch, 2005). Access to these subtle interfaces may help people process realms of experience that are not immediately available to verbalization.

## DANCE MOVEMENT THERAPY

The question of how nonverbal or body-oriented expression of trauma might be useful to people when words fail, and how psychophysical expression might affect health outcomes, remains important to address in research. Therapeutic strategies have emerged based on nonverbal expressive and bodily approaches such as biofeedback, bioenergetics, and somatic therapies (Lowen, 1967; Ogden et al., 2006). Also, expressive approaches involving the creative arts such as dance, art, and drama therapies use a combination of both verbal and nonverbal modes of self-expression. Blanche Evan's dance therapy approach (Evan & Rifkin-Gainer, 1982) involves giving outlet to emotion while actively confronting life transitions and traumas through dance, movement, and words. Dance/movement therapy is based on the assumption of a two-directional interaction between mind and body, such that movement expresses the inner workings of the psyche and also influences physical, emotional, and cognitive states (Dosamantes-Alperson & Merrill, 1980; Evan, 1991a; Grodner, Braff, Janowsky, & Clopton, 1982; Leste & Rust, 1990). The art of dance articulates psychophysical expression, which occurs when an emotion or experience is transmuted into action with feeling.

Dance/movement therapy is also concerned with the bodily manifestations of inhibition and expression. In Evan's model, social and personal inhibitions that restrict spontaneous expressive movement parallel the suppression of emotional expression (Evan, 1991b; Rifkin-Gainer, 1984). Nonverbal expressions of emotion are universal modes of basic communication with others (Ekman, 1965; Ekman & Friesen, 1969). As people learn to inhibit their spontaneous expressive movement, they also learn to hold back and suppress emotional expression and communication (Evan, 1991c). Thus, the inhibitions to move, to feel, to speak, and to show emotions are linked. Conversely, self-directed movement with feeling releases inhibition, allowing self-expression so that active confrontation of problems can take place. In dance therapy, the therapist's verbal cues and directives guide the client's bodily movements to reverse their inhibitions. Bodily expression is then linked to the client's own words, which are spoken and then reconstituted to stimulate further movement work. As the body moves in novel, liberating ways, the client's emotions become accessible to direct experience, first expressed nonverbally and then put into words. This process may be compared to self-disclosure in much the way writing has been used to reverse physiologic inhibition, although it includes a nonverbal subjectively rich component. It may also be analogous to processing vague or presymbolic viscerally felt states into symbolically meaningful communications and expressions. The sensation of one's own body in space, movement, muscular tensions, and visceral rhythms gives a direct, immediate experience of self during self-directed movement (Chambliss, 1982). Reciprocal feedbacks between feelings, ideas, and actions contributes to kinesthetic imagery, evokes muscular memory, and forms ideas and action patterns that in turn feed back to feelings and cognitive processes. Thus, complex emotional and cognitive experiences can be "physicalized" (Evan, personal communication, December 21, 1981), that is, transmuted into action, from passive to active expression.

Dance therapy is an experiential process in which "action precedes insights" (Evan, 1972, p. 8). Through creative methods such as reenactment of situations, physicalization and externalization of feelings, and depth improvisation, connections between meaning and experience are made. Dance improvisation is a process of free association through movement. This is a form of self-disclosure and self-reflection, in which the client expresses emotions, memories, and ideas that have been previously unrecognized and unprocessed. Through self-directed individual improvisation on themes that are personally meaningful, cognition occurs simultaneously with action and emotion. The outlet intrinsic to expressive movement can provide cathartic release of previously unavailable feelings and experiences. After catharsis comes a process of dealing with the feelings, integrating the experiences, and working through the problems.

The use of language is an important component of dance/movement therapy. The client's verbalizations are often used as directives for improvisation or for stimulating further development of thematic material. In addition, verbalization assists in articulating insights to integrate and assimilate the material and relate it to life situations. Words may also be used simultaneously with movement. Words are used selectively as specific and meaningful communication linked to content with an effort to elicit the unspoken word (Evan, personal communication, December 21, 1981), that is, verbal expression which has previously been held back or unreachable by the client, as well as developing the capacity to speak for oneself in truthful and direct ways. To emphasize the importance of meaningful language, Evan eventually referred to her work as "dance/movement/word therapy" (Evan & Rifkin-Gainer, 1982, p.14).

"The integration of dance with therapy" (Evan & Rifkin-Gainer, 1982, p. 10) assumes that by regenerating the body's potential to move, feel, express, and know, emotional, physical, and cognitive states can be changed and integrated. Spontaneous psychophysical expression promotes a dynamic interplay between mind and body. It seems an appropriate nonverbal medium for the study of psychosomatic processes that may be affected by inhibition, repression, dissociation, and expression. Following is a report of a study that looked at dance expression and writing and their effects on health.

### The Dance/Write Study

Pennebaker's paradigm (1997) had the potential to look at nonverbal as well as verbal aspects of expression and their effect on health. The "dance/write study" (Krantz, 1993; Krantz & Pennebaker, 1995) used techniques adapted from dance therapy to examine how bodily expression of personal experiences of emotional upheaval could affect physical and psychological health in a nonclinical population. The design of the study compared three groups of college student subjects. The two experimental groups were asked to dance about personal issues that they had never revealed to anyone, such as traumatic life experiences or emotions they had held inside. To focus on the role of language in the expression of emotions, one of the two expressive movement groups both danced and wrote about emotional experiences. The two expressive dance conditions were compared to an exercise control group that was asked to move continuously but in a nonemotional way.

The main thesis of the project was that people who expressed their emotions about traumatic or troubling experiences through expressive dance (the dance and dance/write groups) would show more improvement in overall health than those who did physical exercise. Since dance therapy combines the benefits of healthful physical activity with the benefits of expression, it was expected that subjects who dance out a trauma would experience more emotional integration and physical well-being when compared to control subjects who do nonexpressive physical exercise. The differential health benefits of verbal and nonverbal expression were expected to shed light on the role of words and body movement in expression of emotion. A related question was whether writing is beneficial because it allows people to put their thoughts and feelings into words, or because it allows people to freely express themselves. The study also hoped to broaden the scope of Pennebaker's paradigm to include nonverbal and artistic modes of expression, as well as verbal and written expression.

The participants were 64 male and female undergraduates with no prior training or experience in dance or dance therapy. They were randomly assigned to one of three conditions in which they were individually given movement instructions on each of the three days. People in the dance group were asked to express their deepest thoughts and feelings about a personally significant issue or traumatic experience in their life through movement. They were told to move their bodies in ways that expressed what they felt inside and to express in movement what they had never been able to say in words. Participants from the dance/write group were given identical movement instructions, to express their feelings and thoughts about a personally significant issue or traumatic experience, but then told that afterward they would write about what they expressed. In their writing, they were encouraged to explore their thoughts and feelings about what they expressed in movement. The exercise group was instructed to work on rhythm and coordination by stepping in place and moving the upper body in different directions in an eight-count rhythm. They were told not to express any thoughts or feelings, but to concentrate on coordination and rhythm.

Participants moved and/or wrote for 10 minutes per day for three consecutive days. Health center illness records, grade point average, self-reports, and selected cardiovascular measures were collected before, during, and after the experiment. Fourteen subjects agreed to be videotaped during the movement session on the third day. Objective and self-report evaluations and responses to subjects' movement and writing, and changes in subjects' physiological levels, mood, and symptom reports, were collected in order to learn about short-term effects of dance and writing. The long-term health effects of the experiment were measured by frequency of health center visits, change in grade point averages, and self-reported health-related habits. Additionally, the videotapes of recorded subjects were rated for expressivity and movement qualities. The results of the study are summarized below.

### Short-Term Effects

Immediately following their movement each day, individuals in the dance/write condition put their movement experience into words. It is important to convey the degree of openness with which the people in the dance/write condition wrote about and/or disclosed in movement their personal experiences. The students vividly portrayed a variety of significant conflicts in their lives, including their interpersonal, emotional, and school-related problems, specific traumatic experiences, and health-related issues. While essays are only available for this group, it is clear from additional written comments that much had been evoked for the subjects in all the movement conditions.

Self-report questions following each day's movement or writing evaluated three dimensions of their performance that indicated significant effects for the expressive movement conditions. As can be seen in Figure 1, subjects in the two expressive movement conditions viewed their movement as more personal than controls. Also intriguing was evidence that writing subjects evidenced a gradual decline in the degree to which their movement was personal for them. A comparable pattern was seen in the way subjects viewed how valuable and expressive their movement was. As with the ratings of how personal their movement was, the interaction is largely attributable to the drop in ratings over time among Dance/Write subjects from Day 1 to Day 3 compared to Dance subjects, whose ratings increased over the same time.

Participants also rated the degree to which they were experiencing each of five physical symptoms (headache, shortness of breath, tired, sweaty hands, and pain) and six negative emotions (sad, guilty, nervous, angry, insecure, difficulty

**Figure 1a**
**Ratings of how personal the movement was in the Dance Study**

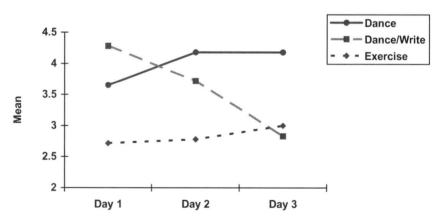

*Note:* After each session, individuals rated the degree to which their movement was personal along a 5-point scale, where 1=not personal and 5=personal.

**Figure 1b**
**Self-ratings of expressiveness of movement in the Dance Study**

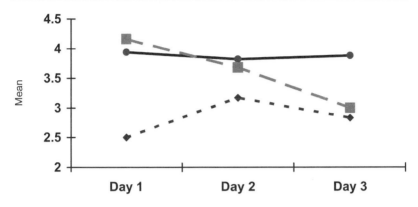

*Note:* After each session, individuals rated the degree to which their movement expressed their thoughts and feelings along a 5-point scale, where 1=not expressive and 5=expressive.

**Figure 1c**
**Ratings of how valuable the movement was in the Dance Study**

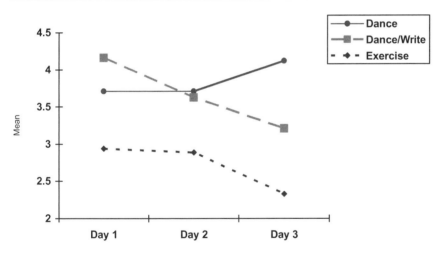

*Note:* After each session, individuals rated the degree to which they felt their movement was valuable and meaningful along a 5-point scale, where 1=not valuable/meaningful and 5=valuable/meaningful.

concentrating). As depicted in Figure 2, people tended to report fewer symptoms and negative moods across the three days of the study. Whereas Dance Only subjects evidenced decreasing negative moods and consistently higher symptom reports across the three days, the Dance/Write participants demonstrated a drop in symptom reporting, relative to their consistently high negative emotion reports. The pattern of decrease in physical symptoms included

**Figure 2a**
**Self-reported physical symptoms at the conclusion of each day's session.**
**The higher the number, the higher the degree of symptom reports**

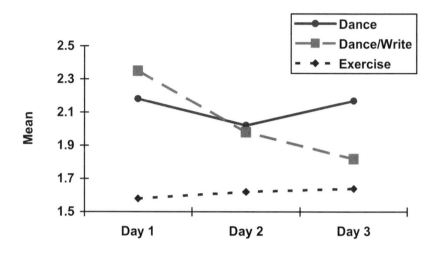

**Figure 2b**
**Self-reported negative emotions by day. The higher the number, the greater the**
**experienced negative effects**

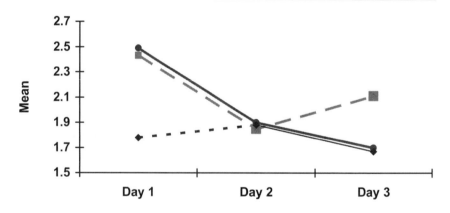

both exercise-related symptoms (e.g., shortness of breath) and symptoms not typically thought to be related to exercise (e.g., headache).

On the last day of the study, a subgroup of 14 participants (5 in each of the dance and exercise groups and 4 in the dance/write group) agreed to be videotaped during their movement. Two independent judges, blind to condition, with training in dance therapy, rated each of the videotapes along six dimensions: degree to which the subject expressed emotion, was personal, let go or opened up, was spontaneous, revealed trauma, and inhibited emotion. The inter-judge agreement was high and showed consistently significant differences among the three conditions despite the reduced sample size. On all rated dimensions, the Dance subjects were viewed as significantly more emotionally expressive, spontaneous, and less inhibited than Exercise controls. Interestingly, the Dance/Write subjects never differed from controls and were consistently less personal than Dance Only subjects.

The experiment was successful in manipulating students' expressions of their thoughts and feelings. Both dance groups initially reported that their dancing was more personal, valuable, and emotion-eliciting than those in the Exercise control condition. An important and consistent difference emerged between the two Dance groups, however. Dance Only participants tended to increase their rates of expressiveness in their movement over the course of the study as evidenced by their self-reports, heart rate levels, and judges' ratings of videotapes. Dance/Write subjects, on the other hand, gradually disengaged from the expressive dance over the three days. By the last day, Dance/Write participants were almost indistinguishable from Exercise subjects in self-reports about their movement, heart rate elevation, and judges' ratings of expressivity.

### Long-Term Effects

Three types of long-term health and adjustment data were collected from the participants: the self-report questionnaire completed 10 weeks after the experiment; changes in frequency of health center visits four months after the experiment compared to six months before; and changes in grade point average for the semester of the experiment compared to the semester before.

At the 10-week follow-up, participants were asked to look back and rate the degree they felt the study had influenced them and complete a questionnaire on a variety of health-related habits. They also were asked to describe any positive or negative long-term effects that the experiment may have had on them. It is clear from their written comments that students in all conditions had experienced a wide range of emotional experiences while moving. Students in the Dance and Dance/Write conditions generally found the movement to be beneficial and thought-provoking. Ironically, two people in the Exercise group indicated that they found movement helpful because they clearly expressed their feelings (contrary to the instructions). Even 10 weeks after a short movement intervention, students continued to be quite affected by what the experience evoked.

Participants were asked a range of questions about the experiment's positive and negative long-term effects, including its meaning and value to them and the degree to which subjects continued to think, talk, and feel about what they had expressed. Students in the two dance groups thought the study was more valuable than those in the exercise condition. Further, both dance groups reported that their movement task was more difficult than control group participants. There were no differences in health-related habits between conditions on reports of their alcohol and caffeinated beverage consumption, cigarette use, and hours of strenuous exercise per week.

As a measure of the participants' physical health, the change in frequency of their visits to the health center from six months before to four months after the experiment revealed a trend in the predicted direction, consistent with results of prior writing studies. As seen in Figure 3, only the Dance/Write group's visits to the health center decreased as compared to the exercise control group.

When each student's grade point average (GPA) for the semester of the study was compared to that of the previous semester, a trend in the direction

**Figure 3a**
**Health center illness visits as a function of condition. Mean health center visits per month in the 4 months after the intervention controlling for pre-experiment health center visits and sex of participant**

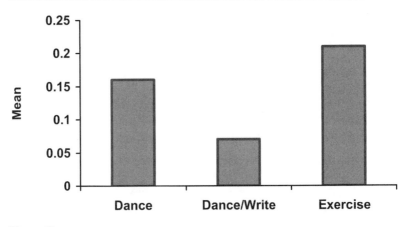

Figure 3b
Grade point averages as a function of condition. Mean grade point average (GPA) in the semester following the experiment controlling for pre-experimental GPA

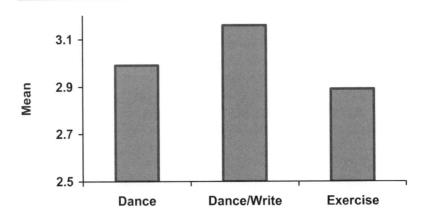

predicted by prior writing studies was visible, as depicted in Figure 3. While marginal, the Dance/Write group showed improvement in GPA as compared to the control group, where the Dance group did not.

### Discussion

This study examined the interplay of a brief exposure to an expressive dance and a language-based intervention. Some inferences may be drawn as to how movement and words interact in the expression of trauma and emotional upheavals. With relatively open-ended instructions and with no prior experience or training, individuals in the Dance Only condition reported increasing expressiveness and value in their movements over the three days of the study. The Dance/Write participants, however, showed a strikingly different trend. On the first day, before writing, Dance/Write subjects were deeply involved in their movement. However, over the remaining days of the study, they became less and less involved in their bodily expression. Indeed, writing about the traumas appeared to overtake the movement experience. By the last day of the study, the Dance/Write participants were no more expressive in their movement than the controls, as assessed by self-reports and judges' ratings of videotapes. The processes of linguistic and bodily expression, then, appeared to be inversely related, perhaps because the subjects found movement expression novel and difficult, whereas writing was familiar to them.

A similar contrast between the experimental groups was evident in the lower negative moods and higher symptom reports of the Dance Only group participants over the three days, perhaps due to their experience of emotional release and heightened bodily focus through movement. However, the Dance/Write group appeared to shift their focus toward verbal expression and evidenced lower symptom reports while maintaining higher negative moods over the three days. It is likely that different pathways of emotional processing of verbal and nonverbal expression determine their unique features, functions, and benefits. Traditionally, the field of dance therapy has viewed the client's use of verbalization as a resistance to experiencing depth in movement work, while verbal psychotherapy has viewed the client's physical action as a defense to symbolizing mental and emotional states. While integrating verbal and movement expression was not a specific goal of this intervention, the complementary roles of body and mind in elucidating and transforming emotional expression are important to understand and put to effective clinical use.

Individuals who expressed their thoughts and feelings through expressive dance found the experience to be positive and generally valuable as compared with people who were simply asked to exercise in a nonemotional manner. Despite the apparent psychological benefits of dance, only the group of participants who both danced and wrote evidenced improvements in physical health and higher college grades. The general pattern in these findings has both theoretical and practical significance for our understanding of the bodily and written expression of upsetting events and, more generally, the therapeutic process.

A central question arising from the present study concerns the degree to which language may be a necessary feature of therapeutic gain. Although reduced health center visits and improved grades were only apparent in the Dance/Write condition, subjects in both dance conditions reported positive psychological benefits. Dance participants' free responses suggest the movement technique was effective in getting individuals to explore, feel, and think about important psychological and life events, to an extent that may have enriched and deepened their cognitive and written expression. It is also interesting that Dance Only subjects reported thinking and talking about their experience more than those in the other conditions. Although unfamiliar with dance, participants found value and meaning both in the nonverbal form alone and in combination with verbal expression.

Admittedly, the study raises more questions than answers. The experiment drew on relatively healthy college students rather than a clinical population. The subjects were familiar with writing and unfamiliar with dance as a medium of expression. There was no Write Only condition run as a comparison group. In addition, participants in the Dance/Write condition participated for an additional 10 minutes each day, during which time they wrote. Despite these shortcomings, the results are encouraging in that measurable psychological and physical health benefits accrued from very brief movement training instructions and only three 10-minute movement periods.

The use of expressive movement and dance is rarely employed in traditional psychotherapy. It should be emphasized that the brief dance intervention was a pale analog of one aspect of a dance therapy method. Indeed, most forms of dance therapy incorporate both movement and subsequent discussions with the client about the movement, so that dance therapy usually incorporates the elements of the Dance/Write condition to a greater degree than the Dance Only strategy. Additionally, as experience is gained over time, one is better able to articulate and process feelings and thoughts through dance and movement, just as a lifetime of writing afforded these college students a capacity to express themselves in writing. Nevertheless, the results of this study point to the potential value of dance and expressive movement as viable techniques of therapeutic value in clinical practice.

## CASE VIGNETTES: WORKING WITH ILLNESS AND TRAUMA USING DANCE AND WORDS

In the following section, three clinical vignettes will illustrate ways in which words and movement are integrated in the therapy process. The case material was chosen to provide insight into the relation between trauma, illness, expression, and health in the clinical setting, and to suggest how movement can be used with verbalization in order to promote healing and change. At times words guide the movement and at others, body experience and movement precede the words, as exemplified in the dance/write study. The idea is that reciprocal feedback between verbal and nonverbal processing can occur at multiple levels of experience with an outcome of greater self-awareness, self-reflection, and emotional integration of the trauma, with possible benefits to physical health.

## LUCY: A HEARTBREAKING TRAUMA

Lucy was a 55-year-old woman of mixed race (Caucasian, Hispanic, and American Indian) and a complicated family history. She came to dance therapy following a heart attack that occurred six months after the murder of her oldest daughter, a drug addict who had been tragically killed by her drug-addicted partner. Lucy came from a family with a history of alcoholism and substance abuse. Although she had never been addicted, she struggled with the effects of the illness on each member of her family, in each generation she had known. When her daughter was murdered, she "shut down emotionally," with the pain being too much to bear. She kept focused on the needs of her teenage granddaughters, who had moved into her home with severe emotional problems, exacerbated by the extraordinarily complicated grief of their mother's murder. When her heart attack occurred, Lucy recognized that the physical trauma expressed a deep spiritual, physical, and emotional reality; her heart was truly broken and needed healing on all levels. That was when our work together began.

It had been almost a year since her daughter's murder, but Lucy could barely talk about her. What she did was to cry and clutch her chest, moaning from the pain inside, felt as "spasms of heart." She was convinced that in order to heal her heart, she would have to deal with the grief of her loss, and the anger and fantasies of vengeance that were constantly with her. Lucy was open to moving her body expressively and had done some art therapy in the past. I directed her to physicalize (e.g., to put into movement) the sensations in her heart and express any feelings that were connected, using movement, sound, and words. She danced a passionate and painful dance in which her whole body cried out in pain. She sighed, gasped, and cried as she enacted the way her daughter's heart had stopped, leaving her alone and bereft. I encouraged

*(Continues)*

*(Continued)*

her to express what she hadn't yet had a chance to let out. In aggressive rhythmic actions, she expressed her anger at her daughter, and the numbness, denial, and loss she felt when she first found out what had happened. The psychophysical impact of the trauma was a clear feeling of not being able to breathe, which had not left her body since that day. As she danced, she felt deep emotional pain, as if she had been stabbed in the heart, as her daughter had been. What emerged in her movement was the image Lucy verbalized as her daughter's heart bleeding into her own, allowing her heart to beat again. She danced this as a healing image, feeling that she was not as alone, and that her daughter was going with other deceased family members into death. I asked Lucy what she felt her heart needed in order to heal. She replied, "Taking care of myself first," and I suggested she move what that meant to her. Her dance signified a more contained sense of stability and self-care, despite many real-life demands and upsets. These dances provided a basis for many subsequent months of therapy work on maintaining her emotional and physical boundaries, making sensible health-oriented decisions, and most of all, allowing her grieving process to take place. Lucy did not have another heart attack and continued to live in good physical health, having worked deeply to allow significant psychophysical healing from the trauma.

## HANNA: A MEDICAL CASE FOR DANCING OUT TRAUMA

Hanna was a 39-year-old Jewish woman who was married with no children. A nurse, she worked as a diabetes manager in a major urban hospital. Her report of her complicated and ongoing medical history was lengthy and of concern. At 12 years she was diagnosed with juvenile diabetes, Type 1, and soon after was diagnosed with hyperthyroidism. At age 18 she contracted Guillain-Barre Syndrome, manifesting in paralysis of her whole body from the neck down for a number of months. Following recovery, at age 21 she was diagnosed with multiple sclerosis, which flared in a bout of blindness from which she subsequently regained her sight. She was placed on medications for all of her medical conditions. She entered dance therapy following her first major depressive episode, in which she just could not keep up with her demanding job. While an initial referral to a cognitive behavior depression group was useful in many ways, she felt a need for long-term treatment. Hanna was interested in dance therapy, as so many of her problems were related to her physical health, and creative dance had been a wonderful outlet for her in high school. Hanna's physical presence was marked by a particular lethargy, apparent in her slow, heavy gait, and apathetic stance. Hanna also reported having taken several falls while walking, sustaining injuries to her hands and wrists.

Hanna took care not to complain about her medical problems, since she believed that doing so would reveal what she considered a deplorable weakness. She was aware that her family members used their medical problems to coerce and control each other with debilitating emotional demands. Her own response was to be emotionally deadened; there was "nothing she could do about it" since her autoimmune diseases were progressive and incurable. She appeared especially unemotional when describing the paralysis and blindness episodes in her young adulthood, which left her temporarily unable to control her body and completely dependent on her family and hospital staff. When I asked her to describe what her depression felt like, she verbalized the image of "a black rock," large, weighted, not very malleable, and pressing down on her. I suggested she move the image, and Hanna began to do forceful outward movements with her arms and torso, saying she was "pushing away painful thoughts and feelings." Hanna associated this movement to her family's style of pushing away emotions with no recognition of feelings. A further directive to dance her own emotions just as she felt them led her to express anger at her family for being so controlling. This was the first time she had let out this feeling that had been held inside for so much of her life. The intensity of her anger moved through her body in powerful thrusts of her arms and her spine; she symbolically lifted the "rock," moved it off her back, and threw it across the room. Her whole body became alive with the vitality of total expression, liberating and changing her psychophysical state significantly. Following her dance, Hanna said that she felt less depressed and more angry, particularly toward her father. His refusal to acknowledge Hanna's MS diagnosis, while he used his diabetes to gain sympathy and attention, was a central dynamic affecting the entire family.

Hanna's therapy proceeded to connect her physical, emotional, and cognitive states, which had been segmented by denial, repression, and neglect of her body. She began a basic exercise regimen for balance and conditioning, and was referred for both neurological and neuropsychological testing. It was determined that objective indications of

*(Continues)*

*(Continued)*

her MS progression were stable. She was better able to cope with life when she recognized and expressed her emotions, such as her sadness about losses, fear about the future, and a deeply embedded sense of lack of control in her life. Her body became a resource for outlet and articulation of these experiences, with movement providing her direct access to emotions, sensations, and potentials. The integration of verbal psychotherapy with dance movement therapy assisted psychophysical, emotional, and cognitive processing related to her illnesses, as she worked through her depression to cope with her illnesses in a constructive and life affirming way.

## RENA: DANCING FOR HER LIFE

Rena entered a dance therapy group for cancer patients at the point at which her breast cancer had metastasized to her bones. At age 45 Rena was a working artist, who had taken dance classes for much of her life. Color was Rena's medium; her paintings were expressive and rich with a bright palette of extraordinary intensity and form. Each week she arrived in brightly colored patterned clothing that she had sewn for herself. Rena was a single mother of a 5-year-old daughter, and was very focused on her healing process. She considered dance therapy an important complement to her chemotherapy treatment, and reported her doctors' and nurses' comments that they knew if she had danced that day by how she looked and responded to treatment. Rena was both comfortable with and understood the creative process. Whether stimulated by verbal, musical, movement, or visual themes, she easily crossed between modalities to create wonderfully articulate dances with highly imaginative content that were later put into words for the group to hear; her cognitive, emotional, visual, and kinesthetic processing worked together in a seamlessly integrated way. Courageous and positive, with a deep personal spirituality, Rena was aware of the seriousness of her medical prognosis. She was fighting for her life.

One session, I suggested that the group members dance their own images of healing and then draw them on paper with markers. Rena danced a rainbow; she began moving through space with her arms outstretched, emphasizing changes in level, from low to high. Her rhythmic strides became dynamic leaps, accented by her arms reaching out as she held colorful scarves in her hands. Rena's rainbow was bold, free, and beautiful, streaking across the room. She then verbalized her intention to connect the earth to the sky as she moved through space. Her drawing further expressed this theme, as the rainbow's meaning to Rena became clear as an expression of her strong spiritual connection to nature. I suggested she dance once more, enriched by the insights of her movement, words, and drawing. The dance poignantly expressed the inspiration and strength she derived from the rainbow's expanse and range, its brilliance made more precious by knowing it would not last long. The dance ended as the rainbow faded, blending imperceptibly into the earth and sky. Rena expressed sadness and a painful acceptance of loss as part of the life cycle. She knew that her cancer was quite advanced with a poor prognosis. Just a few months later, Rena's doctors told her she had about six months to live. Rena was not ready to die, and she fought for survival and quality of life in all the ways she could, including aggressive chemotherapy and radiation treatment. She scheduled her infusions either before or after her weekly dance therapy group, where she revitalized her body, expressed her emotions, reconnected with her spirit, and explored the changing landscape of her deepest thoughts and feelings.

One week, Rena danced the pain of receiving a worsening diagnosis at the same time she was feeling better about herself, in that she felt a greater sense of wholeness from facing her life problems and by doing what she believed in. She danced the image of a willow tree with its gnarled roots deep underground, tangled and crowded, buried deeply in the earth. The roots drew nutrients and water from the earth, weaving and pulling them up so that the tree's trunk and branches could reach toward the sun. Her arms lifted and spread wide as her face opened into a smile. Rena described feeling the warmth of the sun shining down on her as a feeling of peace. She then verbalized her terror at facing death and the turbulent emotions that were always there, underneath all of her coping. By dancing an image that was not directly about her, but with which she could identify, Rena was able to physicalize her unspeakable fear of death and draw strength toward her love for life. Like her rainbow that expanded from the heavens to below the earth, Rena's tree became a metaphor connecting life and death. Rena lived for five more years, dancing weekly with tremendous courage and spirit throughout. She believed that dance therapy prolonged her life; it was clear that unifying her mind, body, and spirit gave her life meaning and depth, and finally, a way of coping with her death.

## SUMMARY AND CONCLUSIONS

The perspective presented here suggests that integrating nonverbal and verbal approaches has relevance and potential in the process of dealing with trauma, and in mitigating the impact of trauma on psychological and physical health. Pennebaker's substantial contributions to the study of verbal and written expression of emotional upheavals on health may be surprisingly powerful and broad, but they also confirm a basic human need for expression of emotion. When people express their emotions and thoughts about extremely upsetting experiences, even when it may be unpleasant for them to do so, it helps them in measurable ways, by improving their physical and psychological health. The verbal process of organizing a meaningful, coherent narrative helps people to make sense out of disruptive experiences, allowing them to attend to other things. This effectively frees up their mental and emotional resources, and correlates to improved physiological as well as behavioral functioning. The key then, is the capacity to put one's deeply emotional and traumatically evoked experiences into words.

Clinicians find that traumatized patients have extraordinary difficulty verbalizing a coherent, meaningful narrative related to their internal experience, and even identifying specific emotions, thoughts, or memories related to the trauma. Instead behavioral, emotional, relationship, and often, physical problems symbolically represent their trauma story, which is defensively dissociated or repressed and cannot be put into words. Verbal psychotherapists learn to understand the symbolic meanings and emotional states, using attunement and other strategies to "read" the patient's nonverbal communications in order to make sense out of them. The therapist's verbal description of the patient's emotional states and interactions then help the patient reconnect to their own experience. Thus, nonverbal and verbal communication between therapist and patient helps the patient learn how to put his or her experiences into words. The point is that even when there are no words, there is always a body that can be brought into the process of making sense out of one's experience. Expanding attention to the body can be very useful in verbal therapy.

Body-oriented clinicians face other challenges. The patient's resistance to movement can be powerful, since the intensity of the immediacy of movement can be overwhelming. Emotions accessed directly through the body are felt as visceral experiences. Not immediately connected to language, movement experiences have qualities of shape, rhythm, intensity, and feeling that may lead to associative content such as visual imagery or memory. Expressive movement modulates and contains emotion, giving it a recognizable form. Following dance, patients often spontaneously speak about their movement experience in their own personal, meaningful, and emotionally expressive words. The dance therapist guides the patient to move bodily and emotional states connected with trauma, and eventually to find the words that best match the experience. Most people new to dance therapy need a basic orientation to their body in action in order to express themselves deeply. They learn to recognize sensations that inform them about their bodily states. The capacity to tolerate physical and emotional states allows access to one's own resources in dealing with life. Putting movement into words helps give perspective to interpret and make sense out of experiences.

The dance/write study raised many questions about the role of nonverbal experience in the formulation of written expression, and the value and meaning of dance and movement in giving outlet to emotion and thought. There is a clear need for well-designed research on dance and other expressive therapies and health, especially looking at how verbalization, basic to any therapy process, works with the process of nonverbal expression. The dance/write study suggests that initially using movement to access feeling states may allow or enhance language processing. A better understanding of the particular contribution of dance would be gained by including a no-treatment control group, and by training subjects to articulate their feelings through dance. Since dance and writing are typically experienced in different settings, the complementary and integrative aspect of this intervention is promising. Further studies that apply Pennebaker's writing paradigm to other nonverbal and creative modalities in relation to verbal expression would help evaluate their effectiveness. Studies of clinical populations are needed to understand their particular limits of language to express overwhelming emotion. As medical centers are integrating movement and other nonverbal techniques into complementary care for people with cancer and other chronic illnesses, it is important to gain more knowledge about how they work and for whom they are most effective.

The power of psychophysical expression in working through trauma can be transformative as meaningful connections are made between dance content and life change, emotion and thought, movement and words. It is hoped that these case vignettes have brought some of these concepts to life, in terms of real human struggles with trauma, illness, and health, by illustrating how dance and words were integral to the process of therapy. The new paradigm of mind/body health suggests that human beings are unified, interactive, complex totalities. Now it is time for clinical models to expand and include verbal and nonverbal approaches that integrate mind and body in order to help people express their traumatic life experiences and promote health.

## TOOL KIT FOR CHANGE

### Perspective of the Healthcare Professional

1. The impact of traumatic life experiences and emotional upsets on the individual's physical, emotional, and mental health often requires psychological and medical intervention.

2. More than 200 studies have demonstrated powerful effects of expression on health. Expressing thoughts and feelings about traumatic events and emotions through writing or talking can be beneficial to psychological and physical health.

3. When the basic research paradigm was extended to expressive dance through bodily expression of personal traumatic experiences, several benefits to psychological and physical health were found. Integrating verbal and nonverbal expression, by combining expressive dance and writing about trauma, resulted in significant improvement in physical and psychological health.

### Perspective of the Patient

1. Dance movement therapy involves expressing emotion while actively confronting life transitions and traumas through dance, movement, and words.

2. Using the body's potential to move, feel, express, and know, dance movement therapy enhances integration and regulation of emotional, physical, and cognitive states and behaviors that accompany them.

3. Case studies illustrate how three individuals were able to use dance therapy to deal with emotions linked to trauma and physical illness. Each patient's own dance expression guided the therapy process and led to a greater sense of personal integration and health.

4. In dance therapy, nonverbal experience is brought into movement and then linked to meaningful words. Traumatic experiences not readily accessed by words can be danced and then verbalized with greater coherence and meaning.

### Interconnection: The Global Perspective

1. The paradigm of mind/body health suggests that human beings are unified, interactive totalities. Complex relationships between extreme states of emotional stress and common mental and physical health problems indicate a need for models that include verbal and nonverbal approaches to integrate mind and body.

2. Coping with trauma relies on individual emotional resilience, the regulation of strong emotion, and a capacity for self-reflection of the experience. Approaches are needed that help people to process potentially overwhelming affects that impact their psychosomatic, emotional, cognitive, and behavioral functioning.

3. Dance movement word therapy promotes a dynamic interplay between mind and body appropriate for the study of psychosomatic processes affected by trauma.

## REFERENCES

Beebe, B., Lachmann, F., & Jaffe, J. (1997). Mother-infant interaction structures and presymbolic self- and object representations. *Psychoanalytic Dialogues, 7*(2), 133–182.

Chambliss, L. (1982). Movement therapy and the shaping of a neuropsychological model. *American Journal of Dance Therapy, 5,* 18–27.

Damasio, A. (1999). *The feeling of what happens: Body and emotion in the making of consciousness.* New York: Harcourt.

Davies, J. M., & Frawley, M. G. (1994). *Treating the adult survivor of childhood sexual abuse: a psychoanalytic perspective.* New York: Basic Books.

Dosamantes-Alperson, E., & Merrill, N. (1980). Growth effects of movement psychotherapy. *Psychotherapy: Theory, Research and Practice, 17,* 63–68.

Ekman, P. (1965). Communication through non-verbal behavior: A source of information about an interpersonal relationship. In S. Tomkins & C. E. Izard (Eds.), *Affect, cognition, and personality: Empirical studies* (pp. 390–442). New York: Springer.

Ekman, P., & Friesen, W. V. (1969). The repertoire of nonverbal behavior: Categories, origins, usage, and coding. *Semiotica, 1,* 49–98.

Epstein, S. (1990). The self-concept, the traumatic neurosis and the structure of personality. In D. Ozer, J. N. Healy, & A. J. Stewart (Eds.), *Perspectives on Personality* (Vol. 3). Greenwich, CT: JAI Press.

Esterling, B. A., Antoni, M. H., Fletcher, M. A., Margulies, S., & Schneiderman, N. (1994). Emotional disclosure through writing or speaking modulates latent Epstein-Barr virus reactivation. *Journal of Consulting and Clinical Psychology, 62,* 130–140.

Evan, B. (1972). *Brochure for the Dance Therapy Centre, New York.* Unpublished manuscript.

Evan, B. (1991a). Jagged tensions and the flow of dance/movement therapy. In R. Benov (Ed.), *The collected works by and about Blanche Evan* (pp. 159–162). San Francisco: Blanche Evan Foundation.

Evan, B. (1991b). Relaxation and resilience. In R. Benov (Ed.), *The collected works by and about Blanche Evan* (pp. 163–166). San Francisco: Blanche Evan Foundation.

Evan, B. (1991c). The child's world: Its relation to dance pedagogy. Article III: The link between. In R. Benov (Ed.), *The collected works by and about Blanche Evan* (pp. 57–60). San Francisco: The Blanche Evan Foundation.

Evan, B., & Rifkin-Gainer, I. (1982). An interview with Blanche Evan. *American Journal of Dance Therapy, 5,* 5–17.

Fonagy, P., Gergely, G., Jurist, E., & Target, M. (2002). *Affect regulation, mentalization, and the development of self.* New York: Other Press.

Foa, E. B., Keane, T. M., & Freidman, M. J. (2000). *Effective treatments for PTSD: Practice guidelines from the International Society for Traumatic Stress Studies.* New York: Guilford Press.

Freud, S., & Breuer, J. (1966). Studies on hysteria. In J. Strachey (Ed.), *The standard edition of the Complete Psychological Works of Sigmund Freud* (Vol. 2). London, Hogarth Press. (Original work published 1895)

Frisina, P. G., Borod, J. C., & Lepore, S. J. (2004). A meta-analysis of the effects of written emotional disclosure on the health outcomes of clinical populations. *The Journal of Nervous and Mental Disease, 192,* 629–634.

Greenberg, M. A., Wortman, C. B., & Stone, A. A. (1996). Emotional expression and physical health: Revising traumatic memories fostering self-regulation? *Journal of Personality & Social Psychology, 71,* 588–602.

Greenson, R. F. (1967). *The technique and practice of psychoanalysis* (Vol. 1). New York: International Universities Press.

Grodner, S., Braff, D., Janowsky, D., & Clopton, P. (1982). Efficacy of art/movement therapy in elevating mood. *The Arts in Psychotherapy, 9,* 217–225.

Knoblauch, S. H. (2005). Body rhythms and the unconscious: Toward an expanding of clinical attention. *Psychoanalytic Dialogues, 15*(6), 807–827.

Krantz, A. M. (1993). *Dancing out trauma: The effects of psychophysical expression on health.* Unpublished doctoral dissertation, California School of Psychology, Berkeley/Alameda.

Krantz, A. M., & Pennebaker, J. W. (1995). *Expression of traumatic experience through dance and writing: Psychological and health effects.* Unpublished manuscript.

Lazarus, R. S., & Folkman, S. (1984). *Stress, appraisal, and coping.* New York: Springer.

Lepore, S. J., & Smyth, J. M. (2002). *Writing cure: How expressive writing promotes health and emotional well-being.* Washington, DC: American Psychological Association.

Leste, A., & Rust, J. (1990). Effects of dance on anxiety. *American Journal of Dance Therapy, 12,* 19–25.

Levine, P. A., & Frederick, A. (1997). *Waking the tiger: Healing trauma: The innate capacity to transform overwhelming experiences.* Berkeley: North Atlantic Books.

Levy, F. J. (1988). *Dance/movement therapy: A healing art.* Reston, VA: The American Alliance for Health, Physical Education, Recreation, and Dance.

Lieberman, A. F., & Van Horn, P. (1998). Attachment, trauma, and domestic violence: Implications for child custody. *Child and Adolescent Clinics of North America, 7*(2), 423–443.

Lowen, A. (1967). *The betrayal of the body.* New York: Macmillan.

Lumley, M. A., & Provenzano, K. M. (2003). Stress management through written emotional disclosure improves academic performance among college students with physical symptoms. *Journal of Educational Psychology, 95*(3), 641–649.

Main, M. (2000). The organized categories of infant, child & adult attachment. *Journal of the American Psychoanalytical Association, 48*(4), 1055–1096.

Main, M., & Hesse, E. (2000). Disorganized infant, child and adult attachment: Collapse in behavioral and attentional strategies. *Journal of the American Psychoanalytical Association, 48*(4), 1097–1127.

Meichenbaum, D., & Fong, G. T. (1993). How individuals control their own minds: A constructive narrative perspective. In D. M. Wegner & J. W. Pennebaker (Eds.), *Handbook of mental control.* New York: Prentice Hall.

Murray, E. J., Lamnin, A. D., & Carver, C. S. (1989). Emotional expression in written essays and psychotherapy. *Journal of Social and Clinical Psychology, 8,* 414–429.

Nichols , M. P. (1974). Outcome of brief cathartic psychotherapy. *Journal of Consulting and Clinical Psychology, 42,* 403–410.

Ogden, P., Minton, K., & Pain, C. (2006). *Trauma and the body: A sensorimotor approach to psychotherapy.* New York: W.W. Norton.

Pennebaker, J. W. (1989). Confession, inhibition, and disease. *Advances in Experimental Social Psychology, 22,* 211–244.

Pennebaker, J. W. (1993). Putting stress into words: Health, linguistic, and therapeutic implications. *Behavior Research and Therapy, 31*(6), 539–548.

Pennebaker, J. W. (1997). *Opening up: The healing power of expressing emotion.* New York: Guilford Press.

Pennebaker, J. W., & Beall, S. K. (1986). Confronting a traumatic event: Toward an understanding of inhibition and disease. *Journal of Abnormal Psychology, 95,* 274–281.

Pennebaker, J. W. & Chung, C. K. (2006). Expressive writing, emotional upheavals, and health. In H. Friedman and R. Silver (Eds.), *Handbook of health psychology* (pp. 263–284). New York: Oxford University Press.

Pennebaker, J. W., Colder, M., & Sharp, L. K. (1990). Accelerating the coping process. *Journal of Personality and Social Psychology, 58,* 528–537.

Pennebaker, J. W., & Graybeal, A. (2001). Patterns of natural language use: Disclosure, personality, and social integration. *Current Directions, 10,* 90–93.

Pennebaker, J. W., Kiecolt-Glaser, J. K., & Glaser, R. (1988). Disclosure of traumas and immune function: Health implications for psychotherapy. *Journal of Consulting and Clinical Psychology, 56,* 239–245.

Pennebaker, J.W., Mayne, T.J., & Francis, M.E. (1997). Linguistic predictors of adaptive bereavement. *Journal of Personality and Social Psychology, 72,* 166–183.

Rifkin-Gainer, I. (1984). Dance/movement/word therapy: The methods of Blanche Evan. In P. L. Bernstein (Ed.), *Theoretical approaches in dance-movement therapy* (Vol. 2, pp. 3–62). Dubuque, Iowa: Kendall-Hunt.

Scheff, T. J. (1979). *Catharsis in healing, ritual, and drama.* Berkeley: University of California Press.

Schore, A. N. (2003). *Affect dysregulation & disorders of the self.* New York: W.W. Norton.

Schore, A. N. (2001). The effects of relational trauma on right brain development, affect regulation, and infant mental health. *Infant Mental Health Journal, 22,* 201–269.

Selye, H. (1956). *The stress of life.* New York: McGraw-Hill.

Sloan, D. M., & Marx, B. P. (2004). Taking pen to hand: Evaluating theories underlying the written disclosure paradigm. *Clinical Psychology: Science & Practice, 11,* 121–137.

Smith, J. (2004). Reexamining psychotherapeutic action through the lens of trauma. *Journal of the American Academy of Psychoanalysis and Dynamic Psychiatry, 32*(4), 613–631.

Spera, S. P., Buhrfeind, E. D., & Pennebaker, J. W. (1994). Expressive writing and coping with job loss. *Academy of Management Journal, 37*(3), 722–733.

Spezzano, C. (1993). *Affect in psychoanalysis: A clinical synthesis.* New York: Analytic Press.

Stern, D. N. (1985). *The interpersonal world of the infant: A view from psychoanalysis and developmental psychology.* New York: Basic Books.

Stern, D. N. (2004). *The present moment in psychotherapy and everyday life.* New York: W.W. Norton.

Sykes Wylie, M. (2004). The limits of talk: Bessel van der Kolk wants to transform the treatment of trauma. *Psychotherapy Networker, 28*(1), 30–41.

van der Kolk, B. A. (1994). The body keeps the score: memory and the evolving psychobiology of posttraumatic stress. *Harvard Review of Psychiatry, 1*(5), 253–265.

van der Kolk, B. A. (2003). The neurobiology of childhood trauma and abuse. *Child and Adolescent Psychiatric Clinics, 12,* 293–317.

van der Kolk, B. A., Roth, S., Pelcovitz, D., Sunday, S., & Spinazzola, J. (2005). Disorders of extreme stress: The empirical foundation of a complex adaptation to trauma. *Journal of Traumatic Stress, 18*(5), 389–399.

Chapter Twelve

# ART THERAPY AND THE SOUL

*Shaun McNiff, PhD, ATR*

Art healing and the professional practice of art therapy are approached in this chapter as ways of harnessing the transformative powers of creative expression. Primary emphasis is placed on an immersion in the creative process, both when making art and when responding to finished objects. This approach to practice recognizes the creative imagination as an intelligence and as a transformative force that can transform difficulties and offer insights in ways that are not accessible when working with more linear and analytic treatments. When immersed in creative expression the artist is led by the process and taken to places that cannot be planned in advance. Life situations and problems are imagined anew, relived from different perspectives, and essentially transformed from conditions of affliction and victimization to sources of creative renewal.

During the early twentieth century C. G. Jung's practice of active imagination anticipated all of today's various forms of expressive arts therapy (Chodorow, 1997) and built upon the nineteenth-century tradition of transformative artistic expression advanced by William Blake (1957), Jean-Paul Richter (1973), Friedrich Nietzsche (1967), and others. Creative imagination was viewed as a primary intelligence with the ability to heal.

This chapter has been adapted and expanded from the following series of essays: "How art heals" (*The Watkins Review, 11,* Summer 2005); "Artistic interpretation as a way of healing" (*Vision Magazine,* May 2005); and "Letting pictures tell their stories" (in Charles Simpkinson and Anne Simpkinson, *Sacred stories: Healing in the imaginative realm,* [San Francisco: Harper Collins, 1993]).

When using the arts to heal, methods of practice focus on disciplined immersion and attentiveness to what happens spontaneously during the process of creative expression. In order to access these medicines the person must "let things happen," as Jung said, and trust that authentic expression will help us transform the conditions of our lives in correspondence with the changes that occur within creative activity. This orientation to letting go and trusting the process, albeit with a clear purpose and rigorous discipline (McNiff, 1998), is well known to artists and contemplative practitioners, but it goes contrary to the more strategic, controlled, and directive orientation that has typically characterized healthcare, the professions, and organizational life.

Rather than trying to fix the typically irreparable conditions of the past and present, the creative and transformative approach encourages living with them in new and more creative ways and re-visioning how they affect us, ideally using our difficulties as sources of creative energy and purpose. I have been closely involved for many years with the discipline of expressive arts therapy, and more specifically art therapy, where professionals work together with individuals, families, and groups in order to help and guide them in accessing the curative powers of all forms of creative expression (McNiff, 1981, 1988, 1989). Over the years there has been a natural progression from what I do within clinical practice to working with people in all sectors of society who desire to access the healing powers of art on their own and in groups of similarly committed people (McNiff, 1992, 1998, 2003, 2004). Art healing is for everyone and it can be effectively used by all healthcare professionals in their practice or by people working alone with the goal of furthering well-being and creative vitality.

Since the variables of professional therapeutic practice are vast, in this chapter I will focus on the core process of artistic expression and how it heals through both the making of art and the process of responding to art objects. This review of the art and healing experience can then be adapted either by professional therapists to the goals of their work, or by readers in need of artistic expression in their personal lives. I view the professional use of the arts in therapy as part of the larger domain of art and healing (McNiff, 2004).

Most expressive arts therapists share a common commitment to the healing aspects of spontaneous artistic expression in varied media. Our differences are more apt to appear in how we respond to art objects. In keeping with the tradition of creative imagination as described above, this chapter will approach the interpretation of images and objects as yet another art form, as a way of responding to the expressions of imagination with more imagination and creative expression, or as Jung suggested, we will imagine them further. On the basis of my experience, these ways of creative interpretation not only take us closer to the original expressions and help us to understand them more completely and deeply, but as with all features of the artistic process, they are inherently transformative and healing in themselves.

Although my practice includes an integrated use of all of the arts, I generally focus on the visual arts as a starting point for art healing, and this chapter reflects that emphasis. This orientation results from my experience as a painter who is committed to all of the arts in therapy. Within the worldwide practice of the expressive arts therapies, professionals and people exploring these processes make use of endless combinations and integrations of the arts depending upon their interests, backgrounds, and opportunities for expression. Others focus on only one art modality. In my opinion, all of the arts are simply materials and different modes of expression that emerge from the same creative source and desire to transform experience and give voice to the urges and needs of the soul.

## HOW ART HEALS

There are many ways that art heals both inside and outside of therapeutic relationships. The creative process furthers sensory awareness; infuses us with creative energy; deepens our appreciation of everyday experience; offers insights that arrive from beyond the limits of linear thought and speech; enhances meaningful communication between people; enables us to express feelings and conflicts that cannot be conveyed in conventional language; and in its most potent forms, art transforms disturbance, and even suffering, into affirmations of life. This alchemical power of transformation characterizes both art and healing. When the two are joined, they make a powerful synergy that is finding its way into many different sectors of healthcare ranging from the psychotherapeutic treatment of trauma, to complementary cancer therapy, and efforts to improve the quality of life for seniors experiencing various forms of dementia.

When I first worked with severely disturbed patients within a mental hospital 35 years ago, I quickly found how for some people the arts offered an expressive lifeline when they could not communicate in other ways. In the hospital, art healed in many ways, from giving voice to deep emotions and realizing personal powers of expression, through spontaneous and authentic gestures and forms, through vital and energizing colors, and through embodiments of inner states that could be witnessed and affirmed by other people. Art animated both the person and the surrounding environment while affirming creative gifts and personal dignity.

These experiences in therapy helped me to see how every community and organizational environment can benefit from infusions of creative expression. In 2003 I published *Creating with Others: The Practice of Imagination in Art,*

*Life and the Workplace* and worked with colleagues throughout the world to expand the focus of our work with art and healing to every conceivable context where there was a willingness to seriously engage the creative spirit. The work of creative transformation and healing cannot be limited to places where people experience serious illness. The enhancement of creative vitality is as much a public health issue as lowering blood pressure, and maybe the two have more in common than some may realize.

Contemporary experience and history show how people everywhere turn to art in times of crisis, discovering how it is uniquely capable of expressing the intensity and depth of complex emotions while furthering a sense of inner balance in response to threatening and potentially overwhelming situations. As Nietzsche said, when we are faced with the most horrendous experiences, "art approaches as a saving sorceress, expert at healing. She alone knows how to turn these nauseous thoughts about the horrors or absurdities of existence into notions with which one can live" (1967, p. 60). Within the context of art, crisis becomes a driving power that energizes and directs artistic expression as it creates light in darkness and gives something to the world in response to devastating circumstances.

In the more public domain of art, Edvard Munch's painting *The Scream* (1893), and Picasso's *Guernica* (1937), demonstrate how the artist evokes emotional states and crafts them into forms that can be experienced by others. Within therapy and when creating alone, the average person can use art in the same way to give form to fears and emotional outrage and turn these conditions into life-affirming creations. Art also heals in less urgent ways through perceptions of beauty and uplifting aesthetic experiences that help us appreciate everyday life and align ourselves with the creative energy that is the basis of health and vitality.

I have emphasized in many previous publications how today's practice of art and healing corresponds closely to traditions of shamanism in all parts of the world (McNiff, 1981; 1992, 2004). Shamanic cultures universally attribute illness to the loss of a person's soul, which is retrieved by the shaman during healing enactments. The metaphor of soul loss applies completely to our contemporary experience with the arts in healing. The arts do not necessarily cure deep-seated emotional problems or physical ailments, but they help people suffering from these conditions to do something meaningful with them, to use the difficulty as a source of creative transformation and soul renewal. Even with the most ordinary anxieties and tension of daily life, the soul becomes alienated, fragmented, and lost in terms of maintaining contact with its core vitality. The arts are our most universal and historically tested way of renewing soul and restoring its creative purpose.

If you were one of the many people who ask me how to start using artistic expression as a way of creative discovery, I would suggest starting with simple and sustained movements on a surface when painting or drawing; connecting physical materials like sticks and other objects from nature into aesthetic arrangements; making a collage, montage, or personal shrine with meaningful personal objects and photos; or going out into nature and arranging stones, earth, sand, shells, sticks, grass, or leaves into configurations that express your aesthetic interaction with the environment. Choose your medium and simply start moving with it without planning too much. Stay with the process with a sense of confidence, belief, and most of all, with a willingness to accept what arrives by surprise. Let the forms and gestures emerge from your most natural and authentic gestures, and allow the different expressions to relate to one another and thus build an overall composition.

Try not to be too clever. Ask your critical aspect to relax, take a seat, and watch how expressions move from your inner source as it interacts with art materials and the environment. I tell people interested in exploring how art heals that the soul medicines of the creative process are as accessible as their breath. If we can get the healing energies of art moving through every fiber of our being, they will find their own way to areas of need. But first people need to become immersed in the creative process. This generally requires changing and demystifying attitudes about what they can and cannot do within the realm of art.

In my experience, a focus on breathing and relaxing the mind is a gateway to art and healing. As trite as this may seem to some, experience garnered from the most challenging situations reinforces an emphasis on breathing, letting go, and opening to a more complete appreciation of the most ordinary and basic gestures, sensations, and forms. When people start to move with art materials in this mindful and responsive way, and stay with it over sustained periods of time, their authentic ways of moving begin to emerge and these expressions become the basis for an expanded commitment to art making. I observe repeatedly how people start to move expressively and then begin to think too much, judge their efforts, belittle them through comparison to others, and lose contact with their most natural ways of expression. I liken this to the loss of soul described in shamanic experiences. Soulful expression is our personal and natural way of moving. It is accessible to us all of the time, but we tend to have difficulty in appreciating this principle and making contact with the creative flow.

"The simpler, the deeper," I repeatedly say to people. If you can begin by focusing on your breath and then move your body without plans, and sustain the pure strain of your spontaneous movement, the creative process will unfold. As simple as this focus may seem, it is difficult for most of us to do because we are blocked and paralyzed by the judging, doubting, fearing, overly controlling mind that keeps the soul medicines of spontaneous creative expression at bay.

People need help in dealing with the resistance, fear, and postponement tendencies that are so closely connected to the creative invitations that life gives us each day. Just about everything in our culture emphasizes the conquest and resolution of problems rather than embracing them as gateways to expression. I have learned through my discipline of art therapy how art heals by accepting the circumstances of our lives and using them as sources of creative transformation.

People everywhere are discovering how they can deal more effectively with crises, trauma, life-threatening illnesses, and the existential angst of the workplace by responding to these experiences through art. Healing occurs when we acknowledge our situation, do something positive with it, and share our creative responses with others. Like the alchemists of ancient times, the artist takes the most leaden substances of daily life and turns them into creative gold.

When you look deeply into your maladies and create with them, you make it possible for creative energy to circulate through your whole being. My experience indicates that art healing happens primarily through this infusion of vitality.

Yet there are many forces keeping us far from these healing and life-enhancing forces. We are hard on ourselves and we construct formidable barriers to our natural ways of creative expression, continuing all of the bad habits of the social institutions that are often blamed for taking away our creativity.

We are all afraid of acting and looking even a little bit "weird" or unusual; of doing something very different from what others do; and so it is no wonder that creativity suffers. Neurosis in relation to artistic quality and life in general comes when we try to present ourselves in ways and according to standards of judgment that are detached from our authentic nature. When an expression bears your inimitable signature, it cannot be judged according to what another person does, and the cultivation of this aesthetic attitude is itself a major source of healing.

But as I have described above, the work of art and healing is not always easy and pleasant, especially if we are dealing with painful and difficult situations and doubts that permeate everything we do. If people feel uncomfortable with their expressions, I suggest staying with the difficulties and getting to know them better. By accepting these conditions we might find that our feelings toward them will change.

Artists throughout history continuously demonstrate how creative expression flourishes in the face of adversity, when all else fails to remedy a situation. As the meditation teachers say, we have to start where we are and work from that place, and do something with it. Healing is all about accepting the conditions of our lives and transforming them. The difficult places, the ones we resist the most, may hold the greatest opportunities for both art and healing.

## RE-VISIONING INTERPRETATION: FROM EXPLANATION TO CREATIVE ENGAGEMENT

It intrigues me how many of my closest and most respected colleagues are apt to view the interpretation of art as "wrong" and as a questionable ethical practice. I am sympathetic with these concerns but feel that they are motivated by the damaging aspects of certain kinds of interpretation that essentially label artistic expressions according to preexisting attitudes and psychological concepts.

In my practice, interpretation is viewed as a core and necessary process. It is our most essential way of responding to artistic expression, either through the basic act of looking, or by communicating responses through language or other forms of expression. Whenever we engage inner and outer experiences through our minds and senses, we are interpreting them. The issue for me has always been how we can interpret the world more creatively, sensitively, and deeply.

When art was first connected to therapy, there was a strong tendency to align the work with the traditional medical model. The pictures that people made were explained according to psychological theories. They were typically reduced to past traumas and conflicts since there was a reasonable assumption that repressed thoughts and instincts may manifest themselves in expressive modalities that fly below the defensive radar of conscious speech. If a child painted with earthen hues, the art diagnosticians attributed this to anal fixations. Red was reduced to anger and the absence of impulse control; black to depression; X configurations to the repression of sexual instincts; lawn mowers to castration fears; and so forth. No matter what a person painted, it was seen as an indicator of some form of unconscious problem, usually of a psychosexual nature.

Well-intentioned clinicians realized that personal symbolic expressions do reflect the interplay of our inner and outer lives. However, the tendency to reduce vacuum cleaners to oral deprivation, and cows to needs for nurturing mothers, is a very sketchy and overly simplistic psychological practice.

These practices of what I call "explanationism" are linked to innate human instincts to understand experience. There is no question that artistic expressions communicate our deepest and most soulful longings. Nonetheless we are too apt to interpret them according to an authoritative doctrine of some kind, searching for meanings and answers to complex problems outside the authority of our own experience. A one-sided focus on what an art object "means" can also block access to its expressive medicines that require a more imaginative way of looking and responding.

Many of our emotional problems can be attributed to ineffective interpretations of experiences. In describing how thought can become a "prison," Hamlet said, "[T]here is nothing either good or bad, but thinking makes it so" (Shakespeare, *Hamlet*, act 2, scene 2). Therefore, we can look inwardly when confronting our greatest difficulties with the external world and ask ourselves whether we are able and willing to interpret our afflictions differently, more creatively, and in ways that move us beyond victimization.

The really hurtful interpretations that people make are often their own judgments about the value of their creative work, dismissals that obscure the unique attributes of a particular expression as well as its medicines. The discipline of healing through art offers an opportunity to relax the grip of our often harsh self-criticism that undermines confidence and expressive freedom.

Within the realm of art and healing we interpret, embrace, and deepen experience by making art from our most spontaneous gestures and movements, and we further our relationship with the resulting creations by welcoming, accepting, and interpreting them in imaginative ways. The deepest and most lasting work tends to occur when we acknowledge the value of disturbing and frightening expressions and transform them into affirmations of life. Paradoxically, people experience a sense of wholeness, vitality, and understanding when they stop trying to explain their difficulties and when they engage them as partners and sources of energy for creative expression.

I find that people get much closer to their art when they interpret it imaginatively by personifying the creations and letting them speak poetically, a method that will be explored in the following section, or by responding to the energetic expressions of art works in more physical ways through movement, vocal improvisation, ritual, and performance. For example, a person might speak empathetically with a frightening figure about its needs, or dance its aggressiveness to achieve a more complete integration of strong emotions. In my experience, the psyche is inherently good and creative, always trying to help. I find that disturbing images in dreams are trying to get my attention. Their provocations invite me to look more closely at things I may avoid. We get into trouble when we fail to take advantage of these opportunities to respond to inner distress signals.

Paintings, movements, and sounds simply cannot be reduced merely to verbal narratives and psychological concepts. Our creative expressions may have narrative aspects but they are so much more. I describe to my students how narrative is important in helping us understand art but how when we stay exclusively within the bounds of the more traditional "talking cure," we overlook how the visual arts are primarily expressive of energy, movement, and other forces that can convey strong medicines if we are able to open ourselves to them.

As important as psychology is within my work, I am increasingly of the opinion that the deepest forms of transformation are connected to the infusions of vitality and energy conveyed by the creative process. Art heals by restoring healthy circulations of creative energy within our bodies and environments.

## IMAGINAL DIALOGUE AS AN INCREASING MAINSTAY OF ART THERAPY

Having just emphasized how surrendering to the process of creation and trusting its innate wisdom leads to the discovery of healing powers that lie outside the lines of verbal description, I want to demonstrate how language can also be used artistically and imaginatively in keeping with the overall dynamics of healing through the creative process. Poetic speech offers the same kinds of spontaneous and dynamic transformations of experience that occur through the other arts, and as I will show in this section, a creative use of language in art therapy can additionally tap into the kinetic energies of the body and voice.

Whenever we make objects in the visual arts and in art therapy, there is an innate tendency to respond to them through words and speech. I found that when we use conventional narrative to describe the art that was made in art therapy, even when speaking from the heart and not within the context of psychological concepts and jargon, there is still an element of distance that ensues. There is a sense that the creative activity happened previously and now we are reflecting on it with what I have called creation stories that try to re-create something that occurred in the past. These descriptions can of course spin into the art of storytelling, which does activate artistic forces operating in the present. I want to affirm imaginative storytelling as yet another way of responding creatively to art objects. But when we start to describe the literal things that we did and how we felt in each phase of a prior process, we tend to leave the realm of art and instead generate a sense of explanation.

As I have emphasized before, these elucidations have an important place within the process of art and healing and I use them all of the time. There are also many instances when we do need distance and an emphasis on reflecting on the past. My purpose here is to show the limits of explanation and how other more artistic ways of talking can enhance the healing process. If our overall purpose is an activation of the healing powers of the imagination, then it makes sense to explore the use of language that sustains and even deepens the process of creative inquiry.

In *Art as Medicine: Creating a Therapy of the Imagination* (1992), I show how this way of responding to art offers many advantages and insights that cannot be accessed thorough more conventional descriptive and literal interpretations. I am pleased to see the method increasingly used as a relatively common way of responding to art objects. More importantly, this trend suggests a wider recognition of the benefits of using the creative imagination in interpreting art.

Jung initiated dialogues with images as a fundamental part of his practice of active imagination. Within the Jungian tradition, James Hillman (1977, 1978, 1979), Mary Watkins (1983), and others have sustained the method as a preferred way of understanding and furthering our relationships with psychic images and artistic expressions. Within the Jungian tradition an image is an invisible and inner psychic phenomenon as distinguished from art objects or pictures, paintings, and photos. I tend to use the word *image* in a broader sense and I refer to different kinds of imagery, both imaginary and physical. In the arts the image can be viewed as "something that is created" (Langer, 1953, p. 47).

Jung established the psychological basis for viewing images and artistic expressions as independent entities with important messages to communicate. These phenomena are real in the psychic sense and they have their own stories to tell, which may be quite different from the way we currently view the conditions of our lives.

In my practice I consistently see how simple methods, such as speaking as a figure or gesture in a painting, meet with considerable feelings of resistance, fear, and ineptitude. Most of us find it very difficult to speak imaginatively from a perspective outside of the habitual ego position. We have to relearn the child's unconscious and instinctual ability to dramatize the figures of the imagination. The process requires that we relax the self and move it out of the way so that imagination can express itself according to its own wisdom.

One of the primary obstacles to what we call imaginal dialogue is the assumption that artistic expressions are essentially printouts of the psyches of the artists who made them. For example, the red that I paint can be likened to my aggressive aspects, but it challenges credibility to say that because I paint red, I am aggressive. Red is not aggression; red is red. If I make comparisons between the color and my emotions, one should not be narrowly defined as expressing the other, or reduced to the other.

I can imagine the red painting saying: "I am not your aggression. You are you and I am me. If we can establish this separateness, maybe we can have a more mature and creative relationship."

Many analogous relations between artistic expressions and the lives of the people who make them can be made without reducing one to the other. We are accustomed to looking at everything in our artistic expressions as parts of ourselves rather than significant others with insights to offer. Rather than encouraging our artistic expressions to speak to us in new ways, we have a tendency to explain them according to what we think they mean or we ask others to tell us what they mean. This ingrained tendency toward literal and reductionistic interpretation makes it difficult to approach artistic image as autonomous entities with a certain degree of separation from the people who made them. I grant that artworks are closely related to their makers, like off-spring that might even carry artistic DNA, but like any other intimate figures in our lives, the artistic expression needs a certain distance from us in order to be fully appreciated. The application of an "I-thou" attitude to our interpretation of artistic expressions is an important starting point.

Jung discovered that the key step to achieving this separation happened when he personified the images of dreams and art objects. He did not literally treat them as people, but he approached them "like" people, giving them a voice as a poet does. I thus introduce imaginal dialogue as poetic speech and distinguish it from the habitual talking we do in the world.

A reluctance to personify is often based on the inability to relinquish control and act as agent for something outside our established concept of who we are. In order to dialogue with an art object I need to speak in a way that is contrary to my most fixed ways of viewing reality and talking. The process may require me to take on a distinctly different persona and be open to expressions that may come from very unfamiliar and uncomfortable places. I may need to risk appearing strange.

Our language structures also reinforce inhibitions since the rules of syntax reinforce the tendency that we all have to approach the self as the center of existence. Objects and things are labeled "inanimate" and we talk about the painting before us via the neuter term, "it." In English, as contrasted to other European languages, nonhuman forms of life and objects are without gender and thoroughly depersonified.

Personifying artistic expressions need not be an upsetting experience. There are times, of course, when spontaneous and unexpected expressions can shake up the existing order. But for many people, personifying involves a subtle shift of consciousness rather than a shattering of worldviews.

For example, people participating in my art therapy groups for the first time frequently make disparaging comments about their pictures—"It's a mess. Those are just childish scribbles."

Rather than give validity to these expressions of insecurity or try to explain how the picture has value, I have found it more effective to ask the artist how the picture might feel about the remark. This simple personification immediately gives the picture dignity; the person who made it invariably begins to respond with compassion to the picture.

Reframing the situation in this way casts the person into an emotional relationship with the art object. Speaking to the picture, the artist might say, "Yes, I see how my comment is offensive to you. Here I am, trying to get in touch with my inner child, and I dismiss you as childish."

Then, responding from the perspective of the picture, the artist might say, "Yes, the child that stopped painting in kindergarten is still intact inside you."

Many artists participating in my art therapy studio for the first time are unable to speak for their paintings. They are stuck in their preconception that paintings do not talk; they are further hampered by the demands that they place on themselves to be imaginative, profound, and psychologically clever while they also fear being too revealing. They are afraid to dialogue, in part because they fear both ineptitude and self-disclosure. Conversely, we have discovered how the same performance anxiety and expectations do not seem as intense when we dialogue with another person's art.

An image may come to the artist's speaker's assistance if simply asked what it needs: "I need to be looked at for what I am. Let go of yourself so that you can see me. If you can experience my unique nature, you will begin to feel emotion within yourself. Articulating my feelings will help you experience yours. You get confused when you try to find something within yourself and use me to present that to another person. I need you to experience me in order for me to enter the world. I need you for this. I come to life through you and maybe I can do the same for you."

It is important to emphasize again how dialoguing with artistic images does not replace visual contemplation or descriptive narratives and more conventional conversations about experience; it is not a more advanced state of experience. It simply engages other aspects of consciousness and expression, more imaginative ones that we do not adequately use.

James Hillman urges us to "doctor" our outmoded and sick stories rather than trying to change the complex and elusive being we call the self (1983, p. 17). In *Healing Fiction* he encourages us to revise and improve the stories by which we organize our lives because the most intractable problems can only be transformed when we approach them with imagination. Furthermore, he says that "healing begins when we move out of the audience and onto the stage of the psyche," actively participating as characters in the play of imagination (p. 38).

Rather than simply functioning as illustrations of the psyches of their makers, the figures in our drawings and paintings can become coparticipants in the life we are making each day. We, in turn, may become concerned for their well-being and protection; we may feel gratitude for their assistance, delight in their presence, and create environments that welcome their visitations, while some may argue, "These persons you are talking about are all parts of your imagination."

I might reply that yes, these are clearly figures of the imagination, but this realm involves more than me alone. Imagination is a different reality from the literal one that we tend to have trouble transcending. Jung actually felt that imagination was the most essential stratum of the psyche. And Hillman emphasizes how the exercise of imagination is not necessarily an introspective pursuit (1983, p. 58). When I personify artistic expressions with a careful sensitivity, I become more attuned to otherness, and perhaps if I listen to what these other figures have to say, they will help me gain a better understanding of experience.

The nineteenth-century European focus on empathy and fellow-feeling reinforced how compassion for others is the basis of morality. Imagination, far from being a frivolous and egocentric activity, is the intelligence that we use to understand others and relationships. The need to develop these sensitivities is greatly overlooked in the world today as people have such a profound inability to go beyond their personal viewpoints. The practice of imaginal dialogue in the personal sphere can thus be a basis for a more comprehensive education of imagination and sensitivity to otherness.

In my experience, the primary challenge that people face when given the opportunity to dialogue with an art object has to do with letting go of control and opening up to spontaneous and unplanned expression. Language and speech are among our most embedded centers of emotional control and it is natural to experience a reluctance to use them in significantly different ways.

For example, the tendency to control open-ended situations often results in people taking on the role of interrogators when they first try to dialogue with a creative expression: "Who are you? What are you doing here? What are you trying to tell me?"

This way of beginning does not exactly put the artistic expression at ease. We act from the perspective of suspicion rather than a generous curiosity about what it may have to say about itself. Why not try approaching the artwork as a person who you really want to meet. Invite the expression into your life with a sense of warmth and hospitality, with a supportive patience that gives it time to speak.

In my practice I find that it is easier for most people to begin talking to artworks as themselves, simply looking at an artistic expression and then telling it what they see in it.

When we act in this way, the object of our dialogue typically begins to speak naturally in response to what we say, just as two might interact in a conversation.

I strongly encourage the most simple and direct speech when introducing imaginal dialogue. We emphasize how depth does not require lots of talking and often has more to do with focus, the quality of attention, openness, and responsiveness. A few words can be transformative. I suggest that people repeat their statements and say them in different ways, discovering how tone has much to do with the content of expression and emotion. When we repeat and restate the words, we are apt to relax, becoming less guarded and more playful, and thus enhance possibilities for discovery. If we are able to expand the range of the voice's expression and connect it to the body and its movement, we feel energized and involved in a whole new world of speaking.

I encourage people to work with whatever words and statements occur rather than thinking too much about what they want to say or trying to be clever or creative. The most common statements can act as gateways to new perspectives on our lives when we totally commit ourselves to them. Ordinary words can take on magical qualities when spoken with conviction and creative energy. In these situations we discover that the way in which we express ourselves, the soulful tone and energy, may have more of an impact than the content of what we say. Healing tends to happen when we transform our feelings toward a problem rather than achieving a conceptual resolution.

An artist in one of my studios found that her picture expressed a desire for autonomy when asked what it needed. It replied, "Let me go! Don't worry, I will be fine."

As the artist continued worrying about whether or not the picture was correct, the painting said, "Put aside your judges. Move like me, in your most natural way. I will support whatever you do. Don't try to be clever. Move from your deep places."

I encouraged the artist to repeat these words over and over since this helped her to internalize them more completely, to say them with more authority, and to listen to the wisdom being generated from her own dialogue.

Her first impulse was to say the words quickly without really letting them penetrate. With the support of our studio group she was able to say the words as she moved and ultimately she used her natural bodily expressions to reinforce the messages conveyed by the dialogue. The authentic way in which she spoke, moved, and related to her painting, and the feelings of sanctity that these expressions generated within our studio, created an atmosphere that transformed everyone who was participating in the experience.

## A NEW MAINSTREAM IN ART THERAPY

During its early stages of growth within the United States the art therapy discipline was primarily identified with psychoanalytically oriented diagnostic practices and it gave less attention to the tradition of healing through creative imagination as developed in Europe by C. G. Jung. Similarly and to this day, there has been a lack of serious consideration of the landmark studies of Hans Prinzhorn, who documented the universal "creative urge" manifested by people afflicted with emotional illness (1972). It is remarkable how Prinzhorn's important work, although now published in an English translation, is still relatively unknown to many art therapists. The same applies to Jung's formative writings on active imagination which, as I have emphasized above, anticipated the best of what people are doing today in the all of the expressive arts therapies.

For example, Jung described how sometimes the hand can help resolve difficulties that the mind and words cannot quite grasp. He also presented a true depth psychology of creative expression that requires a commitment to the unknown, discoveries that can never be planned in advance and that often come upon us suddenly and against our will. These inherently artistic processes do not necessarily accommodate the emphasis on controlled interventions and planned outcomes that characterize so much of contemporary clinical practice.

Over the past decade the discipline of art therapy has moved forcefully and with remarkable consistency toward an embrace of methods based upon the healing powers of the creative process. I am confident that in time the art and healing movement will more completely align itself with the universal forces described by Jung and Prinzhorn at the start of the last century.

The most influential books written in the art therapy field in recent years have embraced soul, spirit, the alchemical depths of the creative process, art making as a primary form of healing, collaboration with other art forms, and a more open view of the discipline grounded in the universal ways in which art heals (Allen, 1992, 1995, 2005; Fryrear & Corbit, 1992; Kapitan, 2003; Knill, Levine, S., & Levine, E., 2005; Knill, Neinhaus Barba, & Fuchs,1995; Levine, E., 1995; Levine, S., 1992; Levine & Levine, 1999; Malchiodi, 2002, 2005; McConeghey, 2003; Moon, B., 1990, 2004; Moon, C., 2001; Robbins, 2000; Rogers, 1993). And in addition, art therapists are significantly expanding the venues of practice to wherever there are people in need, from open studios in urban areas, to healthcare settings where patients are being treated for cancer and other life-threatening illnesses, to refugee camps in the war-torn regions of the world (Kalmanowitz & Lloyd, 1997, 2005).

I predict that these writings will have a lasting impact since they take art and healing beyond the boundaries and trends of contemporary mental health specializations and reconnect us to the universal and reliable power of creative expression to transform afflictions into affirmations of life. The appeal of this new movement lies in its core commitment to healing and renewing the soul through creative expression.

Healthcare professionals, dedicated volunteers, and artists are urged to join us in this work of art and healing. Trained and professionally qualified expressive arts therapists are needed to lead and research this important work, and make it available within clinics and settings where professional credentials are required. But as I mentioned above, the infusion of art and healing into the broad spectrum of society is a public health medicine that needs to be universally accessible. There are no limits to what it can do to repair and improve the world.

## TOOL KIT FOR CHANGE

### Role and Perspective of the Client

1. Art enables the healthcare professional to expand the range of treatment options and access communications and healing forces, as described throughout the preceding chapter, that are not accessible through verbal communication.

2. Patients and participants in art and healing experiences are offered opportunities to become more actively involved in their treatment and to use their most personal expressions as areas of strength.

### Role and Perspective of the Healthcare Professional

1. Therapists and healthcare professionals may support and guide the art experience, but the process largely occurs through the domain of the artist's personal experience, thus making it possible to pursue this way of healing independently as well as within therapeutic relationships.
2. Collaboration with others tends to universally affirm the value of the experience and provides resources that are not available to a person creating alone.

### Interconnection: The Global Perspective

1. Artistic expression is an integrative process where mind, body, and spirit work together within the realm of creative imagination.
2. Healing through art can be considered as offering unique resources for integrating a wide range of experiences and thus able to help transform the most complex and difficult of life's problems and challenges.

## REFERENCES

Allen, P. 1992. Artist-in-residence: An alternative to "clinification" for art therapists. *Art Therapy: Journal of the American Art Therapy Association, 9*(1), 22–29.

Allen, P. (1995). *Art is a way of knowing.* Boston: Shambhala Publications.

Allen, P. (2005). *Art is a spiritual path.* Boston: Shambhala Publications.

Blake, W. (1957). *The complete writings of William Blake with variant reading.* (G. Keynes, Ed.). London: Nonesuch.

Chodorow, J. (Ed.). (1997). *Jung on active imagination.* Princeton, New Jersey: Princeton University Press.

Fryrear, J. & Corbit, I. (1992). *Photo art therapy: A Jungian perspective.* Springfield, IL: Charles C. Thomas.

Hillman, J. (1977). An inquiry into image. *Spring,* 62–88.

Hillman, J. (1978). Further notes on images. *Spring,* 152–182.

Hillman, J. (1979). Image-sense. *Spring,* 130–143.

Hillman, J. (1983). *Healing fiction.* Barrytown, NY: Station Hill Press.

Kalmanowitz, D., & Lloyd, B. (1997). *The portable studio: Art therapy and political conflict: Initiatives in the former Yugoslavia and KwaZulu-Natal, South Africa.* London: Health Education Authority.

Kalmanowitz, D., & Lloyd, B. (Eds.). (2005). *Art therapy and political violence.* London and New York: Brunner-Routledge, 2004.

Kapitan, L. (2003*). Re-enchanting art therapy: Transformational practices for restoring creative vitality.* Springfield, IL: Charles C. Thomas.

Knill, P., Levine, E., & Levine, S. (2005). *Principles and practice of expressive arts therapy: Toward a therapeutic aesthetics.* London: Jessica Kingsley.

Knill, P., Nienhaus Barba, H., & Fuchs, M. (1995). *Minstrels of soul: Intermodal expressive therapy.* Toronto: Palmerston Press.

Langer, S. (1953*). Feeling and form: A theory of art.* New York: Charles Scribner's Sons.

Levine, E. (1995). *Tending the fire: Studies in art, therapy and community.* Toronto: Palmerston Press.

Levine, S. (1992). *Poiesis: The language of psychology and the speech of the soul.* Toronto: Palmerston Press.

Levine, S., & Levine, E. (1999). *Foundations of expressive arts therapy: Theoretical and clinical perspectives.* London: Jessica Kingsley.

Malchiodi, C. (2002). *The soul's palette: Drawing on art's transformative powers for health and well-being.* Boston: Shambhala Publications.

Malchiodi, C. (Ed.). (2005. *Expressive therapies.* New York: Guilford Press.

McConeghey, H. (2003). *Art and soul.* Dallas: Spring Publications.

McNiff, S. (1981). *The arts and psychotherapy.* Springfield, IL: Charles C. Thomas.

McNiff, S. (1988). *Fundamentals of art therapy.* Springfield, IL: Charles C. Thomas.

McNiff, S. (1989). *Depth psychology of art.* Springfield, IL: Charles C. Thomas.

McNiff, S. (1992). *Art as medicine: Creating a therapy of the imagination.* Boston: Shambhala Publications.

McNiff, S. (1998). *Trust the process: An artist's guide to letting go.* Boston: Shambhala Publications.

McNiff, S. (2003). *Creating with others: The practice of imagination in art, life and the workplace.* Boston: Shambhala Publications.

McNiff, S. (2004). Art heals: How creativity cures the soul. Boston: Shambhala Publications.

Moon, B. (1990). *Existential art therapy: The canvas mirror.* Springfield, IL: Charles C. Thomas.

Moon, B. (2004). *Art and soul: Reflections on an artistic psychology.* Springfield, IL: Charles C. Thomas.

Moon, C. (2001). *Studio art therapy: Cultivating the artist identity in the art therapist.* London: Jessica Kingsley.

Nietzsche, F. (1967). *The birth of tragedy and the case of Wagner* (W. Kaufmann, Trans.). New York: Vintage.

Prinzhorn, H. (1972). *Artistry of the mentally ill.* New York: Springer-Verlag.

Richter, J. P. (1973). *Horn of Oberon: School for aesthetics.* Detroit: Wayne State University Press.

Robbins, A. (2000). *The artist as therapist.* London: Jessica Kingsley.

Rogers, N. (1993). *The creative connection: Expressive arts as healing.* Palo Alto, CA: Science & Behavior Books.

Watkins, M. (1983). The characters speak because they want to speak. *Spring,* 13–33.

Chapter Thirteen

# USING THE ARTS TO WORK WITH STRESS AND TRAUMA IN THE ISRAELI CONTEXT

*Vivien Marcow Speiser, PhD, ADTR, LMHC*
*and Phillip Speiser, PhD, RDT, LMHC*

This chapter describes creative arts approaches to working with trauma within the context of the Israeli-Palestinian struggle. While the approaches grew out of a response to a particular situation, they also demonstrate fruitful avenues that can be adapted to other kinds of traumatic situations. Across the globe there are new stresses that include increased threats of terrorism and natural disasters that take place in multicultural settings that can lead to verbal language barriers and miscommunications. The arts offer a nonverbal approach to communication that can address complex actual, symbolic, cultural, and existential issues.

This chapter is coauthored by two expressive arts therapists and academics who live in the United States and who have lived and worked in Israel for many years. As Jews, we needed to do much deep soul-searching and internal confrontation to be able to look at Israel's relationship to the Palestinians, while at the same time understanding and empathizing with the historical, political, and social forces that have brought us to the current moment. Since the time of this work, Israelis and Palestinians have endured more upheaval and torment since the new intifada, which began in October 2000. The need to find effective strategies to cope with the effects of fear and stress is ever more pressing at this time.

In this chapter we will present examples of the work of some groups and individuals who are directly involved in treating the consequences of stress and trauma. We are indebted to the clinicians who shared their work with us, and in particular to the graduates of Lesley University in Israel who are pioneering arts-based approaches to work with traumatic stress. In our conversations with clinicians within Israel and the Palestinian Authority we heard over and over again the personal anguish of these caretakers, who described themselves, their clients, and their societies as all suffering from various degrees of posttraumatic stress disorders. It is within this context that we will present programs and approaches to dealing with the after-effects of war; terror; and the occupation and uprisings in the West Bank and Gaza.

## WORKING IN THE SHADOW OF WAR

Israel has fought the War of Independence of 1948–49; the Sinai Campaign of 1956; the Six Day War of 1967; the Yom Kippur War of 1973; the Peace in Galilee Action in Lebanon in 1982; and the intifada 1987–92 as well as the current intifada. In addition, Israel was attacked in the Gulf War of 1991, and is subject to numerous and ongoing attacks of terror, and sporadic fighting in Lebanon and the West Bank and autonomous regions of Gaza. Given the numbers of Israelis who have served in the armed forces and the impact that this has had upon them and their immediate and extended families, millions of Israelis have been directly affected by the constancy of war and attack. No one is immune to very real danger and risk in this society. In the section that follows, we will describe interventions and programs for working with soldiers and veterans, working with children during the Gulf War, and working with grief. In order to present the painful complexities such work involves, wherever possible we will include clinicians' reactions and feelings.

Menachem Student (1991) attests personally to the painful aspects of doing work with posttraumatic soldiers and their families where: "War is a totally different reality from that of everyday life." He recognizes a real split between everyday reality and the qualities of human connection that operate with the real hell of war. Even though the work he describes takes place subsequent to the traumatic events, the feelings that are evoked in therapist and client alike are intense and painful: "In describing the psychotherapeutic hours included in this book, I am trying to demonstrate the sheer magnitude of pain, loss, and grief and the virtual insanity experienced by my clients and me and demanding from both realities more than they can offer. War can never, by itself, lead to lasting peace. Nor can peace ever heal the wounds war inflicts. Perhaps by calling upon the madness of war and peace, by undergoing the transformations each new crossing demands, and by uniting them in some way, we may achieve peace and sanity" (p. xvi).

At the Community Mental Health Center in Ramat-Chen, Terrie Somekh (1994) describes the feelings she experienced using psychodrama with Israeli veterans suffering from posttraumatic stress disorder:

> For me, working with them was to be overwhelmed by their anger, depression, isolation, and to be caught in the total helplessness of their life experience as second class citizens, a sector of society about whom everyone felt guilty, but also wanted to avoid or forget, indeed deny their very existence. The Israeli male feels that he has to be a warrior, tough and strong, who can always carry on no matter how difficult the situation is (p. 8).

In the Gulf War of January 1991, over a thousand distressed phone calls per day were received in the community center at Ramat-Chen. For Israelis to have to be in a situation where they could not fight back, where their lives and the lives of their families were threatened, was extremely difficult. Israeli citizens were prepared for the possibility of chemical or biological missile attacks. Each person received a gas mask and injections of atropine to use against nerve gas. Each family was asked to prepare a room that could be sealed off with plastic sheets and tapes, which would contain all the family members plus food, supplies, and drinking water. This issuing of gas masks, although necessary, was traumatic for many Holocaust survivors in particular.

Ofra Ayalon (1997) describes the gas masks used during the Gulf War as "a morbid omen." The experience of the gas masks created additional problems, especially for children who had difficulty recognizing their caretakers or hearing their voices through the masks: "The use of gas masks activated the worst fears of total annihilation, and raised, in many cases, panic symptoms which caused approximately one dozen deaths by suffocation or heart attack" (p. 192).

Carmeli, Liberman, and Mevorach (1991) showed that 38 percent of the population demonstrated stress-related symptoms. As many as 43 percent of the people who reached the hospitals after the missile attacks were determined to be suffering from stress reactions. Tamar Zur Weissman (1993) worked with children during the Gulf War using expressive therapy approaches, and summarizes her findings as follows:

> It is important for the intervention to be close to the time the stress was caused and adjacent to the locality of the event. Interventions should be active. It is important to let the person who is affected by stress express his feelings. Returning to dance helped the girls to express their feelings, by sharing it with their friends during the group, and by dancing. Their body and the movement served as a primary means of expression and communication (p. 140).

After the 1973 war the Rehabilitation Department of the Israeli Defense Forces began to run therapy groups for parents and widows whose spouses or children had been killed while serving in the military. Daniella Adam (1993) worked with Druze widows of soldiers who had served in the Israeli army. Her expressive arts therapy group met 26 times over the course of a year in 1990. The group format was very useful since it allowed these women access to expression of feeling and an ongoing support system within Druze society. This group used the arts as expressive tools, including all of the plastic arts, music, and family photographs. Dreams and symbols were discussed and drawn and explored through the use of guided imagery. The group additionally used writing, journaling, bibliotherapy, and literature. All of these interventions proved to be potent tools to help group members with their process of mourning and come to terms with their losses. It helped group members make a transition, from feeling that their lives were over when their spouses died, to finding the will to live. In Druze society, this might take the form of a woman deciding to take driving lessons, which is outside of the norm for women.

Adam also worked for the Ministry of Defense coleading groups for parents who have lost children, children who have lost parents, and adolescents who have lost parents in military action while they themselves are scheduled to be inducted shortly into the Israeli army. Groups for parents tend to be long-term groups that continue for a year or a year and a half, and groups for children tend to be short term and generally continue for three to five weeks. Adam found that time does not make the loss any easier and that over time the loss becomes more difficult. She says: "You can never really overcome this loss when you lose a child" (D. Adam, personal communication, March 3, 1996). The main issue facing parents when they do lose a child in military service is to find ways of continuing to live their lives. The aim of the therapy group is to help parents find these ways. In parallel groups that she runs for children who have lost a sibling, Adam finds that these children often feel neglected by their parents "as if they themselves" had died. In many ways, both parents and the other siblings need to be "brought back to life" in ways where they can once again find meaning.

Adam, who is herself a mother to a son who is serving in the army, talks about her commitment to this work in a personal interview as follows:

> I live in a society which is either at war or threatened by war. I belong to this society, even though deep down I am against conflict. We must do something to help. I can't go to Lebanon so this is my contribution. I try to help people who have made sacrifices in one way or another. I believe that if you help one person you help the whole of Israeli society. (D. Adam, personal communication, March 3, 1996)

Working in the shadow of war, these clinicians are confronting the rawest of wounds in a society where they face the same threats as their clients. They face unique challenges of working with intense transference and burnout. Their work is a testament to the instillation of hope and courage in the face of loss and pain.

## THERAPY GROUP FOR THE ADOLESCENT VICTIMS OF A TERRORIST ACT

In April 1994, a terrorist car bomb parked at a bus stop in the town of Afula exploded and killed 8 people, including 2 children, and injured 30 others. The blast was heard throughout the town, which immediately geared up for emergency action. Rachael Michael was one of the social workers who arrived at the hospital shortly after hearing the explosion. She describes the horrors she witnessed, as she sat with families who were trying to determine whether their family members had survived the blast. Because so many bodies were burned beyond recognition, identification only became possible through fragments of clothing or jewelry, and many of the survivors' bodies were so blackened that it was almost impossible to identify them. In an interview, Michael spoke about her feelings after witnessing such pain and suffering that "I felt that my head was separated from my body." (R. Michael, personal communication, May 6, 1996). Even though her political opinions had been left-wing to start, she has moved even further left in her willingness to work for peace. In a personal interview she described her dilemma as follows:

> We bomb them, they bomb us. We kill them. They kill us. As a therapist I feel unable to help the people who come to me saying that they can't sleep since the bombing. I feel impotent to help. What can I do? How can I help? They are suffering objectively and I feel it too. How can I treat someone when I am feeling the same symptoms? I don't know if we have the professional tools to do so. It's not treating the problem but helping people find comfort in going on living with the same pain. (R. Michael, personal communication, May 6, 1996)

Osnat Segev is an expressive arts therapist who worked with a group of children who had been injured in the bomb blast. The group consisted of seven 13-year-old boys, who had grown up and been schooled together and lost two of their classmates in the blast. The group used art materials as a way of understanding and of coming to terms with their experience, and returning to function, including being able once again to board a bus. As they drew pictures of buses, classmates, and their own feelings of terror and helplessness, they were able to share these with others and begin to come to terms with their grief and losses. They were able to hold memorial services for the classmates they had lost where the following words were said: "I light a candle to your memory, and although I will remember you every day and every minute, I will do everything to keep you as a good memory in my mind and won't feel distressed when I think about you." Or "I know that I have done everything to save you, but there was not much to do because you were killed immediately." At the end of this stage, the teenagers were capable of participating in the unveiling of the monument that was built in the center of town for the memory of the victims, and were able to meet with the bereaved families (Segev, 1998, p. 100).

In questionnaires that were distributed to the group members at the conclusion of the program, all of the participants indicated that the group had been instrumental in helping them to deal with the trauma. Segev elaborated upon some of the issues that came up for her as a therapist dealing with children in this particular situation where she not only had to contain the issues that were coming up for the children, but was called in to support other departments of the hospital in their dealings with the children. Many of these children continue to need further surgical and medical procedures, including cosmetic surgeries, and simply returning to the hospital for any kind of medical procedure was likely to re-evoke the trauma for these them. She talked about how deeply this work affected her and how much anger and depression she has contained as well as feelings of basic helplessness and despair. Both she and the other caregivers in Afula talk about their own reluctance to board buses or let their own children ride the bus.

The continuing work being done in Afula demonstrates the long-term effects that acts of terror perpetrate not only upon immediate victims but upon an entire community. It requires acts of faith for community members to continue to function in the face of such devastation, and great courage for these adolescents and their caregivers to take on, working in the face of such horror.

## COMMUNITY STRESS PREVENTION CENTER

The Community Stress Prevention Center is located in Kiryat Shmona, a small town in the north of Israel, close to the Lebanese border. Kiryat Shmona has been the target of rocket attacks since 1968, and children and adults living there are quite used to spending nights sleeping in shelters. On the day in which we visited the center, there was a general alarm and people were advised to sleep in the shelters that night.

The center was founded by Mooli Lahad. The center had been founded in order to help teachers, parents, and children cope with the psychological effects of being in the shelters. This work has expanded throughout Israel with communities suffering from stress and developed models for caregivers, volunteers, and other community members to cope with stressful situations. The center works systematically to reach the entire community, especially its more vulnerable members. Their approach aims to improve coping mechanisms and to help define what are "normal reactions to an abnormal situation" (Lahad, 1997, p. 1).

Lahad (1997) describes the impact of war and terror on children:

> Childhood is devastated by war. Children who grow up in an environment of continuous, or even intermittent stress are likely to worry about their existence. They may assume that the world is not a safe place, and that parents, the primary source of

children's security, cannot be relied upon for protection at all times, since they leave their children at times of danger. (p. 1)

Following the attack by a Jordanian soldier in which seven girls were killed, the center was called in to help prepare school personnel to deal with the traumatic aftereffects of the attack. The center staff helped the school construct a "critical incident stress debriefing" in which different members of the community worked with different aspects of the incident in order to create as full a picture of the event as possible. In so doing, people got a chance to understand and normalize what they were feeling and were able to develop coping mechanisms and strategies for handling the event. The center also offered services to staff and pupils of the school in the months that followed. Lahad "brought bean seeds painted silver and gave each girl a seed.... Then he told them a story about a forest that was destroyed, but the seeds of which were left behind—the seeds which they were holding in their hands. Then he had them draw group pictures of forests, and they shared what they drew" (p. 14). Lahad was honored at a symposium, "Childhood in the Shadow of War," held at Tel Aviv University in 1998, under the auspices of the Adler Research Center for Social Welfare, for his contribution to the development of resiliency in children in the face of terrorism, war, and violence.

## PALESTINIAN CHILDREN: LIVING WITH VIOLENCE DURING THE INTIFADA

Both Israeli and Palestinian children living in the West Bank and Gaza have had to learn to cope with the stresses of war and the threat of violence. Michele Slone (1998) of Tel Aviv University presented in a symposium on "Childhood in the Shadow of War" in 1998 and reported at that time that the Palestinian children showed a greater incidence of behavioral disorders and Israeli children showed a greater incidence of psychopathology and post-traumatic stress disorders while the Israeli children showed a direct correlation between the a higher the level of political stress and a higher level of distress. The Palestinian children showed a correlation between increased political stress and decreased emotional distress. Slone hypothesized that the Palestinian children were able to "mediate their distress by taking action," even if that was only to throw stones at Israeli soldiers.

Julia Byers used art therapy (1996) in the West Bank and Gaza with Palestinian children under the auspices of the Partnership for Children Project, funded by the Children's Bureau of the Ministry of Health of Canada. Her experience echoes the findings of Slone: "During the author's brief encounter with the people of the West Bank and Gaza, the confusion regarding objective and subjective dangers people experienced was noted. The people felt safe when they should have been afraid, or felt endangered when in fact there was negligible risk" (p. 239).

Working with the arts offers opportunities for the expression of feelings through drawing or use of other media to process and work with those feelings. According to Byers:

> Whether the individual is a child, an adolescent, a parent or an adult mental health worker suffering from burnout, expressing the existential dilemma of war or violence can be extremely empowering when life events leave the impoverished community feeling helpless....Art as communication, therapy, or psychotherapy offers a recontextualized role of validating traumatized people's experiences in a meaningful and healing way. (p. 239)

The psychological impact and consequences of trauma are far-reaching and reach across both sides of the "green line" separating Israel from the Palestinian Authority. Although there are many educators, clinicians, parents, and others who work constantly to ameliorate the effects of war, terror, and occupation, children continue to grow up marked by the shadow side of human experience.

## THE TREATMENT AND REHABILITATION CENTER FOR VICTIMS OF TORTURE

This center was established in the West Bank for the treatment of victims of torture in Israeli and Palestinian jails in 1983 by Dr. Mahmud Sehwail. Sehwail estimates that at least 40 percent of these patients suffer from posttraumatic stress disorder. The Public Committee against Torture in Israel (PCATI) estimates that some 23,000 Palestinians were interrogated by Israel's General Security Services between 1987 and 1993. According to PCATI, these methods of torture include: "Such methods as verbal and psychological abuse, threats against the individual or the individual's family, lack of adequate clothing or hygiene, food and sleep deprivation, tying in painful positions for hours on end, covering the head with a wet or stinking sack, blasting of unbearably loud music, confinement in tiny cubicles, solitary confinement, exposure to cold through outside elements or the blasting of air conditioners, forced physical exercise for excruciating periods, beatings and shaking are all frequently employed by the GSS against Palestinian detainees. These methods have led to irreversible physical and mental damage, and in some cases, even death" (M. Sehwail and the Public Committee against Torture in Israel [PCATI], personal communication, April 26, 1996).

The issue of torture of Palestinian prisoners by Israeli hands is difficult to face. It is a shadow side of the Israeli experience that is deeply at odds with the humanitarian values of the Jewish state. Torture is often explained as a necessary measure to ensure the security of the state. At the same time torture victims are scarred both physically and emotionally by their experience.

## CONCLUSION

It is clear that a heavy toll has been exacted on the Israeli psyche by years of war, acts of terror, occupation, and uprising. The Oslo Peace process and the assassination of Yitzhak Rabin have raised twin banners of hope and despair, and the current deadlock in the peace process is creating a residue and backlog of frustration. Yet many Israelis remain hopeful that there can still be peace with their Arab neighbors.

Yaron Ezrachi (1997) notes:

> [W]hen a growing number of Israelis started to recognize the paradox of the co-existence of our might and limits of our power, to realize how deeply the swords we used cut our own hands, then more and more of us became ready to face the other side as a voice, a subject, an agency in its own right and to hear the counternarratives and memories that have been repressed. It was then that, despite the inner conflicts and divisions, we started to draw a line separating liberation from conquest, our country from theirs, the Palestinian minority in Israel and the Palestinian nation next door, their destiny and ours. (p. 293)

Israelis and Palestinians alike are suffering from the conflict and it is our fervent hope that in being able to look at and confront some of these painful acts and the ways in which clinicians are working with these issues, we can open a doorway into recognizing our common humanity so that future generations may be spared some of the horrors of the past.

## TOOL KIT FOR CHANGE

### Role and Perspective of the Artist/Healer

1. Caregivers often suffer from posttraumatic stress disorders.
2. Active interventions, such as drama therapy, can mediate levels of distress, help people symbolize and understand their feelings, and redirect mourning into reconstruction.
3. The creative arts are especially suited for working with children, who often prefer symbolic or fun ways of telling stories and acting out new possibilities.

### Role and Perspective of the Participant

1. Posttraumatic soldiers can experience virtual insanity via common feelings of terror, helplessness, existential fears of annihilation, pain, and loss.
2. Civilians and families also suffer from stress-related symptoms.

## Interconnection: The Global Perspective

1. Across the globe, new threats from terrorism and natural disasters are growing, and listening to verbal and nonverbal narratives from diverse groups can facilitate communication and understanding.
2. The arts offer a nonverbal approach to communication that can address actual, symbolic, cultural, and existential crises.
3. Individuals' war trauma can awaken and be magnified by previous traumas, such as the Holocaust or being under occupation.
4. This suffering can bring possibilities of transformation.

## REFERENCES

Adam, D. (1993). *Life is not dead: Group work with Druze widows of the Israeli Defense Force.* Unpublished master's thesis, Lesley College Graduate School, Cambridge, MA.

Ayalon, O. (1997). Sealed rooms and gas masks. In M. Lahad & A. Cohen (Eds.), *Community stress prevention* (Vols. 1–2). Kiryat Shmona, Israel: Community Stress Prevention Center.

Byers, J. G. (1996). Children of the stones: Art therapy interventions in the West Bank. *Art Therapy: Journal of the American Art Therapy Association, 13*(4), 238–243.

Carmeli, Y., Liberman, N. & Mevorach, O. (1991). Anxiety related somatic reactions during missile attacks. *Israeli Journal of Medical Science, 27,* 11–12.

Ezrachi, Y. (1997). *Rubber bullets: Power and conscience in modern Israel.* New York: Farrar, Straus and Giroux.

Lahad, M. (1997). Children under stress of war and terror. In M. Lahad & A. Cohen (Eds.), *Community stress prevention* (Vols. 1–212). Kiryat Shmona, Israel: Community Stress Prevention Center.

Segev, O. (1998). *Expressive therapy with post traumatic adolescents.* Unpublished master's thesis, Lesley College Graduate School, Cambridge, MA.

Slone, M. (1998). *Childhood in the shadow of war.* Symposium, Tel Aviv University, Tel-Aviv, Israel.

Somekh, T. (1994). *Art therapy and psychodrama: Their role in the treatment of Israeli veterans suffering from post-traumatic stress disorder.* Unpublished master's thesis, Lesley College Graduate School, Cambridge, MA.

Student, M. (1991). *In the shadow of war: Memories of a soldier and therapist.* Philadelphia: Temple University Press.

Zur Weissman, T. (1993). *Dancing with war.* Unpublished master's thesis, Lesley College Graduate School, Cambridge, MA.

Chapter Fourteen

# MORE THAN WORDS: BRINGING THE ARTS INTO CLINICAL PSYCHOLOGY TRAINING

*Paul M. Camic, PhD*

## INTRODUCTION

How odd and unusual it might seem to think about involving "the arts" in clinical psychology training. Most of us locate the arts as taking place in studios and galleries, on stages, and in concert halls. The practice of clinical psychology, however, occurs in the very different venues of clinics, hospitals, and private offices. Likewise, clinical psychology exclusively involves *talking* and not the range of activities—painting, sculpting, dancing, writing, performing—that are available in the arts. In both North America and the United Kingdom clinical psychology doctoral programs are among the most selective of graduate degrees. Similarly, in many other countries where clinical psychology has risen in popularity and stature, getting accepted into a program is highly competitive and demanding. In such a successful profession, *is* there a need to include something as seemingly esoteric as "the arts" in training schemes? Many would argue that training in clinical psychology seems adequate as it is, but if new areas were to be added to the training curricula, the arts would not be at the top of the list.

Perhaps it might be better to ask what can be gained by including the arts in clinical psychology training. The answer, as I hope this chapter will demonstrate, is that a great deal can be gained. Applied psychology has generally valued the spoken word over other forms of perception. While the privileging of verbal behavior has spawned numerous types of therapies over the last 80 years, it has also limited how we approach clinical work and research. Verbalization of an emotion or feeling state requires certain subsymbolic and symbolic processes to operate. According to Bucci (1985), "To translate emotional experience into words, the massively parallel, analogic, and subsymbolic contents of the non-verbal system must be connected to the single channel, symbolic format of the verbal code" (p. 103). Language, then, is not necessarily the optimal mode of expressing emotion. Sensory and bodily experience, which are the emotional precursors to the spoken word, are subsymbolic and "accessible before the emotional contents themselves can be recognized or acknowledged in symbolic form" (p. 105). Utilizing the arts within a therapeutic context can make subsymbolic emotional content infinitely more accessible.

This chapter begins by addressing where in the doctoral curriculum the arts could be included. It continues by developing a theoretical framework for their inclusion, citing evidence from human evolution, psychological theory, and aesthetics. The arts have been important to the health and mental well-being of many societies throughout history. As central, purposeful, and complex parts of human behavior, the arts can be also be used as tools in the clinical practice of contemporary professional psychology (Sarason, 1990). The arts can engage us emotionally, cognitively, physically, and for some, spiritually. Incorporated within the practice of clinical psychology, they can be part of an interdisciplinary approach to the assessment and treatment of a range of mental health problems in individual, group, and community settings.

## WHAT DO WE MEAN BY *THE ARTS?*

To define what we mean by *the arts* is by no means an easy question as it is laden with inevitable controversy and subject to constant debate. When one thinks about *the arts* one invariably takes into consideration the authors and creators of art and artifacts (Shiner, 2001). Many of these authors-of-arts have attended lengthy university training programs and some have gone on to receive graduate degrees. These people are more easily classified and more readily identified as artists. They perform and exhibit their work and frequently make a living through it. But what of informal artists and the work they do in the basements of community centers and churches, in backyards of neighborhoods (Wali, 2002) and in therapists' offices? Are these people also artists and is their work *art?*

Unfortunately, the classification of who makes art and what may be considered art pervades much of the discussion around the use of the arts in clinical training and in everyday life. The English language does not have a word to describe a person who creates images, sounds, words, and movement other than the word *artist.* Although not legally protected, as is the term *psychologist,* many consider *artist* as a term designated only for properly trained professionals. It is not a declaration that can be as freely used as *gardener* is, for example, to indicate an interest in working the earth. The English language also contains no term to adequately describe art as a *process* and not a product. Yet, it is often the processes, and not the products, of the arts that are the focus of therapeutic art modalities. It has thus become linguistically problematic for us to speak of the arts in the context of clinical practice in psychology.

For the purposes of this chapter, and to separate the professional fine and performing arts with those used in clinical practice, the term *therapeutic arts* will be employed. This author (Camic, 2001) had previously suggested the acronym, *CISMEW* (somewhat seriously, somewhat tongue-in-cheek) to refer to the process of the arts and not the final product, as we are all too accustomed to spotlight in Western culture today. CISMEW—creating images, sound, movement, enactment, and words—while somewhat uneuphonious, helps us move away from associations with formal artistic training, styles of expression, and critical analysis, and places our focus on the creative and therapeutic processes involved within sound making, image producing, movement, ritual, and writing, all of which were the forerunners to the arts as we know them today (Dissanayake, 1988). Therapeutic arts comprise the creative and therapeutic use of the arts within psychological practice, and include the domains of assessment, psychotherapy, consultation, and training.

## Practicalities and Curricula: A Place for the Arts in Clinical Training and Practice

In forming a doctoral curriculum in psychology and the arts one needs to develop a theoretical and evidence-based foundation that considers evolutionary factors inherent in making art, cross-cultural evidence of the arts, emerging brain-behavior research about the arts, and clinical research within psychology and the arts therapies. In addition to these areas of study, I have found it essential to include an art-based experiential component in the curriculum. This is probably the most difficult concept for most psychologists to accept, yet I believe it to be crucial if we are to train clinicians and clinical researchers who will make interdisciplinary contributions to the field.

Doctoral training in clinical psychology is personally and intellectually demanding, time-consuming, costly, and slow to incorporate innovative practices. The curricula of doctoral programs are determined by national accrediting bodies (e.g., American Psychological Association, Canadian Psychological Association, British Psychological Society) and often leave very little room for elective courses, let alone pioneering ones. This traditionalism remains a challenge not only for incorporating the arts but also to initiating other innovative training experiences. The structure of doctoral training in clinical and counseling psychology is organized around three primary components: teaching theory, developing clinical practice (assessment, psychotherapy, and consultation), and research training. While there are opportunities for innovative use of the arts in each of these areas, for the purposes of this chapter I will specifically focus on the clinical practices of assessment and psychotherapy and conclude with some thoughts about training opportunities within the doctoral curriculum.

## Assessment

Assessment in clinical and counseling psychology generally refers to a process of gathering information from (and about) a client, placing that information within a context, developing a formulation, determining the diagnosis, and recommending a treatment plan. Gathering information may take place over a period of a few weeks and includes an interview, review of previous psychological and medical history, and often the administration of psychometric instruments. These paper and pencil tests can be utilized to assess a range of areas such as memory, emotional state, cognitive functioning, intellectual capacity, vocational aspirations, interpersonal relations, unconscious processes, and other related areas of concern to the practicing psychologist.

All clinical and counseling psychology doctoral programs devote class time and time in clinical practica to assessment. Typically organized as a two- to three-course assessment sequence, scheduled concurrently with direct clinical work in a practicum setting, assessment is seen as an important part of training. Therapeutic arts in assessment can be incorporated within the current course structure to complement current assessment topics. Although it is beyond the scope of this chapter to give more than a brief introduction to the many possibilities, there are several areas where therapeutic arts can enhance existing assessment procedures. Within the visual arts, drawing is likely the most accessible medium. It is easily available to a wide range of clients and is not dependent on verbal language skills, making it useful across different cultural groups. Many readers, however, may be aware of the arguable limitations of drawing-based assessment (e.g., House-Tree-Person Test, Kinetic Family Drawing, Bender Gestalt Test) (Lillienfeld, Wood, & Garb, 2000; Wood, Nezworski, & Stejskal, 1996). These visual-based assessment tools often fail to be effective because they ignore an individual's artistic abilities and the visual-spatial, cognitive, and kinesthetic developmental factors that help form these abilities (Lowenfeld & Brittain, 1970). After decades of administering these instruments, psychometric reliability continues to prove elusive.

Drawing can, however, augment routine clinical assessment in children and adults in the following ways:

- As an information gathering tool to complement the initial assessment interview (asking the client to draw a floor plan of his/her office, classroom, or home to further discussion and information gathering) (Jacobson, 1995)

- As a memory assisting tool (helping an adult client recall a particular event or life period through drawing a floor plan of a significant location)

- As a baseline piece of information that can be revisited and revised from time to time during the course of therapy (asking the client to draw a visual representation of the issue[s] they seek to work on in therapy and to write a narrative describing the drawing)

- As a goal-setting device to assess a client's resources and to build a focus for therapy (requesting the client to draw a map of where he or she is currently and where he or she wants to get to; the client can be directed to include obstacles and challenges, resources and strengths, as well as hopes and aspirations)

- A method of program evaluation (Evans & Reilly, 1996)

Other therapeutic arts can also be utilized in the assessment process. They include:

- Assemblage (Elderfield, 1992), collage (Brommer, 1994), and photo collage (Landgarten, 1993) are art forms that are readily accessible in an office or hospital setting and can be used in multicultural environments. These visual art forms share ease of accessibility, are generally seen to be nonthreatening by clients, and can be used in a range of settings.

- The short story is a well-known medium to most children and adults. Beginning with "Once upon a time...." a client is asked to write a one- to two-paragraph story with a beginning, middle, and end about an issue in his or her life. This tool is valuable to help develop a creative narrative that can add a playful, yet useful, element to the assessment process (Vygotsky, 1922/1971, p. 89–117). The story can also be further discussed once therapy begins, if this is appropriate.

- Through the use of movement the client is invited to expand on any feeling or image she or he has at the time of assessment (Rogers, 1993). Although this may not be appropriate for all clients, it can provide the clinician with important information about how a client feels about and perceives her or his body. Asking a client if he or she would like to explore through the use of movement the emotion or issue just mentioned can be a powerful question. It also demonstrates that the therapist is interested in one's entire being and not only what a client can communicate verbally.

## Psychotherapy

Psychotherapy, broadly defined, seeks to heal emotional injuries, increase understanding of self and others, develop a capacity for self-reflection, reduce symptoms, change behavior, alter thinking patterns, inhibit maladaptive emotional responses, and encourage adaptive ones. Although there have been many advances in neuroscience, neuropsychological assessment, and psychopharmacology during the last 25 years, there have been far fewer advances in psychotherapy. The process and procedures of cognitive-behavior therapy, for example, have been well established (Barlow, 1993; Greenberger & Padesky, 1995; Wampold, 2001) in treatment manuals but have remained rather static during this time period. As psychotherapy training within clinical psychology has moved to accept "evidenced-based practice" as the sine qua non of clinical training over the past decade (Sackett, Strauss, Richardson, Rosenberg, & Hayes, 2000), it has also surprisingly ignored the importance of advances in basic science over this same time period (Weston & Bradley, 2005). It is not a matter that pertains only to cognition and behavior—the primary components of evidence-based treatment manuals developed 20 years ago—but also must take into consideration neural mechanisms of learning, underlying vulnerabilities for psychiatric disorders, developmental pathology, emotion, psychoneuroimmunology, unconscious processes, and social and cultural considerations that are not contained in treatment manuals (Knight & Camic, 2004; Weston & Bradley, 2005). Evidenced-based practice has also overlooked the complexities of psychotherapy cases not so easily studied in research paradigms that call for short-term treatment results (Weston, Novotny, & Thompson-Brenner, 2004). Unfortunately, most evidence-based treatments focus on a specific symptom in brief, 8-to-12-session psychotherapy, while ignoring more complex problems and issues that many clinicians routinely face in their day-to-day practices.

Psychodynamic, systemic, group, and art therapies, while often used in clinics, hospitals, and private practice, have mostly eluded the psychotherapy researcher's radar screen. And when they are on the screen they are met either with complaints from researchers (who make adherence to positivist and quantitative methodology more important than asking the challenging questions as to *how* this form of therapy really does help some people) or with resistances from clinicians (who fail to make what happens in therapy explicit enough to research). One exception to this is the case of Cognitive-Analytic Therapy (CAT), an approach that integrates cognitive and psychoanalytic theory in a time-limited framework while also stipulating parameters that can be researched (Ryle, 1990).

Therapeutic arts practices do not offer a panacea in regards to the issue of evidence-based practice. But they do allow the clinician access to additional tools and a creative flexibility to explore complex and challenging problems with a wide range of clients while taking into consideration ethological, biological, and psychological evidence (Camic, 2001). It pushes clinicians to use "clinical practice as a natural laboratory for identifying promising treatment approaches" (Weston & Bradley, 2005, p. 267) developed in the community by clinicians and not a priori by researchers. More recent evolutionary theories, which will be taken up later in the chapter, lend support for the utility of art making as a series of behaviors with emotional and cognitive benefits for the maker of art. Although the function and location of art making may have changed over the millennia, art making remains both a stimulus and a response, coming from and creating emotional responses in the maker. Given that the arts involve kinesthetic, sensory, visual, auditory, memory, and social experience, they seem like ideal additions to a primary-care-oriented biopsy-chosocial approach to health and well-being that makes use of individual, group, couple, family, and community interventions. One such approach, incorporating the therapeutic arts within cognitive-behavior group therapy for chronic pain (Camic, 1999b), drew from behavioral, cognitive, and existential theories to provide a theoretical rationale and a clinical plan to use the arts with this population.

The psychotherapy training core within doctoral level clinical/counseling psychology programs can be expanded to offer a limited range of training in therapeutic arts. In both clinical practica and university course work, therapeutic arts can be introduced and supported as offering additional tools from which the practicing psychologist can draw upon in clinical work.

## Training Models

There are any number of different pathways for a doctoral program to introduce the therapeutic arts. Part of the selection will relate to faculty interest, flexibility of a particular program's course schedule regarding elective options, and the innovative stance held by faculty toward a radical new addition to the psychology curriculum. The latter consideration is an important one as the therapeutic arts will be seen as innovative, but are also likely to be viewed as unconventional and not in the training mainstream that APA, and other national accrediting bodies, mandate for program approval.

One such program that provides extensive training in therapeutic arts is the Chicago School of Professional Psychology, which offers clinical courses utilizing music, drama, visual art, writing, and dance, specifically designed for clinical psychology students. Also offered is an interdisciplinary arts studio class taught by an artist in a studio environment (Wilson, 2001) which introduces these art forms. Additional courses include the psychology of creativity and a capstone course in expressive therapies. This six-course sequence can be completed as electives over a three-year period. The faculty are a team of psychologists, arts therapists, and artists with extensive graduate school instruction within their own disciplines. These courses have produced high levels of student satisfaction, doctoral dissertation research, and expansion of the clinical options available to psychologists (Gaugh, 2001).

In a program where the therapeutic arts are offered as a minor area of concentration in doctoral education, the following areas are important components of any such education: hands-on experience within an interdisciplinary art studio course involving movement, writing, performance, visual art, and music, for without the experience of "playing in the mud," a student will not understand the power and potential of the arts (Wilson, 1998); an ethological-historical overview of the arts (Aiken, 1998; Dissanayake, 1992, 2000); an introduction to applied biobehavioral aesthetics, which examines how the arts can be utilized in psychotherapy practice drawing from work in dance/movement, music, drama, and art therapies (Levine & Levine, 1999; McNiff, 1981, among others); research methods that investigate a variety of approaches to studying the arts in psychotherapy (Camic, Rhodes, & Yardley, 2003; Fedder and Fedder, 1998; Lorenzetti, 1994; McNiff, 1998); supervised clinical practicum work utilizing theories and approaches from the arts therapies and psychology (Warren, 1993; Wiener, 1999).

This extensive offering of therapeutic arts courses may not be possible or desirable within all doctoral programs. Additional training models could include one of the following options:

- A year-long two-course autumn/spring sequence that includes experiential learning, theory, and clinical supervision. This curriculum may be more suited for advanced doctoral students, perhaps to be taken in their final year of classes. Key areas to include in these two courses are evolutionary utility of the arts (Bradshaw, 2001; Dissanayake 1992, 2000; Orians, 2001), experiential learning "labs," psychological aesthetics (Maclagan, 2001), psychological theories and the arts (Dewey, 1934/1980; Freud, 1953/1997; Gardner, 1973, 1982; Long, 2004; Petrie, 1946), and case studies.

- A term-long directed readings seminar where each medium (visual, drama, music, movement, and writing) is discussed within psychological theory and clinical psychology practice. Limited experiential learning can also accompany this seminar.

A description of an above-mentioned term-long seminar, *The Arts in Clinical Practice*, taught by the author in the Clinical Psychology Programme at Canterbury Christ Church University, follows:

Integrating the Arts into Clinical Psychology Practice: Much of the work of clinical psychologists involves the spoken word with little or no attention to other modes of expression. In many ways this has potentially limited the profession to a more or less linear based verbal practice. While respecting the tradition and history of clinical psychology, this seminar will introduce participants to theoretical, historical and empirical perspectives that lend support for including the arts in clinical psychology practice. This support is seen in the evolutionary utility of the arts, in identifiable psychological mechanisms that occur in arts experiences, and in the role aesthetics play in emotion and cognition.

This series of seminars and workshops are designed to provide a "learning laboratory" within which participants can explore how integrating the arts into clinical practice can expand our range of treatment (and research) possibilities with clients. Participation in the seminar does not require previous experience in any of the arts. It does ask however, that you come with a sense of curiosity, exploratory inquisitiveness, and creative openness as to what the arts can offer clinical psychology practice. The seminars will involve discussion, experiential learning, and application, which will allow participants to experience something of how the arts might be applied to clinical work with individuals, families, organisations, and communities.

The focus of each seminar will vary somewhat depending on the interests of participants. Each seminar will be structured using a learning laboratory approach where we will explore the possibilities of the medium, reflect on our responses to it, and discuss how it might be applied to clinical work. The media we will explore include movement, visual images, enactment, sound, and the word. We will also examine how to establish an evidenced based practice using the arts as a part of our clinical repertoire.

Participants will be asked to read 1–3 chapters/papers for each seminar and to actively participate in discussion and experiential learning. This seminar is not an introduction to art (or music or drama) therapy. The focus of our discussion and some of the readings is designed to explore how the arts can be integrated with and incorporated into clinical psychology, alongside other influences and approaches currently utilised by the profession.

## A Theoretical Framework for Integrating the Arts and Clinical Practice

As discussed earlier in this chapter, the evidence of evidence-based practice is often limited to a few specific symptoms and does not address the complexity of issues and problems many people bring into the clinic. Psychologist practitioners are well aware that lack of statistical evidence does not necessarily imply a lack of clinical evidence, and that a therapist's office is often a more valid location to collect data than a laboratory. As a profession, we cannot wait for psychotherapy procedures to be created and validated by a few academic researchers or for government health policy bureaucrats and insurance company executives to be the sole determinates of clinical practice. This is certainly not to suggest we discard those advances, but it is a suggestion that we do not rely solely on results from the academic laboratory. It is equally important that clinical researchers and clinicians document what is created in day-to-day therapeutic work in clinics and offices, taking into consideration the complexity of symptoms and not attending only to discrete disorders.

There is significant theoretical, historical, and empirical evidence to support the inclusion of the arts in psychotherapy training in psychology. This support, which will be discussed in the next section, is seen in the evolutionary utility of the arts, identifiable psychological mechanisms that occur in arts experiences, and the role of aesthetics in emotion and cognition.

## Evolutionary Utility

Although not agreed upon by all ethologists or evolutionary psychologists (Bradshaw, 2001) there is significant evidence that the arts have evolutionary utility (Aiken, 1998, 2001; Dissanayake, 1988, 1992, 2000). Evidence demonstrating the existence of the arts—in various forms using different materials—since the time of *homo erectus* over 200,000 years ago, and well before the appearance of modern *homo sapiens,* is well documented (Bahn, 1998, p. xv).

Every prehistoric, ancient, and contemporary cultural group has developed some form of what we have come to call *the arts* (Bahn, 1998; Dissanayake, 1992; Marshack, 1991). Well before shamans, scientists, or psychologists created their professional roles, the arts existed (Dissanayake, 1988; Pinker, 1997).

The arts' involvement in human evolution, while arguably important to human survival, may provide important insights into how psychologists can use the arts as tools in clinical practice. Dissanayake's hypothesis and her resulting extensive research suggesting the arts came about *to make the ordinary special* (Dissanayake, 1988, 1992) is compelling. Making the ordinary special can be seen as an effort to organize emotional, behavioral, and cognitive responses to environmental and cultural phenomena. For example, the process of synchronizing disparate movements to form an organized pattern of movements (dance), combining sounds in such a way as to create tonal patterns for purposes of emotional remembrance (music), putting words together that seek to evoke, warn, and comfort (poetry and stories), making marks on trees, cave walls, and tools to help expand upon daily experiences (visual art), and integrating sound, movement, and words with visual images to produce rituals and ceremonies (drama) are all examples of how *homo sapiens*, during our 40,000-year history, have needed to mark and to make special important yet ordinary events.

Humans have evolved to create culture and societies for complex reasons. These reasons include the need to socialize and communicate with others for both economic and security purposes, as well as to create what cannot be experienced living alone. The arts, seen ethologically as behaviors that involve the actions of participating, creating, observing, and responding, can also be viewed as psychological identifiers of culture. These identifiers allow humans to recreate initial feelings of mutuality, beginning with the relationship between mother and infant, and go on to encompass many developmental and social events throughout life. They also facilitate the need for belonging, finding, and making meaning, and gaining physical competence, all of which are evolutionarily important (Dissanayake, 2000). These actions and identities, seen here as a biobehavioral foundation for the arts, also provide a conceptual link for incorporating the arts in psychotherapy (Camic, 1999a; Kaplan, 2000).

When considering evolutionary utility of a set of behaviors, such as the arts, most of the attention of evolutionary psychologists and ethnologists has been directed toward the art product or what the art-making activity can gain externally for the artist (e.g., higher status in a social group, better options for mate selection, etc.) (Aiken, 2001; Dissanayake, 2000). In order to understand more fully how the arts can contribute to psychotherapy practice it would be helpful to first examine the emotional and cognitive impact of the art-making process on individuals who make art (Allen, 1995). A better understanding of what occurs cognitively, emotionally, and perceptually for the person making art can help provide needed information regarding how the incorporation of the arts into psychotherapy training can benefit clients. Although it is impossible to establish exactly what emotional responses humans, living thousands of years ago, experienced as they created art, it is likely art making served at least two purposes: the need to understand the unknown and the elaboration of what was ordinary and usual. Emotion and cognition are involved in both of these purposes.

Looking back to the beginning of our species more than 40,000 years ago, we can hypothesize that the tension and anxiety associated with the unknown aspects of life for early *homo sapiens* was managed, in part, through movement and sound making, which in time became ritualized by virtue of the strong emotional response these activities triggered for participants. Likewise, the ordinary things of day-to-day life such as tools and living spaces invited visual elaboration, perhaps with markings, design, and color, which enhanced their emotional-aesthetic appeal through evoking ethological releasers (Coss, 1968). For the arts to have served a psychological function in human development, important emotional and cognitive responses need to have occurred for the art maker and the art viewer from an evolutionary perspective (Kreitler & Kreitler, 1972). For the art maker, these responses include the moments when inspiration coalesces into aesthetic solutions (Aiken, 1998, 2001; Browne, 1980; Csikszentmihalyi, 1988; Piirto, 1992; Rank, 1989/1932; Wilson, 1998). The psychological components involved in these solutions have multiple reinforcing properties that serve to encourage the art maker to continue creating. Working with a client toward an aesthetic response to a problem can build upon existing strengths and help develop new and creative approaches to the challenges of living a full life (Camic, 1999b).

The client-creator (art-maker) is simultaneously making, experiencing, viewing, and evaluating their work in the presence of a therapist. Emotional, cognitive, behavioral, and aesthetic responses occur concurrently in this therapeutic environment. Unlike the professional arts, most of the focus of therapeutic arts lies in attending to the process of creating, with an explicit goal to assist the client in resolving a conflict and gaining greater understanding of a problem, these being the "products" or end result of the work. The end result of present-day arts-oriented psychotherapy may be similar to the benefits early hominids experienced in elaborating and making special thousands of years ago: gaining control over fear; reducing uncertainty; increasing emotional competence; and establishing social relations. Comparing early *Hominid* attempts at elaboration with contemporary clients' use of the arts in psychotherapy provides a link which helps to clarify the important underlying psychological mechanisms and evolutionary role of the arts as a therapeutic practice.

The feelings and emotional responses that are experienced *when creating* are different from the emotional reactions one feels when others respond to one's creative endeavors (Gedo, 1996). I may feel deep satisfaction at completing a poem that expresses my visit to an island off the Maine coast. Working on the poem may allow me to see a new geological formation or observe waves in a neoteric way. Writing the poem may leave me feeling more connected to the island, my sense of self, and my purpose in the world. These are all significant internal (cognitive and affective) responses that make it likely I will write more poetry. After completing a dozen or so poems I may decide to attend the open mike night at the local library and the kindly audience listens to one or two of them. There is some warm laughter, nodding of heads, and a few smiles. While these responses may provoke a positive impact on me—and encourage me to come again or perhaps submit to the local literary magazine—it is my earlier, internal responses that will bring me back to writing. Intermittent reinforcement from others (an external response) may or may not increase the volume of my work. This type of reinforcement is likely to influence whether I publicly recite or publish my poems. It is not likely to affect my emotional responses that come from writing about an early morning sun intermingling with the night's leftover fog, which creates a kind of floating netherworld pierced by the shrill screams of gull-demons. These responses are part of a cognitive-affective "working through" process that involves a client creating an aesthetically influenced solution to a problem.

Evolutionary theory must be seen as limited when psychological needs and emotional responses are considered only as mechanisms or cues that have prompted *homo sapiens* to respond to needs pertaining to food, shelter, or sex (Dissanayake, 2000; Hird, 2006). While understanding these mechanisms is important, a broader understanding of changing evolutionary needs would also unify the biological and the cultural, as E. O. Wilson has done with the concept of consilience (Wilson, 1998). Consilience takes into consideration ethology, biology, economics, sociology, psychology, religion, and the arts in the context of examining a changing environment throughout the evolution of our species. The theory of consilience provides a foundation that allows us to abandon the necessity of reducing ancient or current art-making practices from a separate stimulus-response set, and to see them as behaviors within a broad cultural context. In connecting "making special" or what later she comes to call *elaborating*, Dissanayake (2000) proposes a bioevolutionary theory supporting the interrelatedness of art (elaborating) and love (intimacy) that considers psychological needs and emotional responses as evolutionary evidence for understanding why the arts exist. Her theory lends strong support for the importance of art in human evolution and supplies valuable insights into psychological functions and emotional responses that are seen in all the arts, contributing a theoretical and practical basis in which to make use of the arts in psychotherapy.

## Psychological Mechanisms

In addition to acknowledging the arts as evolutionarily important to human development, psychological mechanisms need to be identified within the art-making process in order for the arts to be a part of psychotherapy practice in professional psychology. This section suggests four such mechanisms and includes psychoanalytic, homeostatic motivation, cognitive orientation, and the experience of mutuality.

Psychoanalytic theories of art, and their inclusion of intrapsychic mechanisms, are likely the most widely known of all psychological theories. These theories, while not unitary, generally share an adherence to seeing artistic work as sublimations of drives or wishes. According to Freud, the created artwork is an attempt to obtain socially sanctioned gratification while screening a hidden wish (Freud, 1953/1997). The hidden wish is an unconscious and socially unacceptable desire that needs to be controlled. This perspective views art as a by-product of sexual and aggressive impulses channeled into socially accepted creative endeavors; by appropriately redirecting the energy of one's id, beautiful works of art can apparently come into being.

Michael Maltby (2003), however, in discussing the creation of poetry as a "basic constructive task," reminds us that the art maker "does not seem to be exclusively dominated by a struggle to overcome repression but is actually seeking to make something by drawing on as full and inclusive access to their emotional life as possible" (p. 55). This is in line with Milner's (1975) description of art making as an attempt to bring to a conscious level of experience what is not graspable by the conscious mind. She regarded painting not as a sublimated form of a repressed drive but as a representation of what cannot be known in other ways (Milner, 1957).

Seeing art making as an undertaking with "the primary aim of creating what has never been radically challenges earlier psychoanalytic theory and demonstrates that the artist's fundamental activity goes beyond the recreation of the lost object" (Anna Freud, quoted in Milner, 1957, p. xiv). Art making becomes something much more than an attempt to recreate a symbolic image of the past, or a defense against unwanted urges and impulses. For D. W. Winnicott, noted British pediatrician and psychoanalyst, art is a form of creativity where "creativity is the doing that arises out of being" (Winnicott, 1971, p. 40). In this view, art making is seen, not as a socially acceptable product of a defense mechanism seeking to keep human drives under wraps, but as a place for creative exploration of what is and what might be. Milner and Winnicott see art as one form of the creative process where the value of knowing and experiencing firsthand becomes a way of pulling together the internal and external. In creating an artifact, a dance, music, a poem or story, one encounters the particularities of the medium as one discovers new parts of the self (Caldwell, 2000).

A second psychological mechanism is described by the model of homeostatic motivation (Kreitler & Kreitler, 1972), which proposes that observing and making art firstly creates tension, then secondly, relief, before bringing about a restoration of emotional balance. For the purposes of psychotherapy I would add it is not always a "restoration" of emotional balance that is possible or desirable, but for some the creation or establishment *of* emotional balance, perhaps for the first time in a person's life. In describing this as a motivational model the authors contend, "The art experience is motivated by tensions which exist prior to its onset, but [is further] triggered through the productions of new tensions by the work of art" (p. 16). The initial tensions are "a major motivation for art…which exist in the spectator of art prior to his exposure to the work of art. The work of art mediates the relief of these preexisting (diffuse) tensions by generating new tensions which are specific [to the art work]" (p. 19). This model proposes that moderate rises in tension, which occur when observing art, are regarded as pleasant but that very high or very low levels of stimulation are unpleasant. Thus, depending on an individual's prior experience with art, cultural background, and knowledge of art, certain art experiences will be under- or overstimulating and not likely to be found pleasant or desirable.

I suggest that this same mechanism is intensified when art is *created* and can be further used as a therapeutic tool in clinical psychology practice (Camic, 1999a). As a client creates visual art, engages in movement and dance, develops a scripted performance, or puts together sounds to make music, specific tensions are increased within the art-making experience. It is through an increase in these art-making-related tensions that solutions to emotional distress can be worked on with the support and insight of the therapist. In a psychotherapy that utilizes any of the arts, attending to the optimal level of activation (Fiske & Maddi, 1961) for the client is a key role of the therapist. According to this model the therapist acts both to restrict sensory stimulation and induce sensory stimulation, as necessitated by the client and his/her problems, hoping to bring about an optimal level of stimulation (Schultz, 1965). It is within this optimal level of stimulation, also seen in many other forms of psychotherapy, where the most productive work is likely to occur. The mechanism of tension reduction through tension induction is not a new concept, first being described by Tinbergen (1951).

The initial motivating tensions that bring a client to therapy can be relieved, in part, by an optimal increase in creative or problem-solving tension through the use of therapeutic arts in the context of psychotherapy. New tensions brought about by art making are specific tensions, as described by Kreitler and Kreitler (1972), which can be addressed within the context of therapeutic art making in psychotherapy. As early *homo sapiens* experienced the tensions of seasonal changes, births and deaths, illness, encounters with wild animals, threats from enemies, the rising sun and the onset of darkness, full moons, and other interactions with their environment, they embellished and elaborated upon their day-to-day lives by creating ritual and ceremony which involved organized movement, rhythmic sound, dramatic performance, and visual display (Dissanayake, 1988; 2000). These emotional and aesthetic responses are also encountered by contemporary psychotherapy clients as they deal with their own burdens, problems, and worries through creating images, sounds, movements, enactment, and writing, likewise engaging in elaboration (art making) to reduce tension from internal and external stresses.

In addition to the psychoanalytic and homeostatic models, which address intrapsychic and motivational principles respectively, the theory of cognitive orientation brings a third dimension to our understanding of art and psychology. This theory postulates "that a stimulus turns into a cue only after it is subjected to a series of (cognitive) processes designed to determine its meaning and the relations of this meaning to the relations of other concomitant stimuli, external and internal" (Kreitler & Kreitler, 1972, p. 23). Stated another way, the theory of cognitive orientation puts forth that "complex structures of beliefs determine, shape, and direct behaviour" (p. 328). Art making, as a part of therapy, allows an individual one way to expand her or his cognitive orientation through confrontation with novel experiences. These novel experiences may cause conflict and be unpleasant as they challenge the status quo. Yet the client's intent to disrupt an unsatisfactory present in order to create an altered future can be enhanced through exposure to the dissonant views and information contained in therapeutic arts through exposure to newness, variety, and optimal complexity. "The motive to expand, elaborate, and deepen cognitive orientation" (Kreitler & Kreitler, 1972, p. 328) is stimulated by a human preference for new information. If humans had only a preference for the recognizable and well-known we might have been extinct several thousand years ago.

In applying the theory of cognitive orientation to therapeutic arts, it is the encounter with the art medium (e.g. clay, paint, movement, development of a character) that is initially experienced as a stimulus by the client. This stimulus disrupts homeostasis and evokes an orientating response (Lynn, 1966). The orientating response includes a number of psychophysiological changes (heart rate, galvanic skin response, pupil dilation, breathing, brain wave activity), which facilitate the obtaining of information about the art medium, the emerging work, and oneself. These initial percepts, originating at the beginning of the client's work, are not likely to be conscious (Bucci, 1995). By continuing to explore the art-making experience (perhaps verbally but not necessarily so), changes in homeostasis occur that will activate additional percepts. The therapist facilitates this process by encouraging further exploration of the work while not placing demands on the client by interpreting the work psychoanalytically or aesthetically. The act of interpreting a client's artwork can have the effect of reducing art created in therapy to a totem or a symbol of an objective external reality. The art making should be seen as a part of the therapy and not as a symbol for a "truth" external to the art. Although this latter concept is open to a great deal of debate among expressive arts therapists as well as psychologists using the arts in therapy, the aim of using therapeutic arts in psychology practice is *not* the creation of a self-styled Rorschach (Exner, 1993).

It is the various sensory qualities of the object (or experience for the temporal arts), if optimally stimulating, that activate percepts. Continuing to create art is inclined to lead to more complex art-making behaviors, triggering further emotional and cognitive responses. These responses require the integration of several meanings, related to both the beliefs of the client and the stimuli of the situation. For example, the client may ask questions such as, What is this that I have painted? What sounds have I formed? Why did I make those spontaneous movements? In answering these questions the client must consider a complex set of meanings drawn from their immediate experience and from their history. Attempting to answer this question further directs the action of the client. The theory of cognitive orientation explains this process as one that emphasizes behavior being guided by what a person believes about self, others, and the world around them. Cognitive development for *homo sapiens* continues to evolve and change over the course of thousands of years for the species, whereas cognitive *orientation* can change over the course of several weeks of psychotherapy for an individual client.

Thus far I have discussed psychoanalytic, motivational, and cognitive mechanisms that are involved in art making within the context of psychotherapy. I will conclude this brief discussion of psychological mechanisms by returning to the work of Ellen Dissanayake (2000). Dr. Dissanayake is neither a psychologist nor an expressive arts therapist, but her work has significant implications for both disciplines. Extending the work of Bowlby (1969), Ainsworth (1989), and Stern (1985), she provides some of the missing conceptual links as to why the arts were developmentally important to early hominids and how they remain so today. Particularly relevant to our discussion is her contention that the arts are evolutionarily rooted in the spontaneous ability of mothers to produce rhythmically coordinated patterns and signals, and for infants to recognize and reciprocate them (Dissanayake, 2000, p. 42). These patterns and signals, referred to as "mutuality" by both Rose (1996) and Dissanayake (2000), and the corresponding affective resonance between mother and infant (Rose, 1996), set the foundation for physical and emotional health throughout life. According to Dissanayake, humans evolved to require the signs of mutuality—respect, affection, comfort, recognition, praise, emotional support, and attention—just as they require water and food. Mutuality is the essential building block of our humanity, she believes, and the essence of cultural development.

The concept of mutuality is made up of two characteristics, rhythms and modes, which are patterns that evolved to help sustain the relationship between mother and infant through years of dependency. The features of rhythms and modes include sounds, facial expressions, and movements. These are vocal, visual, and kinetic signals respectively, which are temporally and spatially patterned, dynamically varied, and multimodally presented and received (Dissanayake, 2000, pp. 129–166). These properties also characterize ritual ceremonies, the precursors to the arts as we know them today. The rhythmic-modal behavior in rituals and in art is also a component of most psychotherapies, manifesting in empathy, reflection, support, mirroring, reinforcement, understanding, and deep caring on the part of the therapist. Incorporating the arts in psychotherapy allows clients to engage in elaboration (Dissanayake, 2000, pp. 129–145), a behavior identified as having psychological significance, within the context of client-therapist mutuality. As clients engage in therapeutic arts, a therapeutic form of elaboration, they find and make meaning through both physical, hands-on behavior and cognitive operations.

## A Role for Aesthetics in Clinical Practice

Discussing the function of aesthetics is likely to be one of the most controversial and challenging components of any discourse involving the arts. Although used for different reasons by art critics and art historians, the importance of aesthetics has not been lost on psychologists (e.g., Arnheim, 1966; Berlyne, 1965; Csiksezentmihalyi & Robinson, 1990; Gardner, 1973), as evidenced by the publication of numerous journals and books relating to psychology and the arts as well as the launch of the American Psychological Association's newest journal, *Psychology of Aesthetics, Creativity, and the Arts,* in 2006. Yet many within the general public seem to associate aesthetics with a form of high-brow judgment, thus deterring many people from participating in the arts. Those who reside in Western countries are well aware of the harsh art critic, taking on the self-appointed role of cultural police, who faults the artist for imperfections and decides what is "good" and "bad" art (Becker, 1982). There is no mystery why more people do not engage in the arts in Chicago, Calgary, or Cardiff!

In part, perhaps because of the association of the term *aesthetics* with external judgment and social acceptability—and what is to be considered "good" art—those using the arts in clinical work tend to ignore aesthetic decision making as an important part of the therapeutic interaction between client, artwork, and therapist. Examining any art medium's aesthetic dimensions has, unfortunately, become associated with assessing its material worth, level of perfection, and acceptability. The meaning, value, and importance of the work become something that is decided externally. This is certainly not a useful process when using the arts therapeutically. Yet to work with the arts in clinical practice, without any reference to aesthetics, is akin to leaving out the sausage when making a *cassoulet*. The stew exists on its own but a key ingredient is missing. Rather than attempting to write the definitive word on aesthetics and therapeutic arts, I would like to use this section to introduce some possibilities for the role aesthetics might play in clinical practice. David Maclagan's (2001) use of the term *psychological aesthetics* is highly apropos for this discussion. He defines psychological aesthetics as "the relation between the aesthetic qualities of an artwork and the psychological effects that those have on the spectator" (p. 7). Within clinical work the spectator is also often the creator of the artwork, and the sensations, feelings, fantasies, thoughts, and other events of mental life that the spectator-creator has about the art also become an integral part of the therapeutic process. It is what Davey (1999) describes as the aesthetic experience: "the occasion of an artwork commencing and recommencing its endless work" (p. 7).

Aesthetic judgment (Winner, 1982), defined here as arranging objects, sounds, movements, or words in some symmetrically pleasing form, predicts a tendency for balance (Lisanby & Lockhead, 1991). In using art within therapy, a mixture of intellectual curiosity and imagination, together with a blend of focused-articulate and unfocused-inarticulate forms of understanding (Maclagan, 2001), form the basis of aesthetic judgment. Although art making involves trying to make sense of something by creating representations that seek an aesthetic balance pleasing to its creator, in a therapeutic process, the concept of "pleasing" holds a wide definition and may include moments that feel unfamiliar, uncanny, reverential, mystical, ecstatic, sensual, and otherwise outside of cognitive coherence. In clinical work, involving any of the arts, the client simultaneously becomes the creator-artist and the observer-spectator where the "aesthetic moment constitutes this deep rapport between subject and object and provides the person with a generative illusion of fitting with an object, evoking an existential memory" (Bollas, 1987). I would also add that this moment may evoke a longing for understanding, emotional connection, and coherence. It is during this experience that the client can come to understand something different about him/herself in a way that goes beyond what can be explained as an unconscious process.

The role for aesthetics within therapeutic arts can be one that helps to explore the triadic relationship between client, therapist, and the artwork. Rather than paying attention only to formal iconographic aspects of the work, the client and therapist can jointly begin to look at the client's efforts as a creative and imaginative attempt to resolve a specific issue or problem. Seeing (or hearing or reading or otherwise experiencing) the work becomes a way of articulating its aesthetic features and exploring normative and symbolic meaning (Bacheland, 1969). The aesthetic features of an artwork will, of course, vary depending upon the medium (e.g., line, color, and texture for visual work; tone, rhythm, and timbre for sound; character development, simile, and metaphor for narrative and poetic writing; rhythm, shape, and gesture for movement). The process of articulating and exploring aspects of the work has numerous processes associated with it including unconscious, cognitive, emotional, and behavioral elements. In creating artwork one plays aesthetically with different media. Playing with different forms, textures, sounds, words, and movements also means being simultaneously played by them (Bollas, 1993, p. 211). Clients shape and form the work but are also affected and informed by arousal, curiosity, and exploration when making and observing their work, as well as by the art medium's stimulus variables such as novelty, complexity, and heterogeneity of elements (Berlyne, 1965, 1967). The importance of emotion in psychotherapy is well established. The biological, physiological, and psychological mechanisms of aesthetic response, seen by Aiken (1998, 2001) as an emotional response, are important to consider in order to gain a richer understanding of the role of art making within psychotherapy for a range of populations that are cared for by psychologists (Long, 1998; Camic, 1999a).

## CONCLUSION

Clinical and counseling psychologists have become two of the most prominent practitioners within mental healthcare in North America. Psychotherapy, one of the competencies of professional psychologists, seeks to heal emotional injuries, increase understanding of self and others, develop a capacity for self-reflection, reduce symptoms, change behavior, alter thinking patterns, inhibit maladaptive emotional responses, and encourage adaptive emotional responses. More recent evolutionary theories lend support for the utility of art making as a series of behaviors with emotional and cognitive benefits for the maker of the art as well as audience. Although the function of art making may have changed from ceremonial ritual to present-day professional art production, art-making remains something that is accessible to all, regardless of training or skill. It is seen as a response to internal and external cues, and a source of spontaneous action simultaneously creating and informing.

The goals of psychotherapy can be enhanced through the arts, and clinical and counseling psychology can develop clinical and research protocols to better understand the psychological, physiological, neurological, biological, and aesthetic components of this process. Developing a curriculum specific to psychological practice is an important step to the achievement of this goal. One way in which the practice of professional psychology can further develop is to move beyond only using verbal-based therapies and consider kinesthetic, visual, and auditory elements as important sources of information for assessment and treatment.

## TOOL KIT FOR CHANGE

### Perspective of the Educator

1. The educator should understand the evolutionary importance of the arts to human development.
2. The arts can make subsymbolic emotional content more accessible.
3. The arts can engage us emotionally, cognitively, physically, and for some, spiritually.
4. The arts can be made part of an interdisciplinary approach to the assessment and treatment of a range of mental health problems in individual, group, and community settings.

### Perspective of the Student

1. The arts provide students with additional tools for helping clients.
2. The arts allow students to facilitate understanding and healing outside of traditional verbal discourse.
3. The arts can be used in both assessment and in therapy for self-reflection and personal growth.

### Global Perspective

1. The arts are part of all cultures and increase our understanding about diversity and communication across cultural groups.
2. The arts are capable of being a component of cross-cultural training and work in different cultures.
3. The arts can help bridge distrust among different ethnic groups.
4. The arts increase options for cross-cultural research in psychology.

## REFERENCES

Aiken, N. E. (1998). *The biological origins of art*. Westport, CT, & London: Praeger.
Aiken, N. E. (2001). An evolutionary perspective on the nature of art. *Bulletin of Psychology and the Arts, 2*, 3–7.
Ainsworth, M. D. S. (1989). Attachment beyond infancy. *American Psychologist, 44*, 709–716.
Allen, P. (1995). Coyote comes in from the cold: The evolution of the open studio concept. *Art Therapy: Journal of the American Art Therapy Association, 12*, 161–166.
Arnheim, R. (1966). *Toward a psychology of art*. Berkeley: University of California Press.
Bacheland, G. (1969). *The poetics of reverie* (D. Russell, Trans.). Boston: Beacon Press.
Bahn, P. G. (1998). *Cambridge illustrated history of pre-historic art*. Cambridge: Cambridge University Press.

Barlow, D. H. (Ed). (1993). *Clinical handbook of psychological disorder: A step by step treatment manual* (2nd ed.). New York: Guilford Press.

Becker, H. S. (1982). *Art worlds.* Berkeley & London: University of California Press.

Berlyne, D. E. (1965). Measures of aesthetic preference. *Sciences de l'Art, 3,* 9–23.

Berlyne, D. E. (1967). Arousal and information. In D. Levine (Ed.), *Nebraska symposium on motivation* (pp. 1–110). Lincoln: University of Nebraska.

Bowlby, J. (1969). *Attachment.* New York: Basic Books.

Bollas, C. (1987). *The shadow of the object.* London: Free Association Press.

Bradshaw, J. L. (2001). Arts brevis, vita longa: The possible evolutionary antecedents of art and aesthetics. *Bulletin of Psychology and the Arts, 2,* 7–11.

Brommer, G. (1994). *Collage techniques.* New York: Watson-Guptill.

Browne, D. F. (1980). Mirroring in the analysis of an artist. *International Journal of Psycho-Analysis, 61,* 493–502.

Bucci, W. (1995). The power of narrative: A multiple code account. In J. W. Pennebaker (Ed.), *Emotion, disclosure and health.* Washington, DC: APA Books.

Caldwell, L. (2000). Continuities in art and psychoanalysis. In L. Caldwell (Ed.), *Art, creativity, living.* Karnac: London & New York.

Camic, P. M. (1999a, August). *Arts-based academic and clinical training in the curriculum of professional psychology.* Paper presented at the annual meeting of the American Psychological Association, Boston, MA.

Camic, P. M. (1999b). Expanding treatment possibilities for chronic pain through expressive arts therapies. In C. Malchioti (Ed.), *Medical art therapy for adults.* London & Philadelphia: Jessica Kingsley.

Camic, P. M. (2001). Creating images, sound, movement, enactment, word: The arts in clinical training. *Bulletin of Psychology and the Arts, 2,* 59–65.

Camic, P., Rhodes, J., & Yardley, L. (Eds.). (2003). *Qualitative research methodology in psychology: Expanding perspectives in methodology and design.* Washington: American Psychological Association.

Coss, R. G. (1998). The ethological command in art. *Leonardo, 1,* 273–287.

Csikszentmihalyi, M. (1988). The dangers of originality: Creativity and the artistic process. In M. M. Gedo (Ed.), *Psychoanalytic explorations in art.* Hillsdale, NJ: Analytic Press.

Csikszentmihalyi, M., & Robinson, R. E. (1990). *The art of seeing: An interpretation of the aesthetic encounter.* Malibu, CA: Getty Center for Education in the Arts.

Davey, N. (1999). The hermeneutics of seeing. In I. Heywood & B. Sandywell (Eds.), *Interpreting visual culture.* London: Routledge.

Dewey, J. (1934/1980) *Art as experience.* New York: Berkley.

Dissanayake, E. (1988). *What is art for?* Seattle: University of Washington Press.

Dissanayake, E. (1992). *Homoaestheticus: Where art comes from and why.* New York: The Free Press.

Dissanayake, E. (2000). *Art and intimacy: How the arts begin.* Seattle: University of Washington Press.

Elderfield, J. (Ed.). (1992). *Essays on assemblage.* New York: Abrams.

Evans, W., & Reilly, J. (1996). Drawings as a method of program evaluation and communication with school-aged children. *Journal of Extension, 34*(6). Retrieved February 3, 2006, from http://www.joe.org/joe/1996december/a2.html

Exner, J. (1993). *The Rorschach: A comprehensive system: Vol. 1. Basic foundations* (3rd ed.). New York: John Wiley.

Feder, B., & Feder, E. (1998). *The art and science of evaluation in the arts therapies.* Springfield, IL : Charles C. Thomas.

Fiske, D. W., & Maddi, S. R. (1961). A conceptual framework. In D. W. Fiske & S. R. Maddi (Eds.), *Functions of varied experience.* Homewood, IL: Dorsey.

Freud, S. (1953/1997). *Writings on art and literature.* Palo Alto, CA: Stanford University Press.

Gardner, H. (1973). *The arts and human development.* New York: John Wiley.

Gardner, H. (1982). *Art, mind and brain: A cognitive approach to creativity.* New York: Basic Books.

Gaugh, L. M. (2001). What will we do today? A clinical psychology graduate student's experience of the creative arts in art therapy. *Bulletin of Psychology and the Arts, 2,* 67–69.

Gedo, J. E. (1996). *The artist and the emotional world.* New York: Columbia University Press.

Greenberger, D., & Padesky, C. A. (1995). *Mind over mood: Change how you feel by changing the way you think.* New York & London: Guilford Press.

Hird, M. J. (2006). Sex diversity and evolutionary psychology. *The Psychologist, 19,* 30–32.

Jacobson, K. (1995). Drawing households and other living spaces in the process of assessment and psychotherapy. *Clinical Social Work Journal, 23,* 305–325.

Kaplan, F. F. (2000). *Art, science and art therapy.* London & Philadelphia: Jessica Kingsley.

Knight, S. J., & Camic, P. M. (2004). Health psychology and medicine: The art and science of healing. In P. Camic & S. J. Knight (Eds.), *Clinical handbook of health psychology: A practical guide to effective interventions.* Seattle, Toronto, & Gottingen: Hogrefe & Huber.

Kreitler, H., & Kreitler, S. (1972). *Psychology of the arts.* Durham: Duke University Press.

Landgarten, H. B. (1993). *Magazine photo collage: A multicultural assessment and treatment tool.* New York: Brunner/Mazel.

Levine, S. K., & Levine, H. G. (1999). *Foundations of expressive arts therapy.* London & Philadelphia: Jessica Kingsley.

Lillienfeld, S. O., Wood, J. M., & Garb, H. N. (2000). The scientific status of projective techniques. *Psychological Science in the Public Interest, 1,* 27–66.

Lisanby, S. H., & Lockhead, G. R. (1991). Subjective randomness, aesthetics and structure. In G. R. Lockhead & J. R. Pomerantz (Eds.), *The perception of structure.* Washington, DC: American Psychological Association.

Long, J. (2004). Medical art therapy: Using imagery and visual expression in healing. In P. M. Camic & S. J. Knight (Eds.), *Clinical handbook of health psychology* (2nd ed.). Cambridge, MA, & Göttingen: Hogrefe & Huber.

Lorenzetti, M. (1994). Perspectives on integration between art therapy areas. *The Arts in Psychotherapy, 21,* 113–117.

Lowenfeld, V., & Brittain, W. L. (1970). *Creative and mental growth* (5th ed.). New York: Macmillan.

Lynn, R. (1996). *Attention, arousal and orientating reaction.* Oxford: Pergamon.

Maclagan, D. (2001). *Psychological aesthetics: Painting, feeling and making sense.* London & Philadelphia: Jessica Kingsley.

Maltby, M. (2003). Wordless words: poetry and the symmetry of being. In H. Canham & C. Satyamurti (Eds.), *Acquainted with the night: Psychoanalysis and poetic imagination.* London & New York: Karnac.

Marshack, A. (1991). *The roots of civilization: The cognitive beginnings of man's first art, symbol and notation* (2nd ed.). New York: Moyer Bell.

McNiff, S. (1981). *The arts and psychotherapy.* Springfield, IL: Charles C. Thomas.

McNiff, S. (1998). *Art-based research.* London & Philadelphia: Jessica Kingsley.

Milner, M. (1957). *On not being able to paint* (2nd ed.). London: Heinemann.

Milner, M. (1975). A discussion of Masud Khan's paper: In search of the dreaming experience. Reprinted in M. Milner (Ed.), *The suppressed madness of sane men.* London: Routledge.

Orians, G. H. (2001). An evolutionary perspective on aesthetics. *Bulletin of Psychology and the Arts, 2,* 25–29.

Petrie, M. (1946). *Art and regeneration.* London: Paul Elek.

Pinker, S. (1997). *How the mind works.* New York: Norton.

Piirto, J. (1992). *Understanding those who create.* Dayton: Ohio Psychology Press.

Rank, O. (1989/1932). *Art and artist: Creativity, urge and personality development.* New York: Norton.

Rogers, N. (1993). *The creative connection: Expressive arts as healing.* Palo Alto: Science & Behavior Books.

Rose, G. J. (1996). *Necessary illusion: Art as witness.* Madison, CT: International Universities Press.

Ryle, A. (1990). *Cognitive-analytic therapy: Active participation in change.* Chichester, UK, & New York: John Wiley.

Sackett, D. L., Strauss, S. E., Richardson, W. S., Rosenberg, W., & Hayes, R. B. (2000). *Evidence based medicine: How to practice and teach EBM* (2nd ed.). London: Churchill Livingstone.

Sarason, S. (1990). *The challenge of art to psychology.* New Haven, CT, & London: Yale University Press.

Schultz, D. P. (1965). *Sensory restriction: Effects on behavior.* New York: Academic Press.

Shiner, L. (2001). *The invention of art: A cultural history.* Chicago & London: University of Chicago Press.

Stern, D. (1985). *The interpersonal world of the infant.* New York: Basic Books.

Tinbergen, N. (1951). *The study of instinct.* London: Oxford University Press.

Vygotsky, L. (1922/1971). *The psychology of art.* Cambridge, MA, & London: MIT Press.

Wali, A. (2002). *Informal arts: Finding cohesion, capacity, and other cultural benefits in unexpected places.* Chicago: Chicago Center for Arts Policy.

Wampold, B. E. (2001). *The great psychotherapy debate: Models, methods, and findings.* Mahwah, NJ: Erlbaum.

Warren, B. (Ed.). (1993). *Using the creative arts in therapy: A practical introduction* (2nd ed.). London & New York: Routledge.

Weston, D., & Bradley, R. (2005). Empirically supported complexity: Rethinking evidence-based practice in psychotherapy. *Current Directions in Psychological Science, 14,* 266–271.

Weston, D., Novotny, C. M., & Thompson-Brenner, H. (2004). The empirical status of empirically supported psychotherapies. Assumptions, findings, and reporting in controlled clinical trials. *Psychological Bulletin, 130,* 631–663.

Wiener, D. J. (Ed.). (1999). *Beyond talk therapy: Using movement and expressive techniques in clinical practice.* Washington, DC: American Psychological Association.

Wilson, E. O. (1998). *Consilience: The unity of knowledge.* New York: Knopf.

Wilson, L. E. (1998, August). *Interdisciplinary arts and the vocabulary of expression.* Paper presented at the annual meeting of the American Psychological Association, San Francisco.

Wilson, L. E. (2001). Erasing the guidelines: An interdisciplinary studio course for therapists who use art. *Bulletin of Psychology and the Arts, 2,* 65–67.

Winner, E. (1982). *Invented words: The psychology of the arts.* Cambridge, MA, & London: Harvard University Press.

Winnicott, D. W. (1971). *Playing and reality.* London: Tavistock Publications.

Wood, J. M., Nezworski, M. T., & Stejskal, W. J. (1996). The comprehensive system for the Rorschach: A critical examination. *Psychological Science, 7,* 3–10.

## ACKNOWLEDGMENTS

Many thanks to Lawrence E. Wilson for his valuable comments on earlier drafts of this chapter.

# AFTERWORD[*]

*Lisa Raimondo, RN, MSN, Rachel Armstrong, RN, MBA, PhD, and Pat DeLeon, PhD, MPH, JD*

The holistic view of health recognizes the integral connection between the mind, body, and spirit of an individual. This holistic view has had to overcome the more traditional perspective of healthcare that associated the level of health with the quality of medicine and the belief that "medicine has been the fount from which all improvements in health have flowed" (Lalonde, 1974, p. 11). The general focus of society has been that the quality of healthcare was related to the quality of the care provided by healthcare professionals or the availability of physicians and hospitals.

Fortunately, health policy experts realize that the traditional perspective of healthcare is inadequate. Good health requires considerably more than access to quality medical care. Marc Lalonde, Minister of National Health and Welfare of Canada, stated, "Good health is the bedrock on which social progress is built. A nation of healthy people can do those things that make life worthwhile, and as the level of health increases so does the potential for happiness. The Governments of the Provinces and of Canada have long recognized that good physical and mental health are necessary for the quality of life to which everyone aspires" (Lalonde, 1974, p. 5). Nonetheless, when we consider that about half the burden of illness is psychological in origin, it is clear that the full impact of mental health on overall physical health has yet to be truly appreciated by many healthcare professionals.

---

[*] The views expressed in this manuscript are those of the authors and do not reflect the official policy or position of the Department of Defense or the U.S. Government.

Moreover, the role of the individual in personal health is slowly gaining support. In 1979, the U.S. Surgeon General concluded that, "In fact, of the 10 leading causes of death in the United States, at least seven could be substantially reduced if persons at risk improved just five habits" (U.S. Surgeon General's Office, 1979, p. 2–3). The Institute of Medicine (IOM) also stressed the importance of personal responsibility in an individual's overall health. As the preeminent advisor to the federal government in identifying issues of medical care, research, and education, the IOM has issued a series of visionary reports. In *Fostering Rapid Advances in Health Care*, the IOM concluded:

> The vast majority of the nation's health care resources are now devoted to the ongoing management of chronic conditions....Fixing the personal health care delivery must be a high priority, but will not be enough. In recent years, it has become increasingly apparent that health outcomes are determined to a great extent by factors in addition to health care, including patterns, genetic predispositions, social circumstances, and environmental exposures. In the 21st century, the health care system must focus greater attention on helping people improve their health-related behaviors, including diet, exercise, and use of nicotine and alcohol. (IOM, 2003a, p. 2)

The need for a more collaborative approach among healthcare providers was also highlighted by the IOM, which stated that, "despite some laudable examples of integrated care, the delivery system consists of silos, often lacking even rudimentary information capabilities to exchange patient information, coordinate care across settings and multiple providers, and ensuring continuity of care over time" (IOM, 2003a, p. 2). In *Health Professions Education*, the IOM concluded, "All health professionals should be educated to deliver patient-centered care as members of an interdisciplinary team, emphasizing evidence-based practice, quality improvement approaches, and informatics" (IOM, 2003b, p.3). If the goal of collaborative practice is to combine the skills and expertise of healthcare professionals in order to maximize the efficiency of both the clinician and the healthcare system, then territorial domains must be replaced with a sense of true collegial spirit.

As Congress explores a universal healthcare system, the need for a more collaborative approach to healthcare will increase in significance. A network of nationwide healthcare services that avail access to all Americans may only be successful when consideration is given to expanding the scope of practice for many healthcare professionals. Many professions, such as psychologists, advanced practice nurses, physician's assistants, and dental hygienists are poised to expand in scope of practice, with the intent of increasing access to healthcare. Advances in the professional scope of practice of those who serve the underserved in geographically remote areas will increase accessibility to healthcare for those individuals whose needs are most often unmet. For when care is comparable in quality and like outcomes are achieved, particularly in a more cost-efficient manner, isn't this a win-win for the healthcare delivery system and the patient alike? Traditional medical interventions must meld with holistic healthcare approaches, as well as the arts—visual arts, music, dance, drama, and poetry therapies—in a collaborative healthcare approach.

Since the early 1970s, the United States has been actively exploring the possibility of ensuring that all Americans have access to necessary healthcare. It was under President Richard Nixon that the Congress enacted far-reaching health maintenance organization legislation with the vision of encouraging interdisciplinary-oriented comprehensive care. The original intent of this legislation was to establish an alternative for fee-for-service practice with the development of coordinated healthcare over an individual's lifetime. A similar perspective was held by the Robert Wood Johnson (RWJ) Foundation, which since its creation in 1972 has become the nation's fifth-largest foundation, with assets of approximately $8 billion. As stated in its initial staff paper:

> the reconstitution of the Robert Wood Johnson Foundation as a national philanthropic organization comes at a unique point in American history. The nation has reached the culmination of a forty-year debate over the need to eliminate economic barriers to access to personal health services. Thus, within three years, we believe we are likely to see the enactment of some form of national health insurance program. National health insurance would address financing, but it would also highlight the health care system's inability to deliver care, especially primary care for the entire population. (RWJ, 2005, p. 184)

As the Democrats prepared for the 110th Congress, former president Bill Clinton met with his former colleagues and highlighted two important underlying issues: the cost and the access to healthcare (B. Dorgan, personal communication, January 11, 2007). The United States spends 16 percent of our income on healthcare, yet no other wealthy country spends more than 11 percent. U.S. companies absorb these healthcare costs—General Motors has $1,500 in healthcare costs per car, while Toyota has $110 per car. Similarly, the United States insures 84 percent of its people, yet no other wealthy nation insures less than 100 percent. These are important and fundamental issues that highlight the problem that the number of uninsured has continued to rise over the years with recent estimates approximating 46 million Americans. The political, economic, and perhaps even moral pressures are steadily building for a national response. At the same time, evolving highly innovative state-based responses, such as those of Maine, Massachusetts, Vermont, and possibly California and Tennessee should remind us of our heritage that the various states can often truly serve as living laboratories of social change. Ultimately, our society must decide where healthcare sits on the national agenda.

Very few health policy experts or elected officials would question the importance of improving access, curtailing ever-escalating costs, and emphasizing the accountability of practitioners and delivery systems through the effective utilization of the unprecedented advances occurring today within the communications and technology fields. And yet, as the authors of the various chapters in this impressive text have suggested in numerous ways, perhaps the most productive next step which we as a nation should take would be to carefully scrutinize what really is quality care. We would rhetorically ask: How can the arts in their broadest conceptualization and utilization have an effective impact on both individual health status and system-wide efforts to improve the overall quality of life of our citizenry? As Minister Lalonde noted: "Good health is the bedrock on which social progress is built." As we enter the twenty-first century, we must be expansive in our vision and willingness to explore nontraditional knowledge and clinical expertise. No single health profession's discipline possesses infinite knowledge or wisdom. Interdisciplinary collaboration will undoubtedly be the key to significant advances. The healing process is above all else, a human process.

## REFERENCES

IOM (Institute of Medicine). (2003a). *Fostering rapid advances in health care. Learning from systems demonstrations.* Washington, DC: The National Academies Press.

IOM (Institute of Medicine). (2003b). *Health professions education: A bridge to quality.* Washington, DC: The National Academies Press.

Lalonde, M. (1974). *A new perspective on the health of Canadians. A working document.* (Cat. No. H31–1374). Ottowa, Canada: Minister of Supply and Services Canada.

RWJ (Robert Wood Johnson). (2005). *To improve health and health care.* Volume 8. San Francisco: Jossey-Bass.

U.S. Surgeon General's Office. (1979). *Healthy people: the Surgeon General's report on health promotion and disease prevention.* (DHEW PHS 79-55071). Rockville, MD: U.S. Government Printing Office.

# ABOUT THE GENERAL EDITOR

Ilene Ava Serlin, PhD, ADTR, is a recognized leader and has been practicing whole person health care for over 35 years. She is a clinical psychologist and registered dance/movement therapist at Union Street Health Associates in San Francisco and Marin County. She is a fellow of the American Psychological Association (APA), past-president of the APA's Division of Humanistic Psychology, and served on APA's Presidential and Division 42 (Independent Practice) Health Care Task Force. She is the founder of the Arts Medicine program at the Institute of Health and Healing at California Pacific Medical Center and of the movement support group at the Integrative Health Care for Women with Breast Cancer at the University of California, and is on the advisory committee for Sutter Hospital's Integrative Health and Healing Services in Santa Rosa. Her videotape called *Dance Movement Therapy for Women with Breast Cancer* was awarded the Marian Chace Award by the American Dance Therapy Association.

Dr. Serlin has taught at Saybrook Graduate School, UCLA, Lesley University, and abroad. She is on the Editorial Board of *PsycCritiques PsycCRITIQUES— Contemporary Psychology: APA Review of Books,* the *American Journal of Dance Therapy,* and *The Journal of Humanistic Psychology* and is a reviewer for APA's *Professional Psychology: Research and Practice* and *Division 32's The Humanistic Psychologist.* Her writings include the following:

Serlin, I. A. (2000). Symposium: Support groups for women with breast cancer. *The Arts in Psychotherapy, 27*(2), 123–138.

Serlin, I. A. (2004a). Religious and spiritual issues in couples therapy. In M. Harway (Ed.), *Handbook of couples therapy* (pp. 352–369).New York: John Wiley & Sons.

Serlin, I. A. (2004b). Spiritual diversity in clinical practice. In J. Chin (Ed.), *The psychology of prejudice and discrimination* (pp. 27–49). Westport, CT: Praeger.

Serlin, I. A. (2005). Year of the whole person. *Psychotherapy Bulletin: Division 29 (APA)*, *40*(1), 34–39.

Serlin, I. A. (2006). Expressive therapies. In M. Micozzi (Ed.), *Complementary and integrative medicine in cancer and prevention: Foundations and evidence-based interventions* (pp. 81–91).

Her Web site is www.ileneserlin.com.

# ABOUT THE VOLUME EDITORS

## VOL. I

**Marie A. DiCowden, PhD,** is a nationally known healthcare psychologist and behavioral medicine specialist. Dr. DiCowden joined the University of Miami/Jackson Memorial Hospital staff in the Department of Orthopedics and Rehabilitation in 1981. She maintains her adjunct faculty position at the medical school in addition to faculty affiliations with Nova University and Saybrook Graduate School. In 1988 Dr. DiCowden founded The Biscayne Institutes of Health and Living, Inc. and The Biscayne Foundation in Miami, Florida. This program was an extension of her work on the medical campus and evolved into the HealthCare Community model. This innovative program provides frontline, integrative care for disabled children and adults in addition to integrative health programs for mind and body for the community at large. She serves as the executive director of this program. Dr. DiCowden is a Fellow of the American Psychological Association and a member of the National Academy of Practice. She writes and lectures extensively, both nationally and internationally, on issues of disability, healthcare, and healthcare policy.

## VOL. II

**Kirwan Rockefeller, PhD,** is the director of arts and humanities continuing education at the University of California, Irvine. His expertise includes psychology, visual and performing arts, humanities, and body-mind modalities. He has taught organizational behavior and social psychology at the doctoral level and has consulted with top national and entertainment organizations on the accurate depiction of social and mental health issues, including the Entertainment Industries Council, ABC, CBS, NBC, FOX, Paramount Pictures, Universal Studios, Warner Bros., Centers for Disease Control and Prevention, National Institute on Drug Abuse, The Robert Wood Johnson Foundation, and Ogilvy Public Relations Worldwide. He is the author of *Visualize Confidence: How to Use Guided Imagery to Overcome Self-Doubt.* He has presented at the Susan Samueli Center for Integrative Medicine and is a member of the American Psychological Association and the California Psychological Association.

**Stephen S. Brown, MA,** is a freelance editor in San Francisco, California. He holds a master's degree in philosophy from San Francisco State University, where he studied with Jacob Needleman and taught philosophy and religion. His interests include contemporary spiritual thought, aesthetics, particularly the philosophy of music, and the philosophy of technology and culture.

## VOL. III

**Jill Sonke-Henderson, BA,** is cofounder and codirector of the Center for the Arts in Healthcare Research and Education (CAHRE) at the University of Florida (UF) and is on the faculty of the School of Theatre and Dance at the University of Florida. She has been an artist in residence in the Shands Arts in Medicine program since 1994, where she founded the Dance for Life program. She has been developing and teaching arts in healthcare coursework and conducting research at UF for over a decade, and is a frequent lecturer throughout the United States and abroad. Jill serves on the board of directors and as a consultant for the Society for the Arts in Healthcare, and is the recipient of a New Forms Florida Award, an Individual Artist Fellowship Award from the State of Florida, and a 2001 Excellence in Teaching Award from the National Institute for Staff and Organizational Development (NISOD).

**Ilene Ava Serlin, PhD, ADTR,** is a nationally known clinical psychologist and registered dance/movement therapist in private practice in San Francisco and Marin County. She is a Fellow of the American Psychological Association, is past president of the Division of Humanistic Psychology, and served on APA's Presidential Task Force on Whole Person Psychology. She is the founder of the Arts Medicine program at the Institute of Health and Healing at California Pacific Medical Center, and has taught at Saybrook Graduate School, University of California at Los Angeles, Lesley University, and abroad. She is on the editorial board of *PsycCritiques, American Journal of Dance Therapy,* and *The Journal of Humanistic Psychology.*

**Rusti Brandman, PhD,** is codirector of the Center for the Arts in Healthcare Research and Education (CAHRE) and is coordinator of dance at the University of Florida. Credits include directorships of professional dance companies, international appearances in Holland, receipt of awards from the Florida Fine Arts Council, the National Dance Association, and the American College Dance Festival Association, and service as a national officer for ACDFA. She was a founder of CAHRE and has served as an artist in residence at Shands Hospital at UF and at Alachua General Hospital. She has presented internationally on the arts in healthcare for the American Holistic Medical Association, the Society for the Arts in Healthcare, the International Institute on the Arts in Healing, the Congress on Research in Dance, and the Hawaii International Conference on the Arts and Humanities. She has received five Scholarship Enhancement grants for her arts in health research, producing the Dancing in Hospitals video.

**John Graham-Pole, MD,** graduated from London University in 1966, and has been on the faculties of London and Case Western Reserve Universities. He is now professor of pediatrics, adjunct professor of clinical and health psychology, medical director of Shands Arts in Medicine, University of Florida, and medical director of Pediatric Hospice of North Central Florida. He has authored or edited five books and made a CD of original poetry and music. He has published about 250 book chapters, articles, and poems in peer-reviewed journals. He has given several hundred presentations across the world on holistic medicine, palliative care, humor, and the healing arts.

# ABOUT THE CONTRIBUTORS

**David Aldridge, PhD,** is a professor at the University of Witten Herdecke and the chair for Qualitative Research in Medicine. He specializes in developing research methods suitable for various therapeutic initiatives, including the creative arts therapies, complementary medicine, and nursing. He teaches and supervises research in medicine, complementary medicine, music therapy, and nursing. He has been active in the early publications on complementary medicine, including the first handbook of research methodologies, *Clinical Research Methodology for Complementary Therapies,* in 1993. Extending his interest in complementary medicine and aesthetics to spirituality is his recent book *Spirituality, Healing and Medicine: Return to the Silence,* published in 2000. His latest book, *Health, the Individual, and Integrated Medicine: Revisiting an Aesthetic of Health Care,* was published in 2004.

**Rachel Armstrong** attended the Ohio State University and completed her Bachelor of Science in Nursing in 1985. In 1986, she joined the U.S. Army Nurse Corps. Her assignments have included Walter Reed Army Medical Center in Washington, DC, Patterson Army Community Hospital in Fort Monmouth, New Jersey, Landstuhl Regional Medical Center in Germany, Brooke Army Medical Center in San Antonio, Texas, and on the faculty of the AMEDD Center and School in Fort Sam Houston, Texas. She also served in the 46th Combat Support Hospital during Operation Desert Storm. She has held a variety of positions in medical-surgical nursing and nursing administration. She completed a Master of Science in Nursing with honors in 1997, and a Master of Business Administration in 1999, both from the University of the Incarnate Word in San Antonio, Texas. In 2004, she completed a Doctor of Philosophy from George Mason University, in Fairfax, Virginia, and later held the position of Deputy Chief of Nursing Research at Walter Reed Army Medical Center. Rachel is currently assigned as the Military Nurse Detailee for Senator Daniel K. Inouye. She is enrolled in the U.S. Army War College through Distance Education. Rachel is certified in nursing administration through the American Nurse Credentialing Center and is a member of Sigma Theta Tau International and the Army Nurse Corps Association. She is married to Colonel Brett Armstrong, U.S. Army and together they have two daughters, Sarah and Anna.

**Rusti Brandman, PhD,** is codirector of the Center for the Arts in Healthcare Research and Education (CAHRE) and coordinator of dance at the University of Florida (UF). Credits include directorships of professional dance companies; international appearances in Holland; awards from the Florida Fine Arts Council, the National Dance Association, and the American College Dance Festival Association; and service as a national officer for ACDFA. She was a founder of CAHRE and has served as an artist in residence at Shands Hospital at UF and at AGH. She has presented internationally on the arts in healthcare for the American Holistic Medical Association, the Society for the Arts in Healthcare, the International Institute on the Arts in Healing, the Congress on Research in Dance, and the Hawaii International Conference on the Arts and Humanities. She has received five Scholarship Enhancement grants for her arts in health research, producing the Dancing in Hospitals video.

**Paul M. Camic, PhD,** is a licensed clinical psychologist in Illinois and a chartered psychologist in Britain. He is clinical research director and reader in clinical and health psychology in the clinical psychology doctoral program at the Centre for Applied Social and Psychological Development, Salomons, Canterbury Christ Church University, Tunbridge Wells, Kent, United Kingdom, and consultant clinical health psychologist in the British National Health Service. He was previously director of the expressive arts therapy concentration at the Chicago School of Professional Psychology and has been on the medical school faculties of the University of Chicago and Northwestern University.

**Pat Deleon, PhD, MPH, JD,** is a former President of the American Psychological Association. He has served on Capitol Hill for over three decades, being principally involved in exploring a wide range of health policy and professional educational issues. He is the former editor of *Professional Psychology: Research and Practice* and is currently the editor of *Psychological Services* (the Public Service Division of APA). A Diplomate and Fellow of APA, he has served as President of three of the practice divisions. He obtained his BA from Amherst College, PhD in clinical psychology from Purdue University, MPH from the University of Hawaii, and JD from Catholic University. He received an honorary nurse degree from the University of Pennsylvania and was elected into Honorary Membership of Sigma Theta Tau International, Inc., the Honor Society of Nursing. Licensed in Hawaii, he has worked for the Peace Corps and State of Hawaii Division of Mental Health. He has approximately 175 publications.

**Dianne Dulicai, PhD, ADTR,** founded the dance/movement therapy program at Hahnemann Medical College and Graduate School in 1974, where she remains a consultant and serves on the Dean's Advisory Committee. She replicated the program at the request of the University of London, Goldsmiths' College, at the Laban Centre in 1984. She served as president of the American Dance Therapy Association and chair of the National Coalition of Pupil Services Organizations. In her retirement she has specialized in research related to children with special needs and their families.

**Jeffrey E. Evans, PhD,** is clinical associate professor in the Department of Physical Medicine and Rehabilitation, Division of Rehabilitation Psychology and Neuropsychology, University of Michigan where he treats patients with brain injuries and other conditions. He also holds an appointment in the Residential College at U of M where he has taught courses on the psychology of creativity, psychology of consciousness, and brain and mind since the 1970s. His dissertation, "The Dancer from the Dance: Meaning and Creating in Modern Dance Choreography" (1980), is a life historical exploration of creative style. Recent research includes executive mental processes involved in task switching.

**John Fox, BA,** is a poet and certified poetry therapist (CPT). He is adjunct associate professor at the California Institute of Integral Studies in San Francisco, California. He teaches in the Graduate School of Holistic Studies at John F. Kennedy University in Berkeley, California, and the Institute for Transpersonal Psychology in Palo Alto, California. He is author of *Poetic Medicine: The Healing Art of Poem-making* and *Finding What You Didn't Lose: Expressing Your Truth and Creativity Through Poem-Making,* as well as numerous essays. John conducts ongoing poetry healing circles in the Bay Area and works throughout the United States. He has taught in Ireland, England, Israel, Kuwait, South Korea, and Canada. John is the past president (2003–2005) of the National Association for Poetry Therapy. He lives in Mountain View, California.

**Sherry W. Goodill, PhD, ADTR, NCC, LPC,** is an associate professor and director of the Hahnemann Creative Arts in Therapy Program at Drexel University. She was the director of dance/movement therapy education for that same program 1990–2004, and also served on the board of directors of the American Dance Therapy Association for 10 years. She received a grant from the National Institutes of Health Office of Alternative Medicine (now the NCCAM) to study dance/movement therapy for medically ill adults, and has recently published the book, *An Introduction to Medical Dance/Movement Therapy: Health Care in Motion.*

**John Graham-Pole, MD,** graduated from London University in 1966, and has been on the faculties of London and Case Western Reserve Universities. He is now professor of pediatrics, adjunct professor of clinical and health psychology, medical director of Shands Arts in Medicine, University of Florida, and medical director of Pediatric Hospice of North Central Florida. He has authored or edited five books and has made a CD of original poetry and music. He has published about 250 book chapters, articles, and poems in peer-reviewed journals. He has given several hundred presentations across the world on holistic medicine, palliative care, humor, and the healing arts.

**Anne Krantz, PhD, ADTR,** is a registered dance therapist and licensed clinical psychologist. For over 30 years she has practiced, taught, researched, and written on Blanche Evan's methods of dance movement therapy in relation to clinical and health psychology. Also trained in psychoanalytic and infant-parent psychotherapy, she has worked with a wide range of chronic illness and trauma and is on the medical staff of UCSF Medical Center. She has created a dance therapy program for cancer patients through the UCSF Cancer Resource Center that has been ongoing since 1996. Her interest has always been integration of the whole person, and of the fields of dance, dance therapy and psychology, while maintaining a primary focus on clinical work with adults and children in her private practice in San Francisco.

**Robert J. Landy, PhD, RDT/BCT, LCAT,** is professor of educational theatre and applied psychology and director of the Drama Therapy Program at New York University. A prolific researcher and writer, Landy has published numerous books, articles, and plays in the fields of drama, musical theater, drama therapy, and related topics. He has been featured in the media in the CBS-TV series *Drama in Education,* the award- winning documentary film *Standing Tall,* and his own production, *Three Approaches to Psychotherapy.* He has received many awards and honors including a Fulbright lecturing grant, the Gertrud Schattner Award for Distinguished Contribution to the Field of Drama Therapy, and the Distinguished Teaching Medal from New York University.

**Shaun McNiff, PhD, ATR,** is past president of the American Art Association, dean of Lesley College, and university professor, at Lesley University in Cambridge, Massachusetts, an internationally recognized figure in the areas of the arts and healing and creativity enhancement, and the author of many acclaimed books that include *Art Heals: How Creativity Cures the Soul; Trust the Process: An Artist's Guide to Letting Go; Art as Medicine: Creating a Therapy of the Imagination; Creating with Others: The Practice of Imagination in Life, Art and the Workplace; Art-Based Research, Depth Psychology of Art;* and *The Arts and Psychotherapy.*

**Dean Ornish, M.D.,** is the founder and president of the non-profit Preventive Medicine Research Institute in Sausalito, California, where he holds the Safeway Chair. He is Clinical Professor of Medicine at the University of California, San Francisco. Dr. Ornish received his medical training in internal medicine from the Baylor College of Medicine, Harvard Medical School, and the Massachusetts General Hospital. He received a BA in Humanities summa cum laude from the University of Texas in Austin, where he gave the baccalaureate address.

For the past 30 years, Dr. Ornish has directed clinical research demonstrating, for the first time, that comprehensive lifestyle changes may begin to reverse even severe coronary heart disease, without drugs or surgery. Recently, Medicare agreed to provide coverage for this program, the first time that Medicare has covered a program of comprehensive lifestyle changes. He recently directed the first randomized controlled trial demonstrating that comprehensive lifestyle changes may stop or reverse the progression of prostate cancer. His current research is focusing on whether comprehensive lifestyle changes may affect gene expression.

He is the author of five best-selling books, including New York Times' bestsellers *Dr. Dean Ornish's Program for Reversing Heart Disease, Eat More, Weigh Less,* and *Love & Survival.* He writes a monthly column for both *Newsweek* and *Reader's Digest* magazines.

The research that he and his colleagues conducted has been published in the *Journal of the American Medical Association, The Lancet, Circulation, The New England Journal of Medicine,* the *American Journal of Cardiology,* and elsewhere. A one-hour documentary of their work was broadcast on *NOVA,* the PBS science series, and was featured on Bill Moyers' PBS series, *Healing & The Mind.* Their work has been featured in all major media, including cover stories in *Newsweek, Time,* and *U.S. News & World Report.*

Dr. Ornish is a member of the boards of directors of the U.S. United Nations High Commission on Refugees, the Quincy Jones Foundation, and the San Francisco Food Bank, and a member of the Google Health Advisory Council. He was appointed to The White House Commission on Complementary and Alternative Medicine Policy and elected to the California Academy of Medicine. He is Chair of the PepsiCo Blue Ribbon Advisory Board and the Safeway Advisory Council on Health and Nutrition and consults directly with the CEO's of McDonald's and Del Monte Foods to make more healthful foods and to provide health education to their customers in this country and worldwide.

He has received several awards, including the 1994 Outstanding Young Alumnus Award from the University of Texas, Austin, the University of California, Berkeley, "National Public Health Hero" award, the Jan J. Kellermann Memorial Award for distinguished contribution in the field of cardiovascular disease prevention from the International Academy of Cardiology, a Presidential Citation from the American Psychological Association, the Beckmann Medal from the German Society for Prevention and Rehabilitation of Cardiovascular Diseases, the "Pioneer in Integrative Medicine" award from California Pacific Medical Center, the "Excellence in Integrative Medicine" award from the Heal Breast Cancer Foundation, the Golden Plate Award from the American Academy of Achievement, a U.S. Army Surgeon General Medal, and the Bravewell Collaborative Pioneer of Integrative Medicine award. Dr. Ornish has been a physician consultant to The White House and to several bipartisan members of the U.S. Congress. He is listed in *Who's Who in Healthcare and Medicine*, *Who's Who in America*, and *Who's Who in the World*.

Dr. Ornish was recognized as "one of the most interesting people of 1996" by *People* magazine, featured in the "TIME 100" issue on integrative medicine, and chosen by *LIFE* magazine as "one of the 50 most influential members of his generation."

**James W. Pennebaker, PhD,** is the Bush Regents Professor of Liberal Arts and the departmental chair in the Psychology Department at the University of Texas at Austin, where he received his PhD in 1977. He has been on the faculty at the University of Virginia, Southern Methodist University, and (since 1997) the University of Texas. He and his students are exploring the links between traumatic experiences, expressive writing, natural language use, and physical and mental health. His studies find that physical and mental health can improve by simple writing exercises. His most recent research focuses on the nature of language and emotion in the real world. The words people use serve as powerful reflections of their personality and social worlds. Author or editor of 8 books and over 200 articles, Pennebaker has received numerous awards and honors.

**Lisa Raimondo** (Captain Raimondo) is a native of Jacksonville, Arkansas. She graduated from the University of Arkansas Medical Sciences, College of Nursing in Little Rock with a Bachelor of Science in Nursing in December 1983. She received a Masters of Science in Nursing from the Catholic University of America in Washington, D.C., in May 2002. Captain Raimondo has over 23 years of diverse military nursing experience, including areas of ambulatory care, health promotion, patient education, staff education, medical/surgical, and critical care. She is a proficient administrator and clinician, exceptionally skilled in coordinating the delivery of high quality health care services to a broad spectrum of beneficiaries to include distinguished members of Congress, the Executive branch, their families, and foreign dignitaries. Well-versed and experienced in working with organizational change at the executive level, she is currently assigned to the Navy Bureau of Medicine and Surgery as the principal adviser to the Director of the Nurse Corps for Policy and Practice. She is a member of the American Academy of Ambulatory Care Nurses and Sigma Theta Tau.

**Ilene A. Serlin, PhD, ADTR,** is a clinical psychologist and registered dance/movement therapist. She is the founder and Director of Union Street Health Associates and the Arts Medicine Program at California Pacific Medical Center. She is a fellow of the American Psychological Association, is past president and council representative of the Division of Humanistic Psychology of the American Psychological Association, serves on the editorial boards of *The Arts in Psychotherapy,* the *Journal of Dance Therapy,* and the *Journal of Humanistic Psychology,* and has taught and published widely in the United States and abroad. Dr. Serlin's approach draws on her extensive background of training and experience in dance and the arts, Gestalt and depth psychotherapy, and behavioral medicine. She has been dancing for 40 years and trained in Labanotation with Irmgard Bartenieff. She studied and taught with Laura Perls at the New York Gestalt Institute, did her predoctoral internship at the Children's Clinic of the C. G. Jung Institute of Los Angeles, and taught at the University of California at Los Angeles, Lesley University, Saybrook Graduate School, and the California School of Professional Psychology.

**Jill Sonke-Henderson, BA,** is cofounder and codirector of the Center for the Arts in Healthcare Research and Education (CAHRE) at the University of Florida (UF) and is on the faculty of the School of Theatre and Dance at the University of Florida. She has been an artist in residence in the Shands Arts in Medicine program since 1994, where she founded the Dance for Life program. She has been developing and teaching arts in healthcare coursework and conducting research at UF for over a decade, and is a frequent lecturer throughout the United States and abroad.

Jill serves on the board of directors and as a consultant for the Society for the Arts in Healthcare, and is the recipient of a New Forms Florida Award, an Individual Artist Fellowship Award from the State of Florida, and a 2001 Excellence in Teaching Award from the National Institute for Staff and Organizational Development (NISOD).

**Vivien Marcow Speiser, PhD, ADTR, LMHC** is director of International and Collaborative Programs, Graduate School of Arts and Social Sciences, Lesley University, Cambridge, Massachusetts. Vivien is a dance therapist and expressive arts educator. She has developed and implemented numerous arts-based training programs throughout the United States and Israel. As former founder and director of the Arts Institute Project in Israel, she has been influential in the development of expressive arts therapy there. She has taught and lectured extensively throughout Scandinavia, Israel, South Africa, and the United States.

**Phillip Speiser, PhD, RDT, LMHC,** is executive director of the Boston Institute for Arts Therapy, a nonprofit mental health and education agency serving over 2,500 children and families annually. Dr. Speiser is a family therapist and expressive arts educator/therapist who has been developing and implementing integrated arts programs since 1980. He has taught and lectured extensively throughout Scandinavia, Europe, Israel, South Africa, and the United States. He is the former chairperson of Very Special Arts Sweden and of the International Expressive Arts Therapy Association.

# ABOUT THE ADVISERS

**Laura Barbanel, EdD, ABPP,** served as professor and program head of the graduate program in the School Psychology at Brooklyn College of the City University of New York for many years. She also served as deputy dean for graduate studies for the School of Education at Brooklyn College. Dr. Barbanel is currently in private practice in Brooklyn, New York. She works with adults and children, couples, and families.

Dr. Barbanel is a fellow of the American Psychological Association (APA) and a diplomate of the American Board of Professional Psychology. She has served in a number of elected and appointed positions in the APA, on its board of directors, and currently on the Committee for the Advancement of Practice. She is president-elect of Division 42, the division of independent practice. In this capacity, she has established a Task Force on Health Care for the Whole Person, which focuses on the collaboration of psychologists with physicians in the delivery of healthcare.

**William Benda, MD, FACEP, FAAEM,** received his professional training at Duke University, University of Miami School of Medicine, Harbor-UCLA Medical Center, and the Program in Integrative Medicine at the University of Arizona. His research and clinical work has focused on patients with breast cancer, animal-assisted therapy, and physician health and well-being. He was principal investigator on two National Center for Complementary and Alternative Medicine–funded investigations of therapeutic horseback riding in the treatment of children with cerebral palsy and is currently extending this research to the field of pediatric autism. Benda is a co-founder of the National Integrative Medicine Council, a nonprofit organization for which he has served as director of medical and public affairs. He is an editor, contributor, and medical advisory board member for a number of conventional and alternative medicine journals and has lectured extensively on a variety of topics in the integrative arena.

**Lillian Comas-Diaz, PhD,** is the executive director of the Transcultural Mental Health Institute, a clinical professor at the George Washington University Department of Psychiatry and Behavioral Sciences, and a private practitioner in Washington, DC. The former director of the American Psychological Association's Office of Ethnic Minority Affairs, Comas-Diaz was also the director of the Yale University Department of Psychiatry Hispanic Clinic. She is the senior editor of two textbooks: *Clinical Guidelines in Cross-Cultural Mental Health* and *Women of Color: Integrating Ethnic and Gender Identities in Psychotherapy*. Additionally, Comas-Diaz is the founding editor in chief of the American Psychological Association Division 45 official journal, *Cultural Diversity and Ethnic Minority Psychology*. She is a member of numerous editorial boards and currently is an associate editor of *American Psychologist*.

**Rita Dudley-Grant, PhD, MPH, ABPP,** is a psychologist currently serving as clinical director of Virgin Islands Behavioral Services, a system of residential services for emotionally disturbed and behaviorally disordered adolescents. She has published and presented extensively on child and adolescent mental health and substance abuse both locally and nationally. A practicing Nichiren SGI Buddhist for the past 26 years, she has presented on Buddhism and psychology as well as spirituality at meetings of the American Psychological Association since 1998. Dudley-Grant is co-editor of *Psychology and Buddhism: From Individual to Global Community*.

**Jeffrey E. Evans, PhD,** is clinical associate professor in the Department of Physical Medicine and Rehabilitation, Division of Rehabilitation Psychology and Neuropsychology, University of Michigan where he treats patients with brain injuries and other conditions. He also holds an appointment in the Residential College at U of M where he has taught courses on the psychology of creativity, psychology of consciousness, and brain and mind since the 1970s. His dissertation, "The Dancer from the Dance: Meaning and Creating in Modern Dance Choreography" (1980), is a life historical exploration of creative style. Recent research includes executive mental processes involved in task switching.

**Joseph S. Geller, JD,** has been active in policy-making, government relations, and community service for many years. He was elected mayor of the City of North Bay Village, Florida, in 2004 and was reelected in 2006. He previously served North Bay Village as an interim city attorney in 2003. He was chair of the Dade County Democratic Party from 1989 to December 2000. He also served as a member of the Democratic National Committee. He was an attorney for the Gore campaign during the recount litigation and represented former Attorney General Janet Reno in regard to the gubernatorial primary in 2002 and the John Kerry campaign in 2004. Geller is a partner in the Hollywood, Florida, law firm of Geller, Geller, Fisher & Garfinkel, LLP. The partners specialize in governmental relations, real estate, land use, civil litigation, municipal law, administrative and appellate practice, and corporate practice. Geller is admitted to practice in the Supreme Court of the State of Florida, the United States District Court, Southern District of Florida, and the United States Court of Appeals for the Eleventh Circuit.

**Marjorie S. Greenberg, MA,** is chief of the Classifications and Public Health Data Standards staff at the National Center for Health Statistics (NCHS), Centers for Disease Control and Prevention, Department of Health and Human Services (DHHS). Greenberg, who has been with NCHS since 1982, also serves as executive secretary to the National Committee on Vital and Health Statistics, which is the external advisory committee to DHHS on health information policy, and as head of the World Health Organization Collaborating Center for the Family of International Classifications for North America. Her areas of interest and expertise include health data standardization, uniform health data sets, health classifications, data policy development, and evaluation policy. She received her bachelor's degree from Wellesley College and a master's degree from Harvard University.

**Stanislav Grof, MD,** is a psychiatrist with more than fifty years of experience in research of nonordinary states of consciousness. He has served as principal investigator in a psychedelic research program at the Psychiatric Research Institute in Prague, Czechoslovakia; chief of psychiatric research at the Maryland Psychiatric Research Center; assistant professor of psychiatry at the Johns Hopkins University; and scholar-in-residence at the Esalen Institute. He is professor of psychology at the California Institute of Integral Studies and Pacifica Graduate Institute, conducts professional training programs in holotropic breathwork and transpersonal psychology, and gives lectures and seminars worldwide. He is one of the founders and chief theoreticians of transpersonal psychology. He has contributed 18 books and more than 130 papers to the professional literature. Among his books are *Psychology* *of the Future, The Ultimate Journey, When the Impossible Happens, The Cosmic Game,* and *The Stormy Search for the Self* (with Chr istina Grof). His Web site is www.holotropic.com.

**Gay Powell Hanna, PhD, MFA,** is the executive director of the Society for the Arts in Healthcare. Through faculty positions at Florida State University and the University of South Florida (USF) from 1987 to 2002, Hanna directed VSA arts of Florida, an affiliate of the John F. Kennedy Center for the Performing Arts, providing arts education programs for people with disabilities including people with chronic illness. In 2001, she established the Florida Center for Creative Aging at the Florida Policy Exchange Center on Aging at USF to address quality of life issues. A contributing author to numerous articles and books, including the *Fundamentals of Arts Management,* 4th edition, published by the Arts Extension Service of University of Massachusetts Amherst, Hanna is noted for her expertise in accessibility and universal design. In addition, she is a practicing artist who maintains an active studio with work in private and corporate collections through the southeastern United States.

**Margaret Heldring, PhD,** is a clinical psychologist whose career spans independent practice to public policy. She has served as a clinical assistant professor in family medicine at the University of Washington and senior health advisors to former U.S. Senators Bill Bradley and Paul Wellstone. In 2000, she founded and is president of a national health policy nonprofit organization, America's Health Together (AHT). Funded by the Robert Wood Johnson Foundation, AHT led a groundbreaking partnership after 9/11 to investigate the mental health effects of that disaster and to build capacity in primary healthcare to respond to natural and manmade disasters. AHT is currently working to strengthen philanthropic activity in mental health, both domestically and globally.

**James G. Kahn, MD, MPH,** is a professor of health policy and epidemiology at the University of California, San Francisco, in the Institute for Health Policy Studies. Kahn is an expert in policy modeling in healthcare, cost-effectiveness analysis, and evidence-based medicine. His work focuses on the use of cost-effectiveness analysis to inform decision-making in public health and medicine. Kahn and colleagues recently published a study in *Health Affairs* entitled "The Cost of Health Insurance Administration in California: Insurer, Physician, and Hospital Estimates." This is the first study to quantify U.S. healthcare administration costs by setting (i.e., insurer, hospital, and physician groups) and within setting by functional department (e.g., billing). It found that insurance-related administration represents at least

21 percent of physician and hospital care funded through private insurance. The research led to the following in Harper's Index: "Estimated amount the U.S. would save each year on paperwork if it adopted single-payer healthcare: $161,000,000,000" (http://harpers.org/HarpersIndex2006-02.html). Kahn was the leader of a team of Physicians for a National Health Program physicians who submitted a single-payer proposal for the California Health Care Options project.

**Gwendolyn Puryear Keita, PhD,** is the executive director of the Public Interest Directorate of the American Psychological Association, where she had previously served as director of the Women's Programs Office for 18 years. She has written extensively and made numerous presentations on women's issues, particularly in the areas of women's health and women and depression, and on topics related to work, stress, and health. She has convened three conferences on psychosocial and behavioral factors in women's health and is coauthor of *Health Care and Women: Psychological, Social and Behavioral Influences.* Keita was instrumental in developing the new field of occupational health psychology, has convened six international conferences on occupational stress and health, and coauthored several books and journal articles on the subject, including *Work and Well-Being: An Agenda for the 1990s* (1992), *Job Stress in a Changing Workforce: Investigating Gender, Diversity, and Family Issues* (1994), and *Job Stress Interventions* (1995). Keita has presented before Congress on depression, violence, and other issues.

**Kenneth Kushner, PhD,** received his PhD in psychology from the University of Michigan in 1977. He is a professor in the Department of Family Medicine of the University of Wisconsin. He has practiced Zen for over 25 years and is a Zen Master in the Chozen-ji lineage. He is founder of the Chozen-ji Betsuin/International Zen Dojo of Wisconsin and the author of *One Arrow, One Life: Zen, Archery and Enlightenment.*

**William Mauk, MBA,** has a long history in public service and in the private healthcare and administrative consulting arena. Graduating from the University of California, Los Angeles, with an MBA degree in finance, Mauk has worked with the Agency for International Development. He was appointed by President Carter to serve as deputy comptroller of that agency in 1977 and in 1979 by President Carter as deputy administrator of the Small Business Administration. Beginning in the 1980s, he was senior vice president of administration for the John Alden Life Insurance Company. From 1995 to 2002, he was chief executive officer for the Health Maintenance Organization, Neighborhood Health Partnership. Since that time he has been active as a business and political consultant. He is currently CEO of VIVA Democracy, providing Internet software consultation for political campaigns.

**Susan McDaniel, PhD,** is professor of psychiatry and family medicine, associate chair of family medicine, and director of family programs and the Wynne Center for Family Research in Psychiatry at the University of Rochester School of Medicine and Dentistry. Her special areas of interest are behavioral health in primary care and family dynamics and genetic conditions. She is a frequent speaker at meetings of both health and mental health professionals. McDaniel is co-editor of the journal *Families, Systems & Health.* She coauthored or edited the following books: *Systems Consultation* (1986), *Family-Oriented Primary Care* (1990 and 2005), *Medical Family Therapy* (1992), *Integrating Family Therapy* (1995), *Counseling Families with Chronic Illness* (1995), *The Shared Experience of Illness* (1997), *Casebook for Integrating Family Therapy* (2001), *Primary Care Psychology* (2004), *The Biopsychosocial Approach* (2004), and *Individuals, Families, and the New Era of Genetics (2007).* Her books have been translated into seven languages.

**Marc Micozzi, MD,** is a physician-anthropologist who has worked to create science-based tools for the health professions to be better informed and productively engaged in the new fields of complementary and alternative (CAM) and integrative medicine. He was the founding editor-in-chief of the first U.S. journal in CAM, *Journal of Complementary and Alternative Medicine: Research on Paradigm, Practice and Policy* (1994). He organized and edited the first U.S. textbook, *Fundamentals of Complementary & Alternative Medicine* (1996), now in its third edition. In addition, he has served as series editor for Medical Guides to Complementary and Alternative Medicine with 18 titles in print on a broad range of therapies and therapeutic systems within the scope of CAM. In 1999, he edited *Current Complementary Therapies,* focusing on contemporary innovations and controversies, and *Physician's Guide to Complementary and Alternative Medicine.* In 2002, he became founding director of the Policy Institute for Integrative Medicine in Washington, DC.

**Geoffrey M. Reed, PhD,** is a clinical and health psychologist who, from 1995 to 2006, was assistant executive director for professional development at the American Psychological Association. He has worked with the World Health Organization (WHO) on the development and implementation of the International Classification of Functioning, Disability, and Health (ICF) since 1995. He continues to lead the development of a multidisciplinary procedural manual and guide for standardized application of the ICF with the official involvement of national professional associations representing psychology, speech-language pathology, occupational therapy, recreational therapy, physical therapy, and social work. He is senior consultant for WHO projects with the International Union of Psychological Sciences and is an international consultant on healthcare issues. He is a member of the WHO International Advisory Group for the revision of the Chapter V: Mental and Behavioural Disorders of the International Classification of Diseases and Related Health Problems. He lives in Madrid, Spain.

**Elaine Sims AB, MA,** is the director of the University of Michigan Hospitals and Healthcare Centers Gifts of Art program. She has worked in arts in healthcare since 1990. Her areas of expertise include the visual and performing arts, healing gardens, caring for the caregiver initiatives, as well as the full spectrum of arts in healthcare offerings including art cart programs, bedside music, artists-in-residence, medical school arts curriculum, and running a full medical center orchestra. Sims is serving her third term on the board of the Society for the Arts in Healthcare (SAH). She is also a consultant for the SAH consulting service. Sims is a member of the Ann Arbor Commission for Art in Public Places. She also serves on the University of Michigan Health System Environment of Care Committee and the Interior Design Standards Committee. She particularly enjoys collaborating with university and community partners in exploring and promoting the world of arts in healthcare.

**Louise Sundararajan, PhD,** received her doctorate in history of religions from Harvard University and her EdD in counseling psychology from Boston University. Currently a forensic psychologist, she was president of the International Society for the Study of Human Ideas on Ultimate Reality and Meaning. A member of American Psychological Association and the International Society for Research on Emotions, she has authored over forty articles in refereed journals and books, on topics ranging from Chinese poetics to alexithymia.

**Tobi Zausner, PhD,** who has an interdisciplinary PhD in art and psychology, is also an art historian and an award-winning visual artist with works in major museums and private collections around the world. Zausner writes and lectures widely on the psychology of art and teaches at the C. G. Jung Foundation in New York. She is an officer on the board of ACTS (Arts, Crafts, and Theatre Safety), a nonprofit organization investigating health hazards in the arts, and was chair of art history in the Society for Chaos Theory in Psychology and the Life Sciences. Zausner is writing a book on physical illness and the creative process of visual artists titled *When Walls Become Doorways: Creativity and the Transforming Illness.*

# CUMULATIVE INDEX